Statistical Concepts

SANDRA ELDRIDGE AND DEBORAH ASHBY

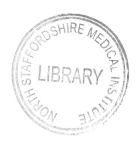

Published by
The Royal College of General Practitioners
2000

The Royal College of General Practitioners
was founded in 1952, with this object:

'To encourage, foster, and maintain the highest possible standards in general medical practice and for that
purpose to take or join with others in taking steps consistent with the charitable nature of that object
which may assist towards the same.'
Among its responsibilities under its Royal Charter the College is entitled to:
'Encourage the publication by general medical practitioners of research into medical or scientific subjects
with a view to the improvement of general medical practice in any field and to undertake or assist others
in undertaking such research.
'Diffuse information on all matters affecting general medical practice and establish, print, publish, issue
and circulate such papers, journals, magazines, books, periodicals, and publications and hold such
meetings, conferences, seminars, and instructional courses as may assist the object of the College.'

© Royal College of General Practitioners

First impression 2000

Published by the Royal College of General Practitioners
14 Princes Gate
Hyde Park
London, SW7 1PU

Printing and binding by BSC Print Ltd, Wimbledon

ISBN 0 85084 250 6

Statistical Concepts

CONTENTS

INTRODUCTION

The primary aim of this workbook is to introduce the statistical methods currently used in primary care research. It is becoming increasingly useful for GPs to have some knowledge in this field, to increase confidence in reading and interpretation of medical literature, and in carrying out their own research.

The workbook was originally designed as course material for a master class in statistical concepts run by the Royal College of General Practitioners. The class was aimed primarily at those who were involved in or wished to become involved in health-related research of some kind, and it was felt that the additional statistical training that this class offered would enable them to be better equipped to pursue their research. Those who wish to teach statistics to similar groups may find the material useful.

In addition, we hope that the workbook will also be useful as a stand alone workbook for GPs and other health professionals who have already gained some knowledge of statistical concepts in previous training but wish to go a bit further in their study of the subject or refresh their distant memories!

It is not intended as a guide through the subject for those starting from scratch although it may be useful as a supplementary text in these circumstances.

The contribution of statistics to research is really twofold. First, statistical ideas help to formulate sensible research designs which can provide useful results. Second, statistical methodology enables us to make sense of the results when they are available.

This workbook deals mostly with statistical methodology for making sense of study results. A constant theme throughout is the importance of good study design, it is not in itself a workbook on study design. Instead we would refer the reader to companion workbooks in this series such as Workbook 4: *Randomised Control Trials and Multi-Centre Research*. In addition, the workbook does not cover statistical theory and calculations in detail. Detail can be found in Bland (1995).

Chapter 1 covers common measures used to summarise study results, one of the important uses of statistics. Another use of statistics is in enabling us to make inferences about wider groups of patients based on results taken from samples of these patients. The ideas behind this are introduced in Chapter 2 and developed in Chapters 3 and 5.

In most studies statistical methodology should be complemented by sound clinical judgement and the importance of this and good study design is covered in Chapters 4 and 6. These chapters also deal with methodology suited to overcoming problems such as confounding which sometimes cannot be fully dealt with in study design.

Chapters 7 and 8 provide guides which will help the reader to use the workbook for the specific purposes of increasing confidence in reading and interpreting medical literature, and carrying out their own research.

The learning objectives for each of the eight chapters are listed below. There are exercises throughout the first six chapters. They are linked to the chapter in which they occur, but also build on and consolidate work covered in previous chapters. The workbook can be best worked through from beginning to end, but each chapter can also be followed independently.

We would be grateful for any feedback as to the usefulness of the text in various circumstances and would welcome any comments which help us to improve it in the future.

LEARNING OBJECTIVES OF EACH CHAPTER:

1. Describing Data
* to understand the concepts of **mean**, **median**, **mode**, **standard deviation** and **inter-quartile range**
* to be able to estimate the mean and standard deviation from a small set of data
* to be able to calculate the mean, median, standard deviation and inter-quartile range from a small set of data
* to know when it is appropriate to use the various measures listed in first point.

2. Introduction to Estimation
* to understand the difference between a measure taken from a **sample** and the likely value of this measure in the **population** from which the sample is drawn
* to understand the idea of an **interval estimate**
* to understand the idea of probability, or chance
* to understand the basic idea of a **randomised controlled trial**.

3. Confidence Intervals and Statistical Significance

- to understand the importance of **confidence intervals**
- to be able to interpret confidence intervals for **proportions**, means, differences between proportions and means, **relative risk** and **odds ratios**
- to be able to calculate a confidence interval for a proportion given basic data
- to understand the basic steps in carrying out a **significance test**
- to be able to interpret the results of significance tests
- to understand the relationship between confidence intervals and significance tests
- to understand when significance tests are needed.

4. Clinical Importance and Sample Size Calculations

- to be able to assess the **clinical importance** of a result using the confidence interval
- to be able to correctly interpret simple computer-generated results
- to understand the importance of **sample size calculations**
- to understand the factors that will increase and decrease the sample size required
- to understand what **cluster randomisation** is, and how it generally affects sample size requirements.

5. Types of Data and Significance Test

- to understand that the appropriate type of statistical test depends on the type of study, the type of data and the question being addressed
- to understand the difference between **paired** and **unpaired data**
- to understand the difference between **parametric** and **non-parametric tests** and when each are appropriate.

6. Confounding and Bias

- to understand what **confounding** is
- to understand the principals of analysis which seeks to deal with confounding
- to be able to identify the commonly used analytic methods of dealing with confounding
- to be able to interpret results from an analysis which deals with confounding
- to understand what **bias** is.

7. Critical Appraisal

- to understand the principles of critical appraisal
- to have a better understanding of how to read and critically assess articles.

8. Conclusion: Doing your own Research

- to understand the essentials skills necessary to undertake statistical analysis of a medical project.

· 1 ·
DESCRIBING DATA

Whenever we are faced with a set of data, our first task is always to describe it. This needs to be done in advance of any more complex analyses so that we get a feel for the data, identify data errors, and can interpret and present the results of these later analyses in a way which makes sense.

Note how often tables in the papers included in this workbook contain simple percentages and means. This chapter describes these basic summary measures and others used to describe data.

While this chapter deals with what to present, read Article 1 for some useful guidance on how to present data, before attempting any exercises.

TYPES OF DATA

Table 1 shows various types of data. A basic distinction can be made between **numerical data** which include all variables that take meaningful numerical values – and **categorical data** which include all variables that can be categorised in some way.

Table 1

Type of data	Type of variable	Variable	Values
categorical	binary	gallbladder disease	yes/no
		survival	dead/alive
		recurrence of convulsion	yes/no
	nominal	occupation	doctor, builder teacher...
	ordinal	health status	good, moderate, poor, v. poor.
		amount drunk	seven ordered categories
numerical	discrete	family size	2, 3, 4...
		list size (general practices)	800... 5000
	continuous	birthweight	in grams or ounces
		blood pressure	in mmhg

There are subdivisions within both numerical and categorical data and these are shown in Table 1 for completeness and also because they are referred to later in chapter five. For the purposes of this workbook, however, the most important distinction is between categorical and numerical variables.

SUMMARISING CATEGORICAL DATA

When summarising categorical data whether it is binary, nominal or ordinal, we can use proportions. For example, in a study looking at how many patients survive a particular treatment, if we have 210 patients of whom eight die, we can say 3.8% (8/210) are dead, and 96.2% (202/210) are alive.

In a study looking at health status, we may be able to summarise our results by saying 15% of patients were in excellent health, 49% in good health, 20% in moderate health, 10% poor and 6% in very poor health.

SUMMARISING NUMERICAL DATA

When summarising numerical data, we have a lot more choice about what sort of summaries to use. The possibilities are **mean**, **median** and **mode**, for giving us some idea of the average value of our data, and **standard deviation** and **inter-quartile range** for giving us some idea of how spread out our data are. For further reading see Bland (1995).

Mean, median and mode

Consider Table 2 containing numerical hypothetical data on length of stay in hospital following a certain operation.

Table 2

Length of stay (days)	Number of patients
1	1
2	5
3	23
4	11
5	9
6	8
7	9
8	5
9	2
10	1
28	1
Total	**75**

We can summarise the data in Table 2 in the following ways:

mode = most common value = three days
median = (middle value when data ordered)
38th value when data ordered = four days
mean = total no. of days/total no. of patients =
376/75 = five days

(The total number of days can be calculated as (1 x 1) + (5 x 2) + (23 x 3) etc, since one person stayed in one day, five people stayed in two days, 23 people stayed in three days etc.)

The three measures have different interpretations. The mean can be interpreted as the average length of time a bed is occupied, the median as the value below which half the patients stayed in hospital (i.e. half the patients stay in four days or less), and the mode as the most likely length of stay.

The mode can be used in this context but cannot be used when we consider a continuous variable such as birthweight. In this case our variable is measured on a continuous scale and very few babies will have identical birthweights – the idea of the most common birthweight does not make sense unless we group birthweight in some way.

Standard deviation and inter-quartile ranges

We may also want to describe the spread of numerical data. This can be done with **standard deviations** and **inter-quartile ranges.**

The **standard deviation** can be thought of loosely as measuring the average distance of a set of values from the mean value. Consider the list of figures given below:

4, 5, 6, 8, 2, 3, 3, 1

EXERCISE 1

a) Calculate the mean value of the figures given above.

b) Given the loose definition of the standard deviation above, guess what the standard deviation might be.

The standard deviation can be calculated as

$$\sqrt{\Sigma(x-\bar{x})^2/(n-1)}$$

where x = individual value
   $\bar{x}$ = mean value
   n = number of values
   Σ = the sum of

The calculation of a standard deviation is shown in Table 3. The steps shown in this table are:
1. Calculate the mean = 32/8 = 4 (column 2)
2. Subtract the mean from each individual value, e.g. for value 1: 4 – 4 = 0 (column 3)
3. Square each of the values in column three (column 4)
4. Add up the values in column four (total = 36)

Table 3

x	$\bar{x}$	$x-\bar{x}$	$(x-\bar{x})^2$
4	4	0	0
5	4	1	1
6	4	2	4
8	4	4	16
2	4	-2	4
3	4	-1	1
3	4	-1	1
1	4	-3	9
total=32			total=36

There are two more steps to finish the calculation:
1. Column 4 total is divided by the number of values less 1 (36/7 = 5.14)
2. Calculate the square root of the answer produced by the previous step – this is the standard deviation.

In this case the standard deviation is 2.27. Using a hand calculator gives the result that the square root of 36/7 is 2.267786838. In this example we have rounded this to two decimal places to get 2.27, but if this were a real example and we were going to present the data, we might round to only one decimal place giving the answer 2.3. For more detail on presentation of results refer to Article 1.

The **inter-quartile range (IQR)** is the range within which the central 50% of the data lie. In other words it is the range between the data point a quarter of the way up from the lowest value and the data point three-quarters of the way up from the lowest value, when the data is ordered from lowest to highest. When the eight data points above are ordered, they look like this (see Table 4).

There are eight points. The lower limit of the inter-quartile range occurs between the second and third data point (i.e. a quarter of the way up the data) and the upper limit between the sixth and seventh data point (i.e. three quarters of the way up the data).

These limits are known as the lower quartile and the upper quartile respectively, and are marked in Table 4 as LQ and UQ. They take the values halfway between the relevant data points and so are at 2.5 and 5.5. Thus the inter-quartile range is (2.5, 5.5). The median is also marked as M.

When to use the different measures

Means and standard deviations are appropriate summaries when the data are roughly symmetrical. Medians and inter-quartile ranges are appropriate when data are **skewed**. For further reading, see Bland (1995).

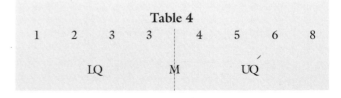

			Table 4				
1	2	3	3	4	5	6	8
	LQ		M		UQ		

Table 5

	Cancer	Not	Odds
Unexposed	500	90,000	500/90,000
Exposed	500	10,000	500/10,000

Odds ratio = 500/10,000 : 500/90,000 = 9

For further reading, see Bland (1995).

Table 6
MRC Vitamin study

Treatment	Outcome		Total
	Neural tube defect	No neural tube defect	
Folic acid	6	587	593
No folic acid	21	581	602

SUMMARISING COMPARISONS

A lot of medical research involves making comparisons, often between treatments or between individuals with and without certain diseases. It is important, therefore, to have some idea of measures that are commonly used to make these comparisons. We can compare means, medians and proportions. Comparisons between means and proportions are more common.

Comparing proportions

When we are comparing proportions, comparisons can be made using relative or absolute differences – e.g. if proportions dying on two treatments, A and B, are 10% and 6% respectively, then **relative risk** = 10%/6% = 1.67, and **the absolute risk difference** is 10% – 6% = 4%

A slightly more complex but often used measure is the **odds ratio**. Consider Table 5 in which, in a population of 101,000, 90,500 have not been exposed to a particular substance, while 10,500 have. In each of the two groups (unexposed and exposed) 500 contract cancer.

Odds ratio = odds of getting cancer if exposed compared to odds of getting cancer if not exposed.

Refer to Article 2

Table 6 shows the results from the MRC Vitamin Study Research Group which is discussed in more detail in Chapter 2. The aim of the study was to determine whether folic acid supplementation around the time of conception could prevent neural tube defects (NTDs). The table shows that the incidence of NTD in both groups was small.

Relative risk, odd ratios, and the difference between proportions are all useful measures for comparing proportions. The odds ratio is particularly useful in situations where we want to deal with additional confounding factors in the analysis (see Chapter 6).

Exercise 2 illustrates that for rare conditions the relative risk and the odds ratio are very similar. The odds ratio can therefore be used as an approximation to the relative risk in these situations, and this is commonly done in case-control studies, which often deal with relatively rare diseases and where the design of the study makes it impossible to calculate relative risk directly.

Comparing mean values

In addition to comparing proportions between two groups, we can compare mean values between two groups.

Refer to Article 3 (Table 2)

The mean change in score for a number of health-related factors as assessed by the SF36 questionnaire were recorded for intervention and control patients. For example, for physical health the mean change in score for the intervention group was 2.28, and for control -1.58, and the adjusted difference between these is 4.33. As this difference is adjusted for other factors (see Chapter 6), it is not identical to the simple unadjusted difference.

EXERCISE 2

Refer to Article 2, Table 6

a) Calculate the proportions with NTDs in each of the two groups.

b) Calculate the relative risk of getting a neural tube defect if treated with folic acid compared with the alternative treatment.

c) Calculate the odds ratio of getting a neural tube defect if treated with folic acid compared with the alternative treatment.

d) What do you notice about your answers to b) and c)?

e) Calculate the difference between the two proportions.

f) In what circumstances would the different measures you have calculated in b), c) and e) be useful?

INTRODUCTION TO ESTIMATION

Any data that we have will usually pertain to a sample of a larger population. Having described our data, we may then want to go on and say something about the population from which our sample was drawn. In other words, we may want to estimate something about our population. In this section we introduce the concepts of **sample** and **population**, and the idea of an **interval estimate**.

There are many different types of study that result in samples of data. In medical research, one of the commonest is the **randomised controlled trial (RCT),** and in this section we outline the basic principle behind an RCT (many of the articles contained in this workbook are based on the results of RCTs).

RCTs

Broadly, an **RCT** is a comparative study in which participants (patients/general practices) are **randomly allocated** to one of several groups, and each group given a different treatment/intervention (which may include placebo or no treatment) for the medical condition/practice under investigation. The effects of the different treatments are then assessed.

Read Article 2

Consider the MRC vitamin study. The aim of this study was to determine whether supplementation with folic acid or a mixture of seven other vitamins around the time of conception can prevent neural tube defects (NTDs) such as spina bifida. This was an RCT in which women were allocated to one of four groups to receive folic acid, other vitamin supplementation, neither, or both.

SAMPLE VALUES AND POPULATION ESTIMATES

The women in the MRC vitamin study are a sample, and measures reported for them are, therefore, **sample measures**. For example, 1% of women given folic acid, and 3.5% of women not on folic acid, had babies with NTDs. The corresponding relative risk is 0.28. This indicates the risk of having a baby with an NTD for women given folic acid compared with women not given folic acid. The values 1%, 3.5% and 0.28 are three sample measures.

Normally we would not be particularly interested in, for example, the relative risk from this one study, but rather in answering the question: What is the relative risk likely to be in the general population of pregnant women, not restricted to those in the study, i.e. what is the likely value of the relative risk in the **population**, and what are the implications of this? As a result of their work on 1195 women, the research group states in the MRC vitamin study:

> 'Folic acid supplementation starting before pregnancy can now be firmly recommended for all women who have had an affected pregnancy, and public health measures should be taken to ensure that the diet of all women who bear children contains an adequate amount of folic acid.'

In other words, the research group makes general public health recommendations about the whole of the population on the basis of their sample. Their recommendations were followed and an extensive educational campaign, advising folic acid supplementation around the time of conception, was instigated.

How do we leap from one single result in one single study to make some kind of inference about what might be going on in the population and, as a result, what changes in policy might we need to make? The answer to this question is contained in the concept of **confidence intervals**.

The MRC study suggests that in the population it is likely that folic acid supplementation will prevent between 29% and 88% of neural tube defects. The range (29%, 88%) is a 95% confidence interval, and it is on the basis of this confidence interval that the authors make the statement quoted above. To understand confidence intervals, you need to have a basic understanding of what an **interval estimate** is, and why it is sensible to use one.

A more difficult issue is that the women in the trial had already had one pregnancy with an NTD. Strictly, the statistical inference relates to this population. It is a wider scientific inference to assume that the reduction in risk will apply to all women.

INTERVAL ESTIMATES

Suppose you were interested in how often GPs visit their own GP. You ask 30 friends how often they have visited their GP in the past year, and find that 50% have done so.

When asked what proportion of GPs you think visit their GP at least once a year, you would probably say about 50%. This is a **point estimate**. You say 'about 50%' because you do not really expect the value in the population to be exactly equal to your result. But how accurate do you think your result might be? What do you mean by 'about'? Perhaps you would be surprised if it is lower than 40% or higher than 70%. The range (40%, 70%) is an **interval estimate**.

Essentially, it is a guess, but you have not found it hard to leap from your sample to the whole population of GPs. You obviously think that your sample of colleagues are a healthier bunch than GPs in general – the interval is not symmetrical around 50% – but nevertheless you have made an attempt to answer the question with respect to all GPs.

PROBABILITY AND CHANCE

The research group of the MRC vitamin study paper also states that:

> 'The result is unlikely to be due to chance and the randomised double-blind design excludes bias as an explanation...'

We do not deal in detail with design issues such as **blinding** in this workbook, but can answer the question: 'How can the authors be sure that the result was not due to chance?' The answer to this question can be obtained using both **confidence intervals** and **significance tests**.

· 3 ·

CONFIDENCE INTERVALS AND STATISTICAL SIGNIFICANCE

We have noted in the previous chapter that most data come from a sample of individuals who are part of a larger population. Many statistical techniques are designed to enable us to say something about a population based on sample results. This is referred to as **statistical inference**.

Confidence intervals enable us to make inferences about population values based on our **sample estimates** and **significance tests** enable us to assess whether any differences or relationships we find in our sample are likely to exist in the population or are just due to chance.

Some caution must be exercised, however, in using statistical inference. Statistical significance tests are widely used but there are a number of situations in which their use is inappropriate.

Significance tests are designed to test a hypothesis, and are therefore only appropriate in circumstances when hypotheses have been formulated. Sometimes data are collected for purely descriptive or exploratory purposes and significance tests are then unnecessary.

In addition, when hypotheses are to be tested these hypotheses should have been formulated in advance of data collection. Formulation of hypotheses once data have been collected – and particularly once they have been examined in any way – can lead to erroneous results, and in particular the overestimation of differences and effects of treatments.

Furthermore, the theory on which statistical testing is based makes assumptions about the way a sample has been drawn from a population and, more relevantly for many medical situations, the way that individuals in a study have been split into two or more comparison groups.

The basic assumption in the latter case is that the individuals are randomly allocated to groups, hence the description of many such studies as randomised controlled trials (see Chapter 2). When individuals in a trial are divided into comparison groups by some method other than random allocation, statistical inference in the form of significance tests is, strictly speaking, inappropriate.

THE CONCEPT OF CONFIDENCE INTERVALS

A **confidence interval** is an interval estimate calculated in a more rigorous way than the interval estimate calculated in Chapter 2, and based on a random sample of the population about which you are interested in generalising. A random sample will give you a better chance of obtaining a sample representative of the whole population. For further reading on random sampling, see Bland (1995).

Confidence intervals occur widely in the literature and tell us something about the possible values in the population based on our sample results.

To illustrate some important points about confidence intervals, we now turn to an hypothetical example. Consider three hypothetical studies in which sample sizes were 20, 200 and 2000. In each study, patients were divided into two equal sized treatment groups using **random allocation**, and all patients were followed up for a specified length of time.

The numbers surviving in each treatment group are shown in Table 1. Each study yields the same result in terms of proportions dying and surviving. However, the table also shows three confidence intervals based on these hypothetical studies.

Number in study	Table 1 Survival rates		Proportions surviving and confidence intervals	
	Treatment group A	Treatment group B	A	B
Study 1: 20	7/10	6/10	70%(56,84)	60%(29,91)
Study 2: 200	70/100	60/100	70%(61,79)	60%(50,70)
Study 3: 2000	700/1000	600/1000	70%(67,73)	60%(57,63)

On the basis of Study 1 which contains only 20 people, we can be 95% certain that if treatment A was applied to the whole population (of people with relevant medical condition), between 56% and 84% would survive.

Two points can be made. First, the confidence intervals are narrower the larger the study. In other words, the larger study, the more accurately we can estimate our population estimate. Secondly, the confidence intervals for the two treatments for the two smaller studies overlap (i.e. 56,84 and 29,91 overlap and 61,79 and 50,70 overlap), while those for the larger study do not.

Thus, while with the smaller study we cannot really be sure whether treatment A is better than treatment B or vice versa, it appears that identical results with the larger study suggest that survival is higher for those on treatment B.

We could also calculate 99% confidence intervals. These are wider than 95% confidence intervals because we are specifying that we want to be more sure that the interval captures the population value. For further reading, see Bland, 1995.

CALCULATING STANDARD ERRORS AND CONFIDENCE INTERVALS

In order to calculate confidence intervals, we first need to calculate **standard errors**.

Any summary measure, such as a proportion, can be assigned a **standard error**.

A **standard error** is a value that can be attached to a summary measure such as a mean, proportion, rate, ratio or difference. It indicates the precision of the sample summary measure as an estimate of the corresponding population value. A small standard error indicates a more precise estimate.

Formulae for calculating standard errors depend on the summary measure under consideration. Here we consider only the formula needed to calculate standard errors for proportions. The standard error of the proportion surviving is calculated using the formula:

$$\text{standard error} = \sqrt{(p(1-p)/n)}$$

where p is the proportion and n is the sample size on which this proportion is based. (Actually, an accurate standard error would be calculated using the proportion in the whole population, but since only the proportion from a single study is usually known, this is used as an estimate, and the standard error calculated is therefore an **estimated standard error**).

To calculate this for treatment group A, Study 1 in Table 1:

p= 0.7, n= 10
Standard error = square root of [(0.7 × 0.3)/10]
$\qquad$ = square root of [0.21/10]
$\qquad$ = square root of 0.021
$\qquad$ = 0.14
as a percentage: 14%

EXERCISE 1

Calculate standard errors for the other proportions given in Table 1.

The standard error can be interpreted loosely as 'the average amount by which a sample measure will differ from the corresponding population measure'.

For example, in samples of size 10 given treatment A, the proportion surviving will be round about the value that would occur if the whole population were to be given treatment A. This proportion surviving will sometimes be lower than the population value, and it will sometimes be higher. On average, the sample value will be about 14% from the population value, sometimes nearer and sometimes further away.

This result is based on statistical theory that it is not important to know for the purposes of this workbook. For more detail see Bland (1995), section 8.2.

Using standard errors we can calculate confidence intervals using the formula:

95% confidence interval = p +/- (1.96 x SE(p))
$\qquad$ = (p − 1.96SE(p), p + 1.96SE(p))

where SE(p) is the standard error of p

Thus, the 95% confidence intervals for Study 1 are (56%, 84%) for treatment group A, and (29%, 91%) for treatment group B.

USING CONFIDENCE INTERVALS FOR ESTIMATION

EXERCISE 2

Read Article 4

In this descriptive study, the aim was to assess the severity of epilepsy and its effect on patients' lives, and to describe patients' use of, and attitudes to, health care. The sample was of 595 people with epilepsy identified from 14 general practices in north west Bristol.

a) What proportion of people with epilepsy do you think experience attacks of epilepsy at least monthly?

b) What sample size is the answer in this study based on, and why is this not equal to the original sample of 595? What are the implications of this?

c) From the paper, identify point estimates and confidence intervals to give answers to the questions:

   i) How many people with epilepsy experience attacks of epilepsy at least monthly?

   ii) What proportion would prefer all or most of their epilepsy care in a general practice setting?

d) Why is the use of confidence intervals important?

USING CONFIDENCE INTERVALS FOR COMPARISONS

Confidence intervals can also be calculated for estimates of comparisons between groups such as those described in Chapter 1. When considering the example from Article 3 the estimated mean change in physical health score was 4.33. The 95% confidence interval for this difference is (2.12, 6.54) indicating that in the population from which this sample was drawn, we are 95% certain that this difference will lie between 2.21 and 6.54.

Other measures of comparison such as differences in proportions, odds ratios, relative risks can all be presented with their associated confidence intervals.

EXERCISE 3

Read Article 5 (an RCT) and Article 6 (an audit)
Using above articles identify estimates with 95% confidence intervals of:

a) relative risk of intervention families using smoke alarms (Clamp)

b) relative risk of intervention families using door slam devices (Clamp)

c) odds ratio of communication by occupational health physician with other medical practitioner if patient had psychiatric illness (de Bono)

d) odds ratio of communication by occupational health physicians with other medical practitioners if patient had long term sickness absence (de Bono)

For each one of these:
e) interpret these confidence intervals in your own words, in each case identifying the two groups that are being compared

f) think about the values that the relative risk and odds ratios would take if there were no difference between the two groups being compared? What are the implications of this for the results you have listed?

EXERCISE 4

Read Article 7 (an RCT)

In this article differences between two proportions are compared.

a) What difference is there between most of the confidence intervals for the diabetes variables, and most of the confidence intervals for the asthma variables?

b) What would you expect the differences to be if the intervention had no effect?

c) What do the results therefore indicate about the effect of the intervention on asthma and diabetes variables respectively?

SIGNIFICANCE TESTS

How do statistical tests assess whether there is a statistically significant difference between two proportions or two means or two medians, or alternatively whether any differences have arisen by chance?

Basically, any significance test, no matter what it is, begins with a **null hypothesis** and ends with a **P-value**.

Null and alternative hypotheses

Normally, a study begins with a study hypothesis i.e. the investigators think their study will show something particular, that treatment A works better than treatment B. When significance tests are used to test hypotheses, however, we stand any study hypothesis on its head and actually test the hypothesis that 'there is no difference', specifically in the case of this example – 'there is no difference between treatment A and treatment B'. This hypothesis is called the **null hypothesis** and the contrasting hypothesis that a difference or relationship exists is called the **alternative**.

In general, the alternative hypothesis includes the study hypothesis, but is broader in the sense that it also encompasses the possibility that, for example, in this case, treatment B works better than treatment A. This is called a two-sided alternative. For further reading, see Bland (1995).

Read Article 8

In this study an educational package, 'Take Care', was introduced into a number of general practices to see whether this could improve the recognition of psychological illness by GPs. Presumably, the investigators expected it would:

> **Null hypothesis**: educational package makes no difference to the recognition of psychological illness by GPs in the general population of GPs
> **Alternative**: package makes a difference.

Outcomes

We need a way of measuring whether the education package makes any difference. Or in other words, we need an **outcome.** In Article 8 the researchers looked at whether GPs missed depressive illnesses in patients before and after the introduction of the educational package. The outcome was therefore, 'proportion of depressive illnesses missed by a GP.'

Statistical test results and p-values

The next step is to choose an appropriate **statistical significance test**. In this case it was the Wilcoxon matched-pair test (see Chapter 5). Then the appropriate calculations are carried out. Since this is usually done by computer, we have not included detail on calculations here. For further reading, see Bland (1995).

The calculations give us a **test statistic** and finally a **P-value**. In this case the P-value is given as <0.05. The **P-value** is a probability which indicates the likelihood that any difference we observe has arisen merely by chance. In more statistical language, the P-value is the probability of obtaining this result or a more extreme result if the null hypothesis is true.

Since the P-value is less than 0.05, the chance of obtaining this result if there really is no effect of the educational package is very small, and we therefore reject the null hypothesis of no effect and conclude that we have evidence that if administered to the population of GPs represented by those in the study, the educational package 'Take Care' would improve the recognition of psychological illness. For further reading, see Bland (1995).

By convention, a P-value smaller than 0.05 is considered statistically significant in the sense that we reject the null hypothesis in favour of the alternative if $P < 0.05$. We then say that our result is significant at the 5% level. We can also consider dignificance at the 1% level (if $P < 0.01$) and 0.1% level ($P < 0.001$).

In Table 2, the flow diagram shows the general procedure to follow when carrying out a significance test, as outlined here.

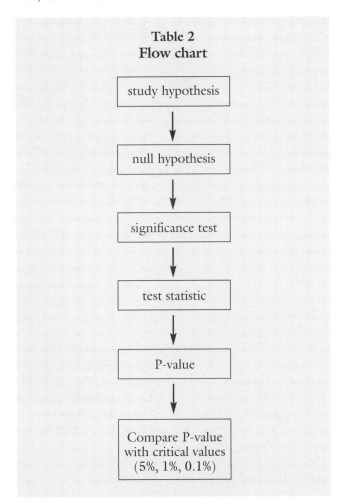

Table 2
Flow chart

study hypothesis
↓
null hypothesis
↓
significance test
↓
test statistic
↓
P-value
↓
Compare P-value with critical values (5%, 1%, 0.1%)

Read Article 3 (an RCT)
In this article, Tables 2 and 3 show differences between mean values, confidence intervals, and P-values. What is the relationship between the confidence intervals and the P-values?

A COMMON STATISTICAL TEST – THE CHI-SQUARED TEST

Read Article 9

One of the most commonly used statistical significance tests is the **chi-squared test**. The chi-squared test is used most frequently for tables of frequencies in which there are two rows and two columns, the example here is taken from Article 9. The aim of this study was:

'to determine the effect on the uptake of breast screening of a personalised letter from the general practitioner recommending mammography, sent to coincide with an invitation from the NHS breast screening programme.'

This was an RCT with two groups of women, one receiving the prompting letter (236 women) and the other not (234 women). The results can be shown in a two by two table of frequencies. See Table 3.

Table 3

Attended for mammography	Received prompt (intervention)	Did not receive prompt (control)
yes	134	120
no	102	114

The null hypothesis is that there is no difference in uptake of breast screening between the two groups of women. This is tested using a chi-squared test which involves calculating a chi-squared statistic.

A chi-squared statistic can be calculated by comparing the actual results of the study with what we might have expected to happen if the proportions attending for mammography were identical in both groups of women. We assume that this proportion is equal to the overall proportion attending:

$(134+120)/(236+234) = 54\%.$

54% attending in each group would give a total of 127.5 in the prompted group and 126.4 in the unprompted group attending, so that the results we would expect would look like this.

Table 4

Attended for mammography	Received prompt (intervention)	Did not receive prompt (control)
yes	127.5	126.4
no	108.5	107.6

The observed (actual) and expected results are then compared using the chi-squared statistic. For further reading, see Bland (1995).

If the differences between observed and expected results are great, the chi-squared statistic is also great. In this case, the differences are not very great and the chi-squared statistic is only 1.43. The P-value which corresponds to this chi-squared test is 0.23.

Thus there is a 23% chance of obtaining this result or a more extreme result if the null hypothesis is true. In other words, if the null hypothesis is true, then the result that we have obtained is quite likely to occur. P>0.05 and we cannot therefore reject the null hypothesis.

What is our conclusion? Although we have no evidence that there is a difference between the groups, it is always a mistake to conclude that this indicates that the null hypothesis is true. There are two reasons for this which will become clear as we deal with clinical importance and sample size.

The first reason is that it is possible to obtain a large P-value such as this simply because the sample size was too small – with a very small sample size it is difficult to pick up important differences even if they exist. The second reason is more pragmatic. In general, it is unlikely that any two groups being compared are identical with respect to whatever we are investigating. There will inevitably be some sort of difference, albeit very small, thus the null hypothesis can generally never be accepted.

In this particular case, therefore, an appropriate conclusion would be that there is no evidence from this study that prompts by GPs would improve the uptake of breast screening among the population of women from which this sample was drawn.

· 4 ·

CLINICAL IMPORTANCE AND SAMPLE SIZE CALCULATIONS

The importance of findings from a study depend not only on their statistical significance but also on their **clinical importance**. A finding can be said to be clinically important if, as a result, some judgement can be made about whether or not to change policy or practice.

In this chapter we show how to assess clinical importance using study results, specifically confidence intervals, once a clinical judgement has been made about what constitutes a clinically important result. At the design stage of a study it is also important to consider clinical importance; a study should be large enough to be able to detect clinically important results. Here we also discuss **sample size calculations**.

CLINICAL IMPORTANCE

Confidence intervals can be used to assess the clinical importance of findings. Look again at Article 9. The difference between the percentage of women in the two groups who attended mammography was 5.5%, and a 95% confidence interval for this difference was -3.5% to 14.5%.

The interpretation of this confidence interval is that we can be 95% certain that (in the population from which the sample was drawn) the difference in the percentage of women attending will lie between these limits, i.e. that we are 95% sure that either the attendance is up to 14.5% better for women receiving prompts, or it is up to 3.5% worse, or somewhere in between.

The authors of this study made a judgement at the start that an increase in attendance of 15% would be considered clinically important, in the sense that if the study could show this sort of difference, or a greater difference, this might result in recommending a change in practice i.e. women should be sent prompts by their GPs.

The study failed to show such a difference, however, in either direction. We are 95% certain of that. Thus the result can be said to be neither statistically significant, nor clinically important.

In general, an examination of the limits of confidence intervals can lead to a judgement about whether a study's result is clinically important. We ask about each of the limits – 'if this was the result in the population, would we recommend a change in practice/change in policy/certain course of action?' If the answer with respect to either limit is 'yes', then the result is potentially clinically important, and this is the case even though it may not be statistically significant.

In Article 3, Table 2, confidence intervals can be examined for their clinical importance. The authors indicate that five point differences are clinically important for all SF-36 domains. The difference in physical functioning is both statistically significant (P<0.001) and clinically important (one of the confidence limits is greater than 5, the value deemed clinically important).

Refer to Article 10

The Randomised Intervention Treatment of Angina (**RITA**) compared the long-term effects of two alternative angina treatments. This is an interim report of follow-up on 1,011 patients after a mean follow-up of 2.5 years.

Comparing CABG and PTCA treatments, the confidence interval limits suggest that deaths and myocardial infarctions could potentially be reduced by 41% or increased by 29% by using CABG rather than PTCA. If the effect in the whole population were near either of these limits it would be considered clinically important.

Here we have a situation where the results are potentially clinically important but not statistically significant. This is largely because these were interim results and the study was not powerful enough to detect statistically significant differences at this stage. Full study results were needed to come to some definitive conclusions.

Table 1			
Study	Point estimate	Interval estimate (95%)	Conclusion
A	7%	5-9%	
B	7%	4-12%	
C	12%	11-13%	
D	12%	-2%-26%	

SAMPLE SIZE CALCULATIONS

Introduction to sample size calculations

Scientific, practical and ethical considerations all contribute to the choice of sample size. The scientific consideration is that the study should be large enough to be able to detect a clinically important difference between treatment groups if one exists. Statistical methods exist to calculate the appropriate minimum sample size to satisfy this consideration – these are often referred to as **power calculations**.

The ethical need to prevent patients receiving an inferior treatment, and practical constraints on resources, tend to limit the size of a trial. In most cases, the size of a study should be justified on scientific grounds. Papers should provide evidence that the study was large enough to detect a clinically important difference if one existed. This is particularly important when no significant differences are found.

Power calculations are often reported in papers as 'a sample of "x" would have a power of 80% to detect a difference of y at the 5% level of significance'. Here, "x" represents the minimum sample size required, and "y" the difference between the groups that is considered clinically important. The determination of the clinically important difference requires a clinical or public health judgement.

The **power** of a study is the probability that the study will detect a significant difference if a given difference (the clinically important difference) exists in the population. A larger study has more power.

For example, in Article 9 it is stated that:

> 'We considered a clinically important increase in attendance to be 15%. To detect such a difference at a 5% significance level with a power of 80%, 209 patients in each group were needed.'

Sample size calculations can also be carried out when our relevant outcome is not a difference in proportions but a difference in mean values. An example of this type of calculation is given in Article 3. Power calculations are not, however, always carried out in general practice research. Read Article 12 for background.

Sample size calculations are based on statistical theory that it is not necessary to know for the purposes of this workbook. The calculations can be done using published tables or computer programmes. Here we concentrate on the steps involved in choosing a suitable sample size (see Table 2). For further reading, see Bland (1995).

Using the table in Article 13

Suppose we have a trial to compare two drugs as described in Exercise 1. We consider 10% to be a clinically important difference, and that with the old drug 50% improve. Then:

$$p_1 = 50\%$$
$$p_2 = 60\%$$

If we wish to have an 80% chance of finding such a difference significant at the 5% level, we set:

$$power = 1 - \beta = 80\%$$
$$and \ \alpha = 5\%$$

We are looking at a two-sided alternative since we are willing to entertain the possibility that the new drug is worse than the old and wish to be able to detect a difference in that direction if one exists. Turn to page 131 of Article 13:

Look at the section of the table headed '$\pi_1 = 0.50$'
($\pi_1 = p_1$, and $\pi_2 = p_2$ in this table)

Find $\pi_2 = 0.6$ in the first column
Find $\alpha = 0.05$ in the second (two-sided alternative) column.
Look across the table until you reach the column headed $1 - \beta = 0.80$. Here you find the sample size required is 388. This is the sample size required in each group.

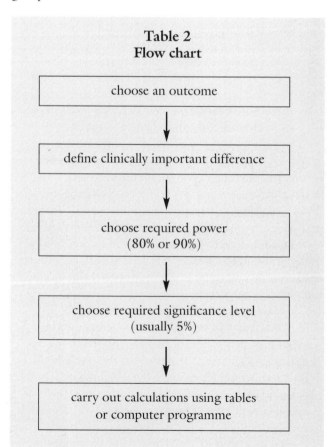

Table 2
Flow chart

choose an outcome

↓

define clinically important difference

↓

choose required power
(80% or 90%)

↓

choose required significance level
(usually 5%)

↓

carry out calculations using tables
or computer programme

EXERCISE 2

Read Article 14

In this article a study was carried out looking at 30 children with atopic eczema (AE) and 30 comparison children, to ascertain whether psychological problems were more common in children with AE. No sample size calculations were carried out initially – this was very much a pilot study. The results given below are produced by STATA, a statistics, graphics and data management package using data on these 60 children.

[Note sex: 1 = male, 2 = female
     group: 0 = no eczema, 1 = eczema
     cutrut: 0 = not disturbed, 1 = disturbed]

Tables 1 & 2 give some background information about the sample of children.

a) What is the main study hypothesis for this study and what is the corresponding null hypothesis?

b) Consider Table 3: what test has been carried out to investigate these hypotheses?

c) Interpret the results given in Table 3.

d) Calculate the proportions psychologically disturbed in each group, and the difference between these two proportions.

e) The standard error of the difference between the two proportions is 0.12 (12%). Using formulae given at the end of Chapter 3 in the workbook, calculate a 95% confidence interval for the difference between the two proportions.

f) Interpret the confidence interval.

g) In the light of the statement 'an excess of psychological disturbance amongst AE children of 20% would lead to a recommendation that psychological input should be considered more frequently as part of the management of children with AE', would you recommend further research in this area? Justify your answer.

Table 1

by group: sum age

-> group = 0

Variable	Obs	Mean	Std. Dev.	Min	Max
age	29	9.980345	2.657053	5.5	14.5

-> group = 1

Variable	Obs	Mean	Std. Dev.	Min	Max
age	30	8.706	2.555629	5.25	13.67

Table 2

tabulate group sex

group	sex 1	2	Total
0	16	14	30
1	13	17	30
Total	29	31	60

Table 3

tabulate group cutrut, chi

group	cutrut 0	1	Total
0	22	8	30
1	15	15	30
Total	37	23	60

Pearson chi2(1) = 3.4548 Pr = 0.063

EXERCISE 3

If the extent of psychological disturbance in the general population of school age children is about 25% (the value found in this study) how large a sample size is needed to have an 80% chance of detecting a difference of 20% significant at the 5% level? Use the table in Article 13.

EXERCISE 4

In fact, other studies have shown the extent of psychological disturbance in the population of school age children to vary a great deal from 6% to 23%.

a) Answer Exercise 3 assuming the proportion in the general population is:
      i) 5%   ii) 10%

b) What are the differences between these results and the result of Exercise 3?

c) Put your results in the second column of the following grid, and complete the grid.

d) What pattern is there in the grid?

	Clinically important change	
Percent in baseline group	10%	20%
5%		
10%		
25%		
50%		

Sample size calculations for cluster randomised studies

Read Article 15 for an introduction to cluster randomisation

When RCTs are undertaken in general practice research, very often general practices (and not patients) are randomised to intervention and control groups.

This occurs, for example, when an intervention such as the introduction of new staff or new guidelines is being investigated and this intervention is at a practice not a patient level. This contrasts with the more familiar type of RCT when any intervention or treatment is carried out at a patient level and patients are randomised.

When an intervention is carried out at a practice level and practices, not patients, are divided into intervention and control groups, the results of the trial may still be assessed via patient outcomes. This sort of trial is commonly referred to as a **cluster randomised trial**, and all the patients from a practice who are included in the trial are referred to as a cluster.

Further allowance for cluster randomisation has to be made in the calculation of sample size. Sample sizes need to be increased when practices not patients are the unit of randomisation.

For further reading refer to Articles 16 and 17

In Article 7:

'Detection of a 50% relative increase in the recording of these two variables [peak flow and blood glucose concentrations] (from 40% to 60%) with a power of 95% at a significance level of 5% required a total sample of 310 patients. A sample size of 390 patients... was sufficient to detect a clinically relevant difference even with a trend towards increased recording in 'control' practices and reduction of power when the practice rather than the patient was taken as the unit of analysis.'

The amount by which sample sizes need to be increased when a group of patients rather than an individual patient forms the unit of randomisation, depends on two factors:

1. The larger the size of the clusters the greater the sample size needed.
2. The sample size needs to be larger, the greater the correlation between clustered individuals compared to non-clustered individuals with respect to the outcome of interest.

This correlation can be measured using the **intra-cluster correlation coefficient (ICC)**, usually denoted by ρ. In theory, ρ can take values anywhere between 0

and 1. It indicates the extent of the variability within clusters compared to the total variability in the data. It takes the value 0 if the value of the outcome is not at all dependent on which cluster an individual comes from. It takes the value 1 if the outcome value can be perfectly predicted for an individual if you know which cluster they are from, i.e. if all the outcome values for individuals from a single cluster are identical. Generally speaking, ρ is usually below 0.05.

If the clusters are all roughly the same size, a fairly simple formula estimates d, the amount by which sample sizes must be increased:

$$d = 1+(\bar{n}-1)\rho$$

where the sample size required is d times what it would be if clustering were not present:

$\bar{n}$ = average cluster size; and
ρ = intra-cluster correlation coefficient

Note that this formula is accurate if all clusters are the same size. If they are not, it is an approximation; d is sometimes referred to as the **inflation factor**. The problem with using the formula above is that ρ is not usually known, unless a previous study has indicated its likely value. Nevertheless with:

$\bar{n}$ (average cluster size) = 100;
and $\rho = 0.02$
$d = 1+(100\text{-}1)0.02 = 2.98$

In the formula above, if $\bar{n} <100$, the value of d will decrease, and if $\rho <0.02$ the value of d will decrease.

In other words, as long as the size of the sample in each cluster can be kept below 100, and $\rho < 0.02$, the sample size required for clustered data will be less than three times what it would be without clustering: ρ is often below 0.02 although larger values do occur.

EXERCISE 5

a) Confirm the sample size calculation carried out in Article 7 and quoted above.

b) As has been noted, the RCT reported in this paper was a cluster randomised study in which practices not patients were randomised. The average number of patients selected from each practice was about 12. Calculate how much bigger the sample size needed to be if the intra-cluster correlation coefficient for peak flow and blood glucose concentrations is 0.01.

c) How much bigger would the sample size have needed to be if a smaller number of practices had been selected with an average number of patients in each practice of 25?

· 5 ·

TYPES OF DATA AND SIGNIFICANCE TESTS

The type of significance test that is appropriate in different situations depends crucially on the type of data being analysed (see Chapter 1), the type of study that has been carried out, and the type of question being asked.

In this workbook we can really only scratch the surface in terms of what type of test to use – there are a great many to choose from. For this reason we have limited our discussion to the very simplest case when comparisons are being made between two groups of data. This will serve to illustrate the major points.

To understand which test to use you need to understand the difference between **Gaussian** and **non-Gaussian** data, and the difference between **paired** and **unpaired** data. These topics are dealt with in the next two sections.

GAUSSIAN AND NON-GAUSSIAN DATA

When we talk about the distribution of a set of data we are talking about the shape and position of the data points.

This can be understood most easily as a description of what the data looks like when put onto a graph. How are the points arranged along a scale? Do the points show bunching (or a peak) in the centre, or towards one end? Is the shape very flat? Are there two peaks or one? While every real data set has its own real distribution, we also make extensive use in statistics of theoretical distributions.

The **Gaussian distribution** is probably the most important theoretical distribution used in statistics. It is symmetrical and bell-shaped, and often also called the normal distribution. But this terminology is misleading in that it appears to imply that this is the distribution that should normally be followed by numerical variables – which is not the case. Very few real life variables follow the Gaussian distribution but this does not diminish the importance of this distribution in statistical theory.

There are many variables which are close enough to a Gaussian distribution that analysis can be undertaken on them which assumes that their underlying distribution is Gaussian. In very crude terms these variables need to have a symmetrical distribution with a peak in the

centre. Significance tests that assume the underlying distribution of variables involved follow a particular theoretical shape (in this case a Gaussian shape) are termed **parametric** tests.

By contrast, significance tests which make no assumptions about the underlying shape of the distributions of the variables involved are called **non-parametric tests**. These tests can be used on numerical variables which have very skewed distributions, but also on ordinal variables, and the chi-squared test is a particular non-parametric test which, we have already seen, can be used for binary data. The chi-squared test can also be used for categorical variables.

PAIRED AND UNPAIRED COMPARISONS

We have already looked at two studies that can serve as examples of paired and unpaired comparisons.

In Article 9 as we have seen in earlier chapters, an RCT was carried out in which a comparison was made between two groups of women, 236 in the intervention group and 234 in the control group. These were two completely separate and independent groups of women. This is an **unpaired** or **unmatched** comparison.

In Article 8 however, a comparison was made between GPs before a particular intervention package was introduced, and GPs after the package was introduced. There was only one group of individuals (the GPs) and the comparison was made between different measurements on the same individual. The 'before package' and 'after package' results are said to be **paired**, or **matched**, in that each 'before package' result has an 'after package' result intrinsically linked with it. This is one of the most common ways in which paired data occurs in a before/after study, but it can also occur in other ways.

WHICH TEST TO USE WHEN?

Table 1 shows five commonly used tests, what sort of data they are used for and where they occur in the articles included in this workbook. (There are very few papers in medical literature which use the McNemar test, sixth in the list, and it is included here for completeness only.)

Table 1

Test	Type of study, data	Study
Paired t-test paired	paired 'Gaussian' numerical data	Campbell, Table 3 (Article 3)
Chi-squared	unpaired, categorical (in most cases binary) data	O'Connor (Article 9)
Unpaired t-test	unpaired, 'Gaussian' numerical data	Bryner (Article 18)
Mann-Whitney U test	unpaired, skewed numerical data or ordinal data	Shepperd (Article 19)
Wilcoxon matched pairs test	paired, skewed numerical data or ordinal data	Hannaford (Article 8)
McNemar's test	paired, binary data	–

EXERCISE 1

Decide which significance test would be suitable for the following situations. In making your decision, consider the type of data, its distribution and whether the data are paired or unpaired. In some situations you may feel that more than one test may be suitable, and you do not have enough information to choose between them.

a) Which aftercare is better?
Data on length of stay in hospital after a particular operation are to be compared for two groups of patients (75 in each group) receiving different forms of aftercare, to see whether one group has a significantly shorter stay in hospital than the other.

b) Are dentists' patient reminders effective?
A dental surgery has recently stopped sending out reminders to patients to attend the surgery. After a year, a random sample of patients are selected and their notes examined to see whether they attended the surgery in the year prior to this, and whether they attended the surgery in the year following (do not copy this study, it has lots of design faults!).

c) Which treatment is better?
In a clinical trial to compare two treatments, patients are to be randomly allocated to two groups and followed up to see how many die and how many survive.

d) Can we reduce anxiety with a drug?
To assess the value of a new tranquilliser on psychoneurotic patients, each patient is to be given treatment with the drug and with a placebo. The order in which the two sets of treatments are given is to be determined at random and the anxiety score is to be recorded following treatment and following the placebo.

e) A matched (paired) case-control study is to be undertaken to find out whether cases have a greater exposure to hairspray (measured as days of exposure per month) than controls.

f) Is oral hygiene related to type of school?
A study classified children according to their oral hygiene (good, fair+, fair-, or bad) and the type of school they attended (above average, average, below average). The aim of the study was to assess whether the type of school affected the oral hygiene of the children.

g) What difference does protein make to growth?
Two groups of rats are to be fed low and high protein diets and their weight gain measured over a period.

h) How satisfied are junior doctors with their training?
The satisfaction levels of junior doctors attending two different types of training for the same area of work are to be assessed using a questionnaire which records satisfaction as:
1 = extremely satisfied, – 5 = extremely unsatisfied.

· 6 ·

CONFOUNDING AND BIAS

Making comparisons between two groups, or looking for relationships between two variables is rarely as straightforward as it sounds. There are often other factors that confuse the comparison being investigated. Our two groups may not be exactly alike in all respects. Two factors may appear to be related to each other, but this may be entirely due to a third factor being related to both.

In this chapter we look at two ways to deal with what is a common problem causing unwanted noise in many studies: **confounding**.

If confounding is not dealt with, the results of a study may be biased. For example, if in a trial of two treatments for a particular disease two treatment groups are being compared and one group starts off with a more severe form of the disease than the other, then obviously our comparison of treatments will be unfair, or biased.

Bias can arise for other reasons. Biased results are less reliable and, at worst, can be positively misleading. Bias should therefore be avoided as much as possible in a study. The last section in this chapter discusses bias in more detail.

INTRODUCTION TO CONFOUNDING

What is **confounding**? A variable is a confounder if it is independently associated with both the outcome and the explanatory variable in a study. In an RCT a variable is a confounder if it is related to the outcome, and also differs between intervention and control groups.

The result of confounding is that it can make some relationships appear that do not really exist, and can mask some relationships that do exist. Therefore, confounding needs to be dealt with in order to obtain an accurate and non-biased result.

The most common confounding factors are age, sex, and time. Confounding can be dealt with at the design stage or the analysis stage. At the design stage of a clinical trial it is important to try and ensure balance between trial groups in terms of potential confounding factors. Potential confounders are then no longer actual confounders in the study. This was done in Article 9 using stratification.

At the design stage of a case-control study, potential confounders are often dealt with by matching. This was done in Article 20 for two potential confounders.

The type of analysis undertaken to deal with confounding is determined by the design of the study and the type of data involved. In general, clinical trials tend to need relatively simple analyses, while observational studies (**cross-sectional studies**, **cohort studies**, and **case-control studies**) require more complex analyses.

The reasons for this are that a greater number of, or more complex, questions may be asked in connection with an observational study, and lack of randomisation in an observational study can lead to more serious confounding.

In the next few sections, we look in more detail at dealing with confounding at the analysis stage. We are going to consider two different types of outcome measure; **binary** and **continuous** (see Table 1, page 9). Generally, when an outcome measure is continuous we use multiple linear regression to deal with confounding, and when it is binary, we use logistic regression.

It is not necessary for the purpose of this workbook to go into detail about the mechanics of multiple and logistic regression. That is done elsewhere, see Bland (1995). Here, we concentrate on the concepts and interpretation.

MULTIPLE REGRESSION

Consider an hypothetical study looking at the relationship between blood pressure and age in a population of adult males, where the **outcome** is blood pressure and the **predictor (explanatory variable)** is age.

We can ask the question: what is the relationship between blood pressure and age? Suppose, however, that weight and sex are potential confounders in the relationship between blood pressure and age. That is, we think blood pressure may depend on sex and weight as well as age and we think that in our sample, weight and sex might be related to age. Let us unravel this a little more in order to clarify what may be happening.

Consider the potential confounder, weight. Being more explicit, we think that blood pressure may go up with weight but also that in our sample, older people will weigh more. If we find a relationship between blood pressure and age, how can we tell how much of this relationship is due to a genuine relationship between blood pressure and age, and how much is due to a relationship between blood pressure and weight and the fact that older people also tend to be heavier?

We can use multiple regression to account for our **potential confounders**. Multiple regression answers the question: what is the relationship between blood pressure and age once we have **controlled for** weight and sex?

We can examine the following relationships as the result of our multiple regression analysis:

1. Blood pressure and age once sex and weight have been controlled for
2. Blood pressure and sex once age and weight have been controlled for
3. Blood pressure and weight once sex and age have been controlled for

We can test the various relationships using significance tests, i.e. one significance test may answer the question: 'once we have controlled for weight and sex, is the relationship between blood pressure and age significant?'. Another answers the question: 'once we have controlled for sex and age is the relationship between blood pressure and weight significant?'.

The answers to these questions tell us both whether the confounder(s) has/have a significant effect, and whether there is any change in the relationship between the explanatory variable that we are interested in and our outcome once we have accounted for the confounder(s).

We can include a lot more explanatory and confounding variables and perform a variety of significance tests.

An example of using multiple regression to account for confounders is contained in Article 21. This study examined the relationship between alcohol intake and coronary heart disease (CHD) in seven countries.

The outcome was CHD monthly rate (over 25 years) and the explanatory variable was alcohol intake. Data were collected from 16 cohorts of men aged 40 to 59 in seven different countries. Alcohol intake varied a great deal from 2g/day in Finland to 91g/day in Croatia.

In a **univariate analysis** (i.e. one which did not take account of confounders) of the relationship between alcohol intake and CHD, a significance test yielded results:

$$b = -3.44, 95\% \text{ CI}:(-5.76,-1.11), \text{P-value} = 0.05$$

The **coefficient** is 'b' which represents the relationship between alcohol intake and CHD, it indicates the amount by which CHD rate increases for every unit increase in alcohol consumption. Since it is negative in this instance and $P = 0.05$, this indicates that the study has provided evidence that as alcohol consumption increases, CHD goes down.

In a **multivariate analysis** (i.e. multiple linear regression) when smoking prevalence, intake of saturated fatty acids, and intake of flavonoids were controlled for, the results were:

$$b = -0.06, 95\% \text{ CI}:(-1.44,1.33) \text{ P-value}>0.05$$

The **adjusted coefficient** is 'b' since it is adjusted for the effect of these other factors and we can conclude that there is no evidence of a relationship between alcohol intake and CHD in these countries. The apparent effect in the univariate analysis was due to the confounding effect of saturated fatty acids – the authors show that there is a significant inverse relationship between alcohol intake and saturated fatty acid intake in these cohorts.

ODDS RATIOS AND LOGISTIC REGRESSION

Logistic regression is similar to multiple linear regression as described above except that it is used when the outcome variable is binary rather than continuous. Because many outcome variables in medicine are binary (e.g. dead/alive) logistic regression is more common than multiple linear regression in medical research.

Results of a logistic regression model are often given in terms of **odds ratios** (see Chapter 1) and their confidence intervals (Chapter 3). The odds ratios from a logistic regression analysis will be adjusted odds ratios in the sense that they have been adjusted for the effect of other variables entered into the logistic regression.

Odds ratios are calculated by comparing odds in one group with odds in another group. Therefore it is necessary for one category of a predictor variable to be identified as the base category so that comparisons can be made of odds in other categories with the odds in this **base category**.

EXERCISE 1

Read Article 20

This is a report of the confidential inquiry into stillbirths and deaths in infancy. This study was a case-control study carried out over two years. The investigators were interested in whether the following 'sleep environment' variables were related to sudden infant death. See below:

- sleeping position
- tog value of bedding
- using duvet
- bedding tucked in or loosely covered
- covers over head of infant
- whether mother ever breast fed
- bed-sharing with parents
- using dummy
- heating on all night
- wearing a hat

They collected a great deal of information, and decided to control for the following confounding variables in the analysis:

- maternal age
- parity
- gestation
- birth weight
- whether family received family income supplement
- exposure to tobacco smoke

a) Take two of the factors listed above and explain how they could be confounders in this study

b) From Article 20, Table 1:
i) why is there an odds ratio of 1 for the 'back' category?
ii) which sleeping position was the least common?
iii) which sleeping position carried the most risk?
iv) how can you assess from this table whether the increased risk due to various sleeping positions was likely to have arisen by chance or not?

c) From Article 20, Table 2:
i) which tog ratings carried the most/least risk?
ii) in general, what has been the effect of controlling for socio-economic status on the odds ratios presented in this table?
iii) explain why controlling for socio-economic status has had this effect.

d) From Article 20, Table 3:
i) interpret the odds ratios and confidence intervals in this table.
(NB: a chi-squared test on which the analyses in this table are based can only be carried out when the cell sizes in the table being analysed are large enough – for the 'where in bed' data, one cell has only three babies in it, and a chi-squared test could not therefore be carried out – instead Fisher's exact test was used.)

e) From Article 20, Table 4:
(i) interpret the odds ratio and confidence interval for using a dummy.

BIAS

What is bias? Bias is any systematic influence that means that an estimate from a study tends to over or underestimate its true population value.

Epidemiological studies are very susceptible to bias. In a survey of alcohol consumption in the general population, non-responders may be more likely to be heavy drinkers and so average alcohol consumption is underestimated. This is termed **response bias**.

In case-control studies, people with the disease may be more likely to recall particular exposures than controls, as they have spent time reflecting on why they got the disease. This is termed **recall bias**. In a cohort study of workers, disease rates may be lower than the general population because those with existing problems are less likely to join the workforce. This is called the **healthy worker effect**.

In epidemiological studies, good design can sometimes help, but otherwise we need to think carefully about possible sources of bias, and how they might affect interpretation of the study.

Clinical trials are less susceptible to bias if they are planned properly. **Allocation bias** is where the clinician systematically puts certain types of patients on a particular treatment, but good randomisation procedures guard against this.

Assessment bias may mean the clinician or patient tends to rate the results on the new treatment better than on the old. Blinded assessment can protect against this. Further biases can arise because, for example, patients may drop out of the placebo group due to lack of efficacy and the remaining patients are then the ones doing better. Analysis by intention to treat, where all patients are included regardless of whether they completed treatment, can guard against these biases.

Other kinds of bias are **publication bias,** where significant findings may be more likely to reach publication, and **citation bias**, where certain studies get referred to because of 'exciting' results but other more cautious studies get ignored.

Some kinds of bias have predictable consequences, others may be harder to tell even which way the biases go. Sometimes studies will have biases operating in different directions, but unfortunately there is no guarantee that such biases will cancel out!

Although the above examples include some very important sources of bias, they are by no means exhaustive. However, when critiquing a study, ask yourself whether any systematic influences in the design, conduct or analysis of the study could be a source of bias. If you are designing a study, ask the same questions, and then try to think of ways to guard against them.

· 7 ·

CRITICAL APPRAISAL

A great deal of medical research is currently being undertaken. Over recent years there has been a growing awareness that to be able to answer important questions such as 'how effective is a particular treatment?', 'should a patient be treated with a new drug or an existing treatment?', and 'how safe is the new drug?', GPs need to be able to assess and evaluate this literature rather than just ingest it.

Questions need to be asked about the validity and reliability of the research being undertaken, so that medical practice is based on sound evidence and critical appraisal provides the tools to do this.

There are standard guides for appraising different types of study. The guide shown in Exercise 1 is for use in the critical appraisal of a therapy paper, i.e. one that has tried to evaluate one or more therapies (or interventions) using a randomised controlled trial.

The first five questions deal largely with the design of these types of trial. This workbook has not dealt with design issues, they are covered in Workbook 4 of this series.

Further Reading
More detail on the interpretation and use of the guide is given in Eldridge and Naish (1998).

EXERCISE 1

Read Article 10 and use the following guide to critically assess this paper (this workbook has not covered all the information that you might need to answer all the questions in full but there are answers given on page 36).

1. Were the patients randomly allocated to treatment groups?

2. Were all the patients who entered the trial properly accounted for at the conclusion? Was follow-up complete? Were patients analysed in the groups to which they were allocated?

3. Were patients, health workers and study personnel (researchers) 'blind' to the treatments?

4. Were the patients in the groups similar at the start of the trial?

5. Apart from the experimental investigation, were the patients in the groups treated equally?

6. How large was the treatment effect between the groups?

7. How precise was the treatment effect?

8. Can the results be applied to <u>my</u> patient care?

9. Were all clinically important outcomes considered?

10. Are the likely benefits worth the potential harms and costs?

· 8 ·

CONCLUSION: DOING YOUR OWN RESEARCH

In this workbook, we have largely concentrated on reading, understanding and critiquing published research. However, many readers will have been motivated by the desire to do some research of their own.

For those who are trying to design a study well or who find themselves needing to use unfamiliar techniques, it is worth getting to know your local statistician. Although few can take on analyses, many are prepared to talk with a health professional for an hour or so, and this can be very valuable. Occasionally such conversations can result in collaborations.

We offer some pointers:

1. Be clear about the main questions you are trying to answer.
2. Good analysis cannot rescue bad design.
3. Always plot your data, to help you understand it and explain it to others.
4. Calculate appropriate descriptors (e.g. means, relative risks) that are clinically meaningful.
5. Confidence intervals help show how accurate your estimates are.
6. Hypothesis testing should be used sparingly, if at all.
7. Regression can help to understand and quantify the relationship between variables.
8. Computing power can make life easier, although your hand calculator can be your best friend.
9. Sample size estimation requires hard thought, but is an essential part of planning any study.
10. Most doctors' appreciation of statistics comes from analysing their own studies, or thinking hard and critically about other people's work.

Glossary

a **baseline** group is a comparison group, such as non-smokers. Typically, the **relative risk** of disease in other groups will be calculated relative to this group.

bias is any systematic influence that means that an estimate from a study tends to over or underestimate its true population value.

a **binary** variable or outcome is one with two categories such as male and female, or dead and alive.

a **case-control study** is an **observational study** in which a group of individuals who have a particular disease or disorder (cases), and another group who do not (controls) are investigated to see if they were exposed to the study factor.

categorical data is data that can be grouped such as male/female, or occupation, e.g. builder, teacher, doctor.

a **chi-squared test** is a **hypothesis test** used for comparing **categorical data**. It is most often seen in medical applications when the data can be summarised in a 2 by 2 table, but is also applicable to larger tables.

a **clinical trial** is an experiment on humans to compare two or more treatments or other procedures.

a **clinically important difference or change** is a difference (e.g. between the survival rates from two different treatments) that it would be important to know about should it exist. It is important for **power calculations**.

a **cluster** is the unit of randomisation in a **cluster randomised trial** e.g. practices or schools.

a **cluster randomised trial** is one where **randomisation** is by **cluster**, such as GP practice, or school, rather than by individual.

a **cohort study** is an **observational study** in which people are followed up over time.

a **confidence interval** shows the range of values that will be expected to include the true value with a particular degree of confidence. It shows how precise an estimate actually is.

a **confounding factor** is one that is independently associated with both the disease and with the study factor.

a **continuous** variable or outcome is one that can be measured on a continuous scale to whatever the accuracy of the measurement instrument, such as blood pressure, height or weight.

a **control group** is a group taking standard therapy (or **placebo**) to act as comparator for an **intervention group** taking the test therapy.

a **correlation coefficient** is a measure of linear association between two continuous variables. A value of 1 (or -1) indicates that a plot of the data would fall on a straight line, 0 indicates no linear association at all.

critical appraisal is a systematic approach to reading and interpreting journal articles focusing on whether the study design and analysis was appropriate to the question being asked.

a **cross-sectional** study is a study carried out at one point in time.

a **difference in means** is calculated by subtracting the mean of one group from the mean of another, e.g. in a clinical trial to quantify the average extra drop in blood pressure on one treatment compared to another.

a **difference in proportions** is calculated by subtracting the proportion with a characteristic in one group from the proportion in another group, e.g. in a clinical trial to see what extra proportion of people could expect to suffer a particular side-effect on one therapy compared to another.

discrete data are observations taking distinct values but no values in between these, such as the number of patients visiting a GP on a particular day, which can take values such as 0, 5, 33, etc, but not 5.33 or 0.54.

an **epidemiological study**, such as a **case-control** or a **cohort study**, is designed to describe the relationship between incidence of disease and one or more putative **risk factors**.

epidemiology is the study of the pattern and distribution of diseases in human population.

explanatory variables (also called **predictors**) are used in **regression** as the variables which might explain or predict the **outcome measure**.

a **Gaussian distribution** is a symmetrical bell-shaped curve whose area sums to one. It is often used to model observations such as blood pressure. It also plays a central role in statistical theory, cropping up, for example, in the calculation of **confidence intervals**.

an **hypothesis test** is a statistical procedure for testing how likely we are to have observed the actual data, such as a difference between groups, given a **null hypothesis** of no true difference between the groups. It can be thought of as a measure of surprise, and is used to gauge whether data are compatible with random chance or whether we have to reject this explanation and conclude there could be a real effect.

an **inter-quartile range** is a measure of spread of a set of observations. It is calculated by finding the point above which the top 25% of observations lay, and the point beneath which the bottom 25% of observations lay.

an **interval estimate** gives a range of values within which the true value is likely to fall, e.g. a **confidence interval**.

an **intervention group** in a **clinical trial** is the group getting the new therapy or procedure, so their **outcome** can be compared with that of the **control group**.

an **intra-cluster correlation coefficient** is a measure of how similar the individuals within a **cluster** are to each other rather than to a randomly chosen member of the whole population.

linear regression is a technique to describe the relationship between two continuous measures, such as height and FEV1, where one, the **explanatory variable** (e.g. height), is thought to be predictive of the other the **outcome** (e.g. FEV1). It summarises the rate of change of one with the other.

logistic regression is the analogue of **linear regression** when the **outcome** is **categorical**, most often **binary**.

a **Mann-Whitney U test** is a **non-parametric hypothesis test** to compare two unpaired groups of observations.

matched data: see **paired data**.

a **matched case-control study** is a **case-control study** in which the controls are individually matched to the cases e.g. by age and sex.

a **McNemar test** is a hypothesis test for **paired categorical data**.

the **mean** is the average of a set of observations.

the **median** is the middle value of a ranked set of observations. It is better than the **mean** to summarise **skewed** data.

the **minimum sample size required** is the smallest sample needed for a study to stand a reasonable chance of detecting the **clinically important difference or change** if it exists.

the **mode** is the most frequently occurring value in a set of observations.

multiple regression is the extension of **linear (or logistic) regression** to **multiple explanatory variables**.

multivariate analysis is, strictly speaking, the analysis of several **outcomes** simultaneously and requires complex statistical techniques. It is often used, however, to refer to analyses using more than one explanatory variable. The most important aspect is sorting out what questions it is important to ask of such data.

nominal data is **categorical** data, in which the categories are not ordered and there are more than two categories. An example is blood group. There is no intrinsic order in blood groups and more than two categories.

non-parametric tests are **hypothesis tests** that do not make distributional assumptions. They typically work with the ranks of data rather than the raw values.

normal distribution see **Gaussian distribution**.

A **null hypothesis** is a formal statement that there is no true difference between groups, or no true association between variables. It is used in a **hypothesis test**.

numerical data is data which is interpretable quantitatively and includes **continuous** data and **discrete** data.

An **observational study** is a general term for non-experimental studies and includes **cross-sectional, case-control** and **cohort studies**.

an **odds ratio** is a measure of comparing the rates in each of two groups. For rare events it approximates the **relative risk** and are often used interchangeably in the medical literature.

a **one sample t-test** is an **hypothesis test** to see whether a sample of values come from a population with a specified mean value.

ordinal data are data where the data can be ordered, but the values do not have a quantitative interpretation, such as much improved, improved, no change, worse, much worse.

an **outcome** is a term used in a clinical trial for the end-points by which the new therapy will be judged. For an anti-hypertensive, for example, the main outcome will be blood pressure.

paired data are data arising from particular study designs leading to linkages of data points. Examples arise from **matched case-control studies** where each case is paired with a control, and cross-over **clinical trials**, where each patient's observations on the two treatments form a pair. If the pairing is ignored in analysis, information can be lost.

a **paired t-test** is a **one sample t-test** where the sample consists of paired differences. It is the equivalent of the **two sample t-test** when the data are **paired**.

parametric tests are **hypothesis tests** based on assuming distributional forms for the data, such as a **Gaussian** distribution.

a **placebo** is a dummy tablet or treatment used in a **randomised controlled trial** to preserve blinding.

a **point estimate** is a single estimate of a quantity such as a **proportion** or a **difference in means**. The uncertainty associated with the estimate can be described using **confidence intervals**.

a **potential confounder** is a variable that would be a **confounder**, but is dealt with by matching (see **matched case-control study**) or some other design strategy which ensures that it does not have a confounding effect in the study.

the **power** of a study is the probability it has of detecting a **clinically important difference** to be **statistically significant** at a particular level should such a difference truly exist.

power calculations see **sample size calculations**.

the **P-value** is the probability of observing such extreme data (or more extreme) as that observed, were the **null hypothesis** to be true.

random allocation is a method of allocating patients to treatments in a **clinical trial** to avoid systematic **biases** between groups. (see also **randomisation**).

a **random sample** is a subset of a population who are studied in order to learn about the whole population, where each person has an equal probability of being in the sample.

randomisation is a procedure for **randomly allocating** patients (or groups of individuals in a cluster randomised trial) to treatments in a **clinical trial** as if by the toss of a coin. The purpose is to avoid any systematic differences between groups. Typically randomisation lists are computer generated.

a **randomised controlled trial** is a **clinical trial** in which treatment assignation is at random and the new therapy (or therapies) is compared to a **control group**.

RCT see **randomised controlled trial**.

regression see **linear regression** and **logistic regression**.

the **relative risk** of a disease in relation to a particular exposure is the incidence of diseases among exposed persons divided by the incidence of disease among the unexposed persons.

a **risk factor** for a disease is a factor whose presence means a person is more likely to get that disease.

sample size calculations are used to determine how large a study needs to be to have adequate **power** to detect a **clinically important difference**.

SD see **standard deviation**.

SE see **standard error**.

significance level is a term to decide at what level a study will be judged to be **statistically significant**.

significance test see **hypothesis test**.

a **significant difference** is a term used where the **P-value** for the difference lies beyond a pre-specified cut-off such as 0.05.

skewed data is data where the bulk of the observations are low but with a long tail of high values (or a mirror image of this).

standard deviation is a measure of spread of **continuous data**. A useful guideline is that 95% of observations are expected to lay within 2 standard deviations of the **mean**.

standard error is a measure of accuracy of an estimate, and is used in the calculation of **confidence intervals**.

statistical significance is a term used to refer to the **P-value**, or whether the **P-value** is less than some critical value such as 0.05.

a **study hypothesis** is a prediction that is to be tested in a study. Pre-specification of study hypotheses helps guard against *post hoc* data dredging.

a **two sample t-test** is a hypothesis test used to compare two groups of observations with **continuous variables** thought to approximately follow a **Gaussian distribution**.

the **unit of randomisation** is often the patient, meaning that each patient is individually randomised, but can be, for example, the practice, if all patients within a practice must get the same procedure. See **cluster randomised trial**.

univariate analysis looks at one factor at a time.

unpaired data are independent samples with no linkage between individual observations in the samples.

unpaired t-test see **two sample t-test**.

the **Wilcoxon matched pairs test** is a **non-parametric hypothesis test** used when the data are paired.

95% CI is an abbreviation for 95% confidence interval, see **confidence interval**.

Answers

Chapter 1

Exercise 1 (see text)

Exercise 2

a) Folic acid group: 6/593 = 0.0101

No folic acid group: 21/602 = 0.0349

b) Relative risk = $\dfrac{6/593}{21/602}$ = 0.290

[0.289 if you have used $\dfrac{0.0101}{0.0349}$]

c) Odds ratio = $\dfrac{6/587}{21/581}$ = 0.283 to 3 decimal places.

(If you are using a calculator this figure is obtained by rounding up the fourth figure after the decimal point.)

d) The answers are very similar, but the relative risk is closer to one than the odds ratio

e) Difference between proportions = 0.0349 – 0.0101 = 0.0248.

f) The relative risk tells us how much less likely the risk of NTD is on treatment.

The odds ratio is interchangeable with the relative risk. The difference in proportion tells us more directly how many NTDs will be prevented by this strategy, but it assumes the underlying rate will be the same.

Chapter 3

Exercise 1
Study 1
If p = 0.6   n = 10
standard error = square root of [0.6 x 0.4/10]
               = square root of 0.24/10
               = square root of 0.024
               = 0.155 to 3 decimal places
as a percentage 15.5%

Study 2
If p = 0.7   n = 100
standard error = $\sqrt{0.7 \times 0.3/100}$
               = $\sqrt{0.0021}$
               = 0.0458 or 4.6%

If p = 0.8   n = 100
standard error = $\sqrt{0.6 \times 0.4/100}$
               = $\sqrt{0.0024}$
               = 0.0490 or 4.9%

Study 3
If p = 0.7   n = 1000
standard error = $\sqrt{0.7 \times 0.3/1000}$
               = $\sqrt{0.00021}$
               = 0.0145 or 1.5%

If p = 0.6   n = 1000
standard error = $\sqrt{0.6 \times 0.4/1000}$
               = $\sqrt{0.00016}$
               = 0.0155 or 1.5%

Exercise 2
a) Your guess!

b) 365 – Not everyone responded (394 to questionnaire and only 365 to relevant question).
- Sample may not be truly representative.

c) (i) 20.4% (17.0 – 23.7%) (results section)
  (ii) 74.1% (70.3 – 77.8%) (abstract and Table 3)

d) Confidence intervals are important because they remind us that the simple ('point') estimate is not precise, and they indicate where the true value is likely to be.

Exercise 3
a) 1.14   (1.04 to 1.25)
b) 3.60   (2.17 to 5.97)
c) 3.17   (1.69 to 5.97)
d) 10.58   (8.13 to 27.08)

Smoke alarm
e) Intervention families are being compared with controls. Intervention families are about 14% more likely to use a smoke alarm, but this could be just a 4% increase or it could be a 25% increase. (Read Article 22 for more detail on interpreting relative risks.)

f) If there is no difference both the relative risk and the odds ratio will be 1. All of the confidence intervals exclude this, with a high degree of confidence. Thus we are pretty confident that the intervention has had a positive effect (Clamp).

Exercise 4

a) The diabetes variables exclude zero, whereas the asthma variables mainly include it.

b) These refer to a difference in proportions. When there is no difference, this value will be zero.

c) This indicates evidence of an effect of intervention on diabetes but not on asthma.

Exercise 5

Confidence intervals and P-values are closely related. When looking at differences, a value of zero indicates no difference between the groups. If the 95% confidence interval excludes zero, then the P-value will be significant at $P < 0.05$. 'Role Emotion' (Table 2, line 4) illustrates this well. The P-Value is only just less than 0.05, and the lower limit is only a little higher than zero.

CHAPTER 4

Exercise 1

Study A shows benefit which is not clinically worthwhile. (The confidence interval does not cover 0, but is also is wholly below the clinically important difference of 10%, so it does not look likely that this difference could be achieved.)

Study B shows benefit which could be clinically worthwhile.

Study C shows benefit which is definitely clinically worthwhile.

Study D is highly inconclusive – we cannot tell if the benefit is extremely good, or even slightly harmful. The confidence interval is extremely wide – this may indicate that the study was rather small.

Exercise 2

a) The main hypothesis is that psychological problems are more common in children with AE. The null hypothesis is that there is no difference in the rate of psychological problems between children with AE and children without AE.

b) An x^2 test – this is indicated by the syntax 'chi' in the line above the table and the 'chi^2' in the line below.

c) We cannot reject the null hypothesis. We would only expect to see such extreme results about six times in 100.

d) Group 0 $p_1 = 8/30 = 0.27$ or 27% (here the rounding has been carried out to only two decimal places, not three because of the small sample size).
Group 1 $p_2 = 15/30 = 0.5$ or 50%
difference = 0.5 – 0.27 = 0.23 or 23%

e) Standard error = 0.12
95% CI = $(0.23 – (1.96 \times 0.12), 0.23 + (1.96 \times 0.12)$ = $(-0.01, 0.47)$ or (-1%, 47%) (Again rounding to two decimal places.)

f) We are 95% sure the true difference in proportions lies somewhere between a 47% increase or a 1% decrease in AE compared controls.

g) Although the difference could be in excess of 20%, it could be much less. Further research is needed to establish more precisely the magnitude of any such difference.

Exercise 3

$p_1 = 0.25$ $p_2 = 0.45$
Significance 5%, power 80% requires 89 in each group.

Exercise 4

a) (i) 49
(ii) 62 (Different tables and programmes will often give slightly different answers!)

b) Smaller numbers are required.

c) clinically important change

% in baseline group	10%	20%
5%	141	49
10%	199	62
25%	329	89
50%	388	93

d) Sample sizes required increase as % in baseline group increases and decrease as clinically important change increases.

Exercise 5

a) $p_1 = 0.4$ $p_2 = 0.6$, power 95%, significance 5% gives 160 in each group or 320 in all.
(Different tables and programmes will often give slightly different answers!)

b) d = 1 + (12 – 1) 0.01
    = 1 + (11 x 0.01)
    = 1 + 0.11
    = 1.11

total sample size = 320 x 1.11 = 355

c) d = 1 + (25 – 1) 0.01
    = 1 + (24 x 0.01)
    = 1 + 0.24
    = 1.24

total sample size = 320 x 1.21 = 390

CHAPTER 5

Exercise 1

a) Data unpaired. Choice of test depends on distribution of days. A two sample t-test depends on distribution of days. A two sample t-test is probably reasonable, although if data are very skew, a Mann Whitney U-test could be used.

b) Data are paired (before/after) and binary (did/did not attend). A McNemar's test could be used.

c) Groups are unpaired. If follow-up is for a fixed period and complete, then an x^2 test could be used, otherwise some kind of survival analysis.

d) Data are paired as each patient has both active and placebo. The test to be used depends on the distribution of the (differences in) scores, but either a one sample t-test or a Wilcoxon (non-parametric) test should work.

e) Data are paired because of the matching and the 'outcome' continuous, so a one sample t-test could be used. More formally, for a matched case control study, conditional logistic regression is often used.

f) These data can be summarised by a 3 x 3 contingency table. An x^2 test can be used, although modifications may be needed to take account of the ordering.

g) The groups are unpaired. Provided the gains in weights are reasonably distributed, a two sample test should suffice.

h) These data could be summarised with a 5 x 2 contingency table. An x^2 test to trend would probably be the best test (this has not been covered in the workbook) but a Mann-Whitney U test could also be used.

CHAPTER 6
Exercise 1
a) Gestation – early babies may be more vulnerable to SID and more likely to have heating on all night because parents want to keep them warm.

b)
(i) Because this is base category.
(ii)) Position put down: front, position found: side.
(iii) Front.
(iv) No confidence intervals cover 1 so increased risk unlikely to have arisen by chance.

c)
(i) Most ≥ 10, least<6.
(ii) Slight decrease in OR = decreased effect.
(iii) Socio-economic status associated with warmth of bedding.

d)
(i) SID more likely if duvet used, 95% confident that in population odds of SID if duvet used between twice and four times odds if no duvet.
(ii) More likely if bedding loose, 95% confident odds in pop.1.5 to 2.75 times greater etc.
(iii) Where in bed makes no difference.
(iv) More likely if covers often/always over head etc.
(v) More likely if covers over head in last sleep etc.

e)
(i) Univariate: 95% certain that odds of SID if using dummy is 42% to 82% that if dummy not used i.e. using dummy is good.

CHAPTER 7
Exercise 1
1) Yes. (**abstract** and **patients and methods** sections.)
2) Yes. 98% of those assigned CABG and 97% of those

assigned PTCA successfully completed the trial protocol; the assigned procedures were carried out on them. 12 individuals were crossovers; 5 from CABG to PTCA and 7 the other way round. There were six dropouts (refused treatment) among the CABG patients and 3 among the PTCA patients (**patients and methods** section).

Yes, follow-up was complete for survival (**extent of follow-up** section). Follow-up not quite so complete for other outcomes: '11 patients have withdrawn, and a few patients fail to attend each planned visit'.

Yes, patients were analysed in the groups to which they were allocated (**randomised procedure** section) 'on the intention-to-treat principle, these patients (i.e. those for whom intended treatment was not carried out) have been included in the original randomised groups for the follow up results'. See also **statistics section**.

3) Patients and health workers could not be blind to the treatments because of the nature of the treatments themselves.

By 'study personnel' question referring to those who assessed the outcomes – not necessary for all those involved in the study to be blind to treatments and impossible for those analysing the results or holding the allocation list to be blind. The paper makes clear that those who assessed outcomes were 'blind to the patient's assigned treatment' [**data collection** section].

4) Yes (**Table 1**). Differences between the two groups do occur. For example, 41% (207/501) of CABG patients are aged 50-59 compared with 44% (225/510), but these differences are a matter of two or three percentage points; usually not important.

5) No. There were approximately four times as many subsequent interventions in the PTCA group than in the intervention group [**subsequent interventions** section], and patients in the PTCA group made much more use of anti-anginal drugs. Although subsequent interventions can be seen as part of treatment. The important question here is what effect this may have on the results?

6) This question is asking about both statistical significance and clinical importance. It is usual to consider the primary outcome first, although other outcomes may also be considered. The primary end point was 'the combined 5-year incidence of death and definite non-fatal myocardial infarction.' [**data collection** section.] 43 out of 501 CABG patients had reached the primary end point, and 50 out of the 510 PTCA patients had (**abstract**). The treatment effect is presented as 'relative risk 0.88 [95% confidence interval 0.59-1.29]'. In Article 10, 'logrank p=0.47' [**deaths and myocardial infarctions during follow-up** section.] The logrank test compares two survival curves. (For more detail, see Bland.) Test is not significant at the 5% level (because p>0.05), and confidence interval for the relative risk covers 1. Thus the result is not statistically significant.

Is the treatment effect clinically important? The confidence interval limits suggest that deaths and myocardial infarctions could potentially be reduced by 41% or increased by 29% by using CABG rather than PTCA. If the effect in the whole population was near to either of these limits it would be clinically important.

The present study has not been large enough to give a definitive answer as to which of the treatments is better, but it seems to indicate that there may be a difference between the two, only we do not know which direction it is in. In this case we can say that the difference is potentially clinically important.

7) The confidence interval for the relative risk tells us we can be 95% certain that the RR in the population lies between 0.59 and 1.29 – not particularly precise.

8) There are clear selection criteria [**patients and methods** section], your patients would have to be similar to those entered into the study.

Note that in the end only 4.8% of those for whom 'myocardial revascularisation was considered necessary' were randomised in the trial. This is a very small subset, and so might consider that there is no reason to think they are representative of the much larger group of patients requiring revascularisation.

However, in the discussion the authors state that 'in the RITA trial many angiographically eligible patients were not randomised for non-clinical reasons (e.g. consent refused). The trial patients are therefore likely to be representative of the relatively large subgroup of patients who are suitable for either CABG or PTCA, particularly patients in whom equivalent revascularistion is considered feasible by either treatment method.' No

substantial justification is given for this statement, however. We are left to trust the investigators!

9) Yes. Mortality was considered as part of the primary outcome. Morbidity was considered via subsequent interventions and angina. Quality of life was considered via physical activity, employment status, and exercise testing. Side effects were considered (see Table 3).

10) We have already established that for the primary outcome we cannot really be certain which is the better treatment, therefore the answers to this question are not as relevant or as useful as the might be if one treatment had really been shown to be significantly better than the other.

Nevertheless, the calculations can be carried out for illustrative purposes. In this context the question becomes: are the likely benefits of CABG (on balance the better treatment) worth the potential harms and costs of CABG? Harm is measured via side effects, and costs are often measured in terms of the numbers needed to treat (NNT) to prevent one adverse effect. In this case NNT=1/ARD= $1/(0.98-0.86) = 83$, so 83 people need to be treated with CABG in order to save one death. A major side effect is stroke and Table 3 gives details of this indicating 10 strokes amongst CABG patients and 9 amongst PTCA.

The timing of these strokes, however, is somewhat different between the two groups, being much earlier on average in CABG patients. Arrhythmia and cardiac failure have both been more common amongst the PTCA patients, so no extra harm in terms of these side effects will come to a patient on CABG. However, the extra harm in terms of a slightly higher level of stroke and possible earlier stroke must be considered.

REFERENCES

Absolon CM, Cottrell D, Eldridge SM et al. (1997) Psychological disturbance in atopic eczema: the extent of the problem in school-aged children. *British Journal of Dermatology* **137**: 241-5

Altman DG, Bland JM (1996) Statistic notes: presentation of numerical data. *British Medical Journal* **312** (7030): 572

de Bono AM (1997) Communication between an occupational physician and other medical practitioners – an audit. *Occupational Medicine* **47**(6): 349-56

Bryner CL (1995) Learning as a function of lecture length. *Family Medicine* **27**(6): 379-82

Campbell NC, Thain J, Deans HG et al. (1998) Secondary prevention clinics for coronary heart disease: randomised trial of effect on health. *British Medical Journal*: **316**: 1434-7

Clamp M and Kendrick D (1998) A randomised controlled trial of general practitioner safety advice for families with children under 5 years. *British Medical Journal* **316**: 1576-9

Donner A (1982) An empirical study of cluster randomisation. *International Journal of Epidemiology* **11**(3): 283-286.

Feder G, Griffiths CJ, Highton C et al. (1995) Do clinical guidelines introduced with practice-based education improve care of asthmatic and diabetic patients? A randomised controlled trial in general practices in east London. *British Medical Journal* **311**: 1473-8

Fleming PJ, Blair PS, Bacon C et al. (1996) Confidential enquiry into stillbirths and deaths regional co-ordinators and researchers. Environment of infants during sleep and risk of sudden infant death syndrome: results of 1993-95 case-control study for confidential inquiry into stillbirths and deaths in infancy. *British Medical Journal* **313**: 191-5

Fox N and Mathers N (1997) Empowering research: statistical power in general practice research. *Family Practice* **14**(4): 324-9

Hannaford PC, Thompson C and Simpson M (1996) Evaluation of an educational programme to improve the recognition of psychological illness by general practitioners. *British Journal of General Practice* 1996 **46**: 333-7

Kerry SM and Bland JM (1998) Trials which randomise practices I: how should they be analysed? *Family Practice* **15**(1): 80-3

Kerry SM and Bland JM (1998) Trials which randomise practices II: sample size. *Family Practice* **15**(1): 84-7

Kromhout D, Bloemberg BP, Feskens EJ et al. (1996) Alcohol, fish, fibre and antioxidant vitamins intake do not explain population differences in coronary heart disease mortality. *International Journal of Epidemiology* **25**(4): 753-9

Lam TH (1997) Relative risks are inflated in published literature. *British Medical Journal* **315**(7112): 880

Machin D, Campbell MJ, Fayers P et al. (1997) Table 3.1 Sample sizes for comparison of proportions. In *Sample Size Tables for Clinical Studies.* Oxford, Blackwell Science

Mills N, Bachman M, Harvey I et al. (1997) Patients' experience of epilepsy and health care. *Family Practice* **14**(2): 117-23

MRC Vitamin Study Research Group (1991) Prevention of neural tube defects: results of the Medical Research Council vitamin study. *The Lancet* **338**: 131-7

O'Connor AM, Griffiths CJ, Underwood MR et al. (1998) Can postal prompts from general practitioners improve the uptake of breast screening? A randomised controlled trial in one east London general practice. *Journal of Medical Screening* **5**: 49-52

RITA Trial Participants (1993) Coronary angioplasty versus coronary artery bypass surgery: the randomised intervention treatment of angina (RITA) trial. *The Lancet* **341**: 573-80

RITA-2 Trial Participants (1997) Coronary angioplasty versus medical therapy for angina: the second randomised intervention treatment of angina (RITA-2) trial. *The Lancet* **350**: 461-8

Shepperd S, Harwood D, Gray A et al. (1998) Randomised controlled trial comparing hospital at home care with in patient hospital care. II cost minimisation analysis. *British Medical Journal* **316**(7147): 1791-6

SUGGESTED FURTHER READING

Bland JM (1995) *An Introduction to Medical Statistics.* 2nd edition, Oxford Medical Press

Eldridge S and Naish J (1998) Workbook 3: What the papers say. *Evidence-based Primary Care.* London, Radcliffe Press Ltd

Carter Y, Shaw S and Thomas C (2000) Workbook 4: *Randomised Controlled Trials and Multi-Centre Research.* London, RGCP.

READING MATERIAL

1 Altman DG, Bland JM (1996) Statistic notes: Presentation of numerical data. *British Medical Journal* **312**(7030)

2 MRC Vitamin Study Research Group (1991) Prevention of neural tube defects: Results of the Medical Research Council Vitamin Study. *The Lancet* **338**: 131-7

3 Campbell NC, Thain J, Deans HG et al. (1998) Secondary prevention clinics for coronary heart disease: randomised trial of effect on health. *British Medical Journal* **316**: 1434-7

4 Mills N, Bachman M, Harvey I et al. (1997) Patients' experience of epilepsy and health care. *Family Practice* **14**(2): 117-23

5 Clamp M and Kendrick D (1998) A randomised controlled trial of general practitioner safety advice for families with children under 5 years. *British Medical Journal* **316**: 1576-9

6 de Bono AM (1997) Communication between an occupational physician and other medical practitioners – an audit. *Occupational Medicine* **47**(6): 349-56

7 Feder G, Griffiths CJ, Highton C et al. (1995). Do clinical guidelines introduced with practice based education improve care of asthmatic and diabetic patients? A randomised controlled trial in general practices in east London. *British Medical Journal* **311**: 1473-8

8 Hannaford PC, Thompson C and Simpson M (1996) Evaluation of an educational programme to improve the recognition of psychological illness by general practitioners. *British Journal of General Practice* 1996; **46**: 333-7

9 O'Connor AM, Griffiths CJ, Underwood MR et al. (1998) Can postal prompts from general practitioners improve the uptake of breast screening? A randomised controlled trial in one east London general practice. *Journal of Medical Screening* **5**(1): 49-52

10 RITA Trial Participants (1993) Coronary angioplasty versus coronary artery bypass surgery: the Randomised Intervention Treatment of Angina (RITA) Trial. *The Lancet* **341**: 573-80

11 RITA-2 trial participants (1997) Coronary angioplasty versus medical therapy for angina: the second Randomised Intervention Treatment of Angina (RITA-2) trial. *The Lancet* **350**: 461-8

12 Fox N and Mathers N (1997) Empowering research: statistical power in general practice research. *Family Practice* **14**(4): 324-9

13 Machin D, Campbell MJ, Fayers P et al. (1997) Table 3.1 Sample sizes for comparison of proportions. In *Sample size tables for clinical studies*. Oxford: Blackwell Science

14 Absolon CM, Cottrell D, Eldridge SM et al. (1997) Psychological disturbance in atopic eczema: the extent of the problem in school-aged children. *British Journal of Dermatology* **137**: 241-5

15 Donner A. (1982) An empirical study of cluster randomisation. *International Journal of Epidemiology* **11**(3): 283-6.

16 Kerry SM and Bland JM (1998) Trials which randomise practices I: how should they be analysed? *Family Practice* **15**(1); 80-3

17 Kerry SM and Bland JM (1998) Trials which randomise practices II: sample size. *Family Practice* **15**(1); 84-7

18 Bryner CL (1995) Learning as a function of lecture length. *Family Medicine* **27**(6): 379-82

19 Shepperd S, Harwood D, Gray A et al. (1998) Randomised controlled trial comparing hospital at home care with in patient hospital care. II cost minimisation analysis. *British Medical Journal* **316**(7147): 1791-6

20 Fleming PJ, Blair PS, Bacon C et al. (1996) Confidential Enquiry into Stillbirths and Deaths Regional Coordinators and Researchers. Environment of infants during sleep and risk of sudden infant death syndrome: results of 1993-95 case-control study for confidential inquiry into stillbirths and deaths in infancy. *British Medical Journal* **313**: 191-5

21 Kromhout D, Bloemberg BP, Feskens EJ et al. (1996) Alcohol, fish, fibre and antioxidant vitamins intake do not explain population differences in coronary heart disease mortality. *International Journal of Epidemiology* **25**(4): 753-9

22 Lam TH (1997) Relative risks are inflated in published literature. *British Medical Journal* **315** (7112): 880

This article was first published in the BMJ and is reproduced by permission of the BMJ

EDUCATION AND DEBATE
Statistics Notes: Presentation of numerical data

Douglas G Altman, J Martin Bland

Douglas G Altman, head, *IRCF Medical Statistics Group, Centre for Statistics in Medicine, Institute of Health Sciences, PO Box 777, Oxford OX3 7LF,* J Martin Bland, professor of medical statistics, *Department of Public Health Sciences, St George's Hospital Medical School, London SW17 0RE*

Correspondence to: Mr Altman.

BMJ 1996;312:572 (2 March)

The purpose of a scientific paper is to communicate, and within the paper this applies especially to the presentation of data.

Continuous data, such as serum cholesterol concentration or triceps skinfold thickness, can be summarised numerically either in the text or in tables or plotted in a graph. When numbers are given there is the problem of how precisely to specify them. As far as possible the numerical precision used should be consistent throughout a paper and especially within a table. In general, summary statistics such as means should not be given to more than one extra decimal place over the raw data. The same usually applies to measures of variability or uncertainty such as the standard deviation or standard error, though greater precision may be warranted for these quantities as they are often used in further calculations. Similar comments apply to the results of regression analyses, where spurious precision should be avoided. For example, the regression equation[1]

birth weight=-3.0983527 + 0.142088xchest circumf + 0.158039 x midarm circumf, purports to predict birth weight to 1/1000000 g.

Categorical data, such as disease group or presence or absence of symptoms, can be summarised as frequencies and percentages. It can be confusing to give percentages alone, as the denominator may be unclear. Also, giving frequencies allows percentages to be given as integers, such as 22%, rather than more precisely. Percentages to one decimal place may sometimes be reasonable, but not in small samples; greater precision is unwarranted. Such data rarely need to be shown graphically.

Test statistics, such as values of t or x^2, and correlation coefficients should be given to no more than two decimal places. Confidence intervals are better presented as, say, "12.4 to 52.9" because the format "12.4-52.9" is confusing when one or both numbers are negative. P values should be given to one or two significant figures. P values are always greater than zero. Because computer output is often to a fixed number of decimal places P=0.0000 really means P<0.00005—such values should be converted to P<0.0001. P values always used to be quoted as P<0.05, P<0.01, and so on because results were compared with tabulated values of statistical distributions. Now that most P values are produced by computer they should be given more exactly, even for non-significant results—for example, P=0.2. Values such as P=0.0027 can be rounded up to P=0.003, but not in general to P<0.01 or P<0.05. In particular, the use of P<0.05 (or, even worse, P=NS) may conceal important information: there is minimal difference between P=0.06 and P=0.04. In tables, however, it may be necessary to use symbols to denote degrees of significance; a common system is to use *, **, and *** to mean P<0.05, 0.01, and 0.001 respectively. Mosteller gives a more extensive discussion of numerical presentation.[2]

The choice between using a table or figure is not easy, nor is it easy to offer much general guidance. Tables are suitable for displaying information about a large number of variables at once, and graphs are good for showing multiple observations on individuals or groups, but between these cases lie a wide range of situations where the best format is not obvious. One point to consider when contemplating using a figure is the amount of numerical information contained. A figure that displays only two means with their standard errors or confidence intervals is a waste of space as a figure; either more information should be added, such as the raw data (a really useful feature of a figure), or the summary values should be put in the text.

In tables information about different variables or quantities is easier to assimilate if the columns (rather than the rows) contain like information, such as means or standard deviations. Interpretation of tables showing data for individuals (or perhaps for many groups) is aided by having the data ordered by one of the variables—for example, by the baseline value of the measurement of interest or by some important prognostic characteristic.

References

1 Bhargava SK, Ramji S, Kumar A, Mohan MAN, Marwah J, Sachdev HPS. Mid-arm and chest circumferences at birth as predictors of low birth weight and neonatal mortality in the community. *BMJ* 1985;**291**:1617-9.
2 Mosteller F. Writing about numbers. In: Bailar JC, Mosteller F. eds. *Medical uses of statistics.* 2nd ed. Boston: NEJM Books, 1992:375-89.

This article was first published in the Lancet and is reproduced by permission of the Lancet.

PREVENTION OF NEURAL TUBE DEFECTS:
RESULTS OF THE MEDICAL RESEARCH COUNCIL VITAMIN STUDY

Lancet 1991; **338**: 131–37

MRC Vitamin Study Research Group*

*This report was prepared by Nicholas Wald, with assistance from Joan Sneddon, James Densem, Christopher Frost, and Rossana Stone. For membership of steering committee, data monitoring committee, trial office staff, and representation of participating centres, see end of paper. Correspondence to Prof Nicholas Wald, Department of Environmental and Preventive Medicine, Medical College of St Bartholomew's Hospital, Charterhouse Square, London EC1M 6BQ, UK.

A randomised double-blind prevention trial with a factorial design was conducted at 33 centres in seven countries to determine whether supplementation with folic acid (one of the vitamins in the B group) or a mixture of seven other vitamins (A, D, B^1, B^2, B^6, C, and nicotinamide) around the time of conception can prevent neural tube defects (anencephaly, spina bifida, encephalocele). A total of 1817 women at high risk of having a pregnancy with a neural tube defect, because of a previous affected pregnancy, were allocated at random to one of four groups — namely, folic acid, other vitamins, both, or neither. 1195 had a completed pregnancy in which the fetus or infant was known to have or not have a neural tube defect; 27 of these had a known neural tube defect, 6 in the folic acid groups and 21 in the two other groups, a 72% protective effect (relative risk 0.28, 95% confidence interval 0.12–0.71). The other vitamins showed no significant protective effect (relative risk 0.80, 95% CI 0.32–1.72). There was no demonstrable harm from the folic acid supplementation, though the ability of the study to detect rare or slight adverse effects was limited. Folic acid supplementation starting before pregnancy can now be firmly recommended for all women who have had an affected pregnancy, and public health measures should betaken to ensure that the diet of all women who may bear children contains an adequate amount of folic acid.

INTRODUCTION

It has long been suspected that diet has a role in the causation of neural tube defects, which are among the most common severe congenital malformations. The possibility that folic acid (a vitamin in the B group) might be involved was raised in 1964[1,2] In 1980 and 1981 the results of two intervention studies were published in which vitamin supplementation around the time of conception was given to women who had had a pregnancy with a neural tube defect.[1,4] These suggested that folic acid or other vitamin supplementation might reduce the risk of a recurrence. In the first study,[3] which was not randomised, participating women were given a mixture of eight vitamins which included folic acid (0.36 mg/day), and women who were already pregnant

or had declined to take part in the study served as controls. The risk of a recurrence in supplemented women was about one-seventh that in the unsupplemented women.

The second study was a small randomised trial of folic acid supplementation alone (4 mg/day).[4] It yielded inconclusive results when analysed according to randomly allocated treatment group (so avoiding bias), but when analysed after the transfer of women in the folic acid group who did not take their capsules to the control group (ie, ignoring the randomisation and so introducing the possibility of bias) the supplemented women had a significantly lower recurrence rate.

The lower recurrence rate in the supplemented women in these two studies is unlikely to have arisen purely by chance. Two explanations were possible. One is that folic acid or possibly the other vitamins can prevent some cases of neural tube defects. A second plausible explanation is that women who chose to take the vitamins represented a selected group, perhaps with a more affluent or health-conscious diet, who were therefore at low risk of having a further affected pregnancy. Indeed, it is likely that such selection was operating; however, it was not known whether there was also a genuine preventive effect, and, if so, its magnitude and whether the responsible component was folic acid or one of the other vitamins.

Neither further statistical analysis of the results of these studies nor the accumulation of further results without appropriate controls would have solved the problem.[5] The issue could be resolved only by performing a large trial in which, to avoid bias, women at risk would be randomly allocated to various groups, including a control group that did not receive the extra vitamins. Furthermore, such a study would also permit the unbiased detection of any major adverse effects. A trial was launched in July, 1983, with the aim of recruiting women known to be at high risk through having had a previous affected pregnancy. It was the intention to obtain information on the outcome of at least 2000 pregnancies unless a sufficiently clear result emerged sooner. By April, 1991, sufficiently conclusive results had emerged to warrant ending the trial. The results at that time are the subject of this paper.

Table I

Number of women randomised and number with informative pregnancies according to centre

Centre	No of women randomised	Informative pregnancies*
UK		
Glasgow	383	287
Cardiff	64	40
St Bartholomew's Hospital	61	46
Newcastle	54	28
Oxford	49	38
Edinburgh	32	19
Queen Charlotte's	25	21
Sheffield	15	7
Dundee	13	8
East Birmingham	11	9
The London Hospital	10	9
Southampton	5	5
St George's Hospital	5	3
University College Hospital	3	3
Aberdeen	3	0
Ashton-under-Lyne	1	0
Leicester	1	0
Total UK	**735**	**523**
Hungary		
Budapest	284	201
Debrecen	149	86
Miskolc	111	65
Pecs	88	56
Szombathely	62	47
Szeged	54	33
Gyor	21	2
Israel	140	107
Australia		
Adelaide	31	19
Melbourne	24	8
Sydney	20	14
Canada		
Hamilton	23	19
Halifax	10	2
Vancouver	8	8
USSR,		
Moscow	53	5
France, Lyon	4	0
Total non-UK	**1082**	**672**
Grand total	**1817**	**1195**

*An informative pregnancy was one in which the fetus or infant was known to have or not have a neural tube defect by the time the trial was stopped.

METHODS

The study was an international, multicentre, double-blind randomised trial involving 33 centres (17 in the UK and 16 in six other countries). Women with a previous pregnancy affected by a neural tube defect, not associated with the autosomal recessive disorder Meckel's syndrome, were eligible for the study if they were planning another pregnancy and were not already taking vitamin supplements. Women with epilepsy were excluded in case the folic acid supplementation adversely affected their treatment. Antenatal diagnosis of neural tube defects was available at all centres in the study. The effect of supplementation both with folic acid and with a selection of other vitamins was investigated by use of a factorial study design. Women were allocated at random to one of four supplementation groups, the supplements containing folic acid, other vitamins, both, or neither, in the following way:

Group	Folic acid	Other vitamins
A	Yes	No
B	Yes	Yes
C	No	No
D	No	Yes

Comparison of the outcomes in groups A and B with those in groups C and D tested the effect of folic acid supplementation; comparison of the outcomes in groups B and D with those in groups A and C tested the effect of the other vitamins. Separate sets of random allocations were used for each centre to ensure that there would be approximately equal numbers of women in each supplementation group at each centre.

The capsules used in the study were prepared by the Boots Company and packaged in 2-week calendar "blister" packs. Women in the trial were asked to take a single capsule each day from the date of randomisation until 12 weeks of pregnancy (estimated from the first day of the last menstrual period). Capsules for those in the folic acid groups contained 4 mg of folic acid — the larger of the two doses used in the previous studies being chosen because a negative result with the lower dose would have left the matter open. Capsules for those in the multivitamin groups contained vitamin A 4000 U, D 400 U, B_1 1.5 mg, B_2 1.5 mg, B_6 1.0 mg, C 40 Mg, and nicotinamide 15 mg. The control substance in the capsules was dried ferrous sulphate 120 mg and di-calcium phosphate 240 mg. The potency of the capsules was independently checked every three months by Hoffmann La Roche in Basel, Switzerland. The trial was double-blind, in that neither the doctor nor the patient knew which regimen had been allocated. It was agreed that the groups to which patients were allocated would normally be revealed only at the end of the trial. The randomisation was carried out through the Clinical Trials Service Unit in Oxford.

Women invited to join the trial were given a week to decide if they wished to take part, so that they could consider the matter at leisure and discuss the matter further with others if they wished. All patients were given a printed information leaflet about the trial.

No special advice was specified regarding diet. On entry into the trial, samples of blood and urine were collected

Table II

Mean age, mean number of previous births, and mean number of previous neural tube defect pregnancies among all women randomised according to randomisation group

Randomisation group		No. of women	Mean age (yr)	In previous pregnancies, mean no of:				Mean no of previous NTD pregnancies
Folic acid	Other vitamins			Total births	Live births	Miscarriages and other intrauterine deaths*	Terminations of pregnancy	
A +	–	449	27.0	2.05	0.88	0.43	0.74	1.03
B +	+	461	27.4	2.12	0.94	0.48	0.70	1.04
C –	–	454	26.8	2.05	0.91	0.43	0.71	1.01
D –	+	453	26.5	1.88	0.81	0.39	0.68	1.01

*Including ectopic pregnancies.

Table III

Outcome of all pregnancies according to randomisation group and whether the pregnancy was informative

Randomisation group		No. of women randomised	Number of completed pregnancies									
			Not informative				Informative				
Folic acid	Other vitamins		Miscarriage	Ectopic Pregnancy	Termination of pregnancy	Total	Livebirth	Miscarriage	Stillbirth	Termination of pregnancy	Total
A +	–	449	39	1	0	40	290	3	2	3	298
B +	+	461	41	3	0	44	285	4	2	4	295
C –	–	454	41	4	1	46	283	3	3	11	300
D –	+	453	33	2	2	37	287	6	0	9	302
Total		1817	154	10	3	167	1145	16	7	27	1195

and sent to the central trial office in the Department of Environmental and Preventive Medicine at St Bartholomew's Hospital for folic acid analysis, performed by radioimmunoassay [6] (Amersham International). Patients were then given capsules and requested to attend every three months so that a note could be made of their general health and how many capsules they had taken. Blood and urine samples were collected at each visit for despatch to the trial office laboratory and a further supply of capsules was given. The last visit took place in the 12th week of pregnancy. The outcomes of all completed pregnancies were recorded, including details of any fetid malformation, sex, birthweight, and head circumference. In the event of a termination of pregnancy or miscarriage the fetus was examined if possible. A woman remained in the trial until she had had a pregnancy in which the fetus could be classified as having a neural tube defect or not ("informative pregnancy"). If, for example, she had a miscarriage and the fetus was not examined, she remained in the study in the same randomisation group until the end of the trial or until she had an informative pregnancy. In this way each woman contributed no more than one informative event to the study. The final results are based on the outcome of all informative pregnancies. Whenever a neural tube defect (anencephaly, spina bifida cystica, or encephalocele) was reported, independent corroboration was sought, with a necropsy report if one was performed, or a description of the lesion for independent review at the trial centre in London (done without knowledge of the allocated group). To monitor possible toxicity associated with the supplementation, forms were provided for the notification of any medical event arising among the women in the trial irrespective of whether this was thought to be associated with the capsules. The health of each child born into the study was ascertained annually by sending a questionnaire to the mother on the infant's first, second, and third birthday. This part of the study is continuing. The results of the study, available only to the principal investigator, the study administrator, and the data monitoring committee, were reviewed every six months to enable the study to be stopped early if, as indeed occurred, a clear result emerged.

RESULTS

Table I shows the numbers of women randomised and the numbers of informative pregnancies according to centre. Just over half were from outside the UK. All four groups were similar with respect to age and the outcome of previous pregnancies; thus randomisation had ensured that like was being compared with like (table II). Women in the UK centres were also categorised according to social class as defined by the Registrar General; the proportions in social class distributions were similar in the four groups — for example, the proportions in classes IV and V combined were 25%, 29%, 29%, and 28% in groups A, B, C, and D, respectively. Table III gives the outcome of all pregnancies according to randomisation group and

Table IV

Prevalence of neural tube defects (NTD) according to randomisation group: Main analysis based on all women randomised who had an informative pregnancy classified according to randomisation group (intention-to-treat analysis)

Randomisation group		All women		Women not already pregnant at randomisation*	
Folic acid	Other vitamins	NTD/all	Relative risk: folic acid *vs* non-folic acid (95% CI)	NTD/all	Relative risk: folic acid *vs* non-folic acid (95% CI)
A +	–	2/298 } 6/593 (1.0%)		2/258 } 5/514 (1.0%)	
B +	+	4/295	} 0.28 (0.12–0.71)	3/256	} 0.28 (0.11–0.75)
C –	–	13/300 } 21/602 (3.5%)		11/260 } 18/517 (3.5%)	
D –	+	8/302		7/257	

*First day of last menstrual period was 14 days or more after date of randomisation.

whether or not the pregnancy was informative. The miscarriage rate was similar in the four groups. Most (23/30) of the terminations were performed on account of antenatal diagnosis of a neural tube defect.

Table IV shows the prevalence of neural tube defects in each of the four groups. Among women allocated to the groups receiving folic acid the rate was 1.0% and among those allocated to the other groups it was 3.5%, yielding a relative risk of 0.28 (95% confidence interval 0.12 to 0.71). The relative risk among women allocated to the "other vitamin" groups compared with the remaining groups was 0.80, a result that was not statistically significant (95% CI 0.37–1.72). Table IV also provides data after exclusion of the 164 women who may have been pregnant at the time of randomisation (ie, the first day of the last menstrual period occurred less than 14 days after the date of randomisation). The results of these analyses are virtually identical. In table V we give the results after excluding women who reported that they had stopped

taking the capsules before their last scheduled visit (an "on-treatment" analysis). The recurrence rate among such women in the folic acid groups of the trial was 0.7 % and in the groups without folic acid the recurrence rate was 3.4%, yielding a relative risk of 0.21 (95% CI 0.07–0.62). The relative risk among women allocated to the "other vitamin" groups, excluding those who stopped taking capsules, was 0.93 (95 % CI 0.41–2.12). There is no indication that the vitamins other than folic acid conferred any preventive effect nor that they enhanced the effect of folic acid, although the power of the study to detect an interaction is limited. The effect of folic acid on the risk of anencephaly was not significantly different from that on spina bifida/encephalocele (the relative risks were 0.44 [3/593 *vs* 7/602] and 0.22 [3/332 *vs* 14/602], respectively), nor did it differ significantly between the UK centres and the other centres (the relative risks were 0.38 [3/261 *vs* 8/262] and 0.24 [3/332 *vs* 13/340], respectively).

Table V

Prevalence of neural tube defects according to randomisation group among women with informative pregnancies: subordinate analysis excluding women who stopped taking capsules (on-treatment analysis)

Randomisation group		All women		Women not already pregnant at randomisation*	
Folic acid	Other vitamins	NTD/all	Relative risk: folic acid *vs* non-folic acid (95% CI)	NTD/all	Relative risk: folic acid *vs* non-folic acid (95% CI)
A +	–	1/280 } 4/588 (0.7%)		1/242 } 3/483 (0.6%)	
B +	+	3/278	} 0.21 (0.07–0.62)	2/241	} 0.17 (0.05–0.59)
C –	–	11/281 } 19/558 (3.4%)		10/243 } 17/477 (3.6%)	
D –	+	8/277		7/234	

*First day of last menstrual period was 14 days or more after admission.

Table VI

Informative pregnancies: Abnormalities other than neural tube defects according to randomisation group

Randomisation				
Folic acid	Other vitamins	Total non-NTD	No with abnormal outcomes other than NTD	All reported abnormalities as notified (T = termination of pregnancy; M = miscarriage)
A + −		296	7	Agenesis of corpus callosum and hydrocephalus (T); Down's syndrome; tetralogy of Fallot; severe asphyxia with low birthweight and cleft palate; pes varus; intrauterine growth retardation; polydactyly
B + +		291	12	Lethal multiple pterygium syndrome (M); trisomy 15 (M); Adams-Oliver syndrome; Turner's syndrome (T); talipes; hypospadias; pyloric stenosis; dislocatable hips; persistent fetal circulation; pectus excavatum; purple birthmark/lump between eyes; unexplained neutropenia
C − −		287	5	Partial deletion chromosome 18 (M). Down's syndrome; bilateral talipes (2); cardiac murmur
D − +		294	8	Hydropic fetus with cervical cystic lymphangioma, complex cardiac malformation, and ganglioneuroblastic hamartoma of adrenals; hydropic fetus and cervical hygroma (T); Klinefelter's syndrome (T); congenital nystagmus and dilated ventricles; arthrogryposis; pes equinovarus; mongolian blue spot; skin tag at base of spine
Total		1168	32	—

The trial results were regularly reviewed. The figure shows the results of a sequential analysis up to April 12, 1991, when the data monitoring committee recommended that the trial be stopped — a decision that was endorsed by the steering committee. The difference between the number of neural tube defects in the non-folic-acid groups and in the folic-acid groups is plotted sequentially against the total number of neural tube defects in the trial. The boundaries define the limits for stopping the trial early at values calculated to give 75% power to detect a halving in the relative risk (at $p = 0.05$). It can be seen that the boundary was crossed after the 27th case. This sequential analysis was used as a guide, in the decision whether to terminate the trial, rather than as an absolute indication.

The observed relative risk estimate of the effect of folic acid supplementation will tend to be exaggerated, since the trial was stopped early because of the results. An estimate of the relative risk allowing for early stopping,[7] itself an approximation that is influenced by the exact choice of the boundaries in the figure, was 0.33 ($p=0.013$, 95% CI 0.06–0.80) — close to the directly observed estimate of 0.28. The use of alternative reasonable boundaries yields similar results. Early stopping has not, therefore, distorted our measure of effect to any material extent.

Possible adverse effects of folic acid to the fetus and the mother were examined. Table VI shows the number of reported congenital abnormalities other than neural tube defects (together with any reported details) according to randomisation group. The details of the abnormalities are as notified, irrespective of severity. There were more reports in the vitamin groups, but this excess could readily have arisen by chance. In addition two of the disorders in the vitamin groups were inherited single gene defects — Adams-Oliver syndrome (autosomal dominant) and lethal multiple pterygium syndrome (autosomal recessive). Examination of the individual disorders did not reveal any excess that provides grounds for concern. The mean birthweights and head circumferences of infants with notified abnormalities born in the study were similar in all four randomisation groups (3387, 3376, 3344, and 3382 g and 34.2, 34.1, 34.1, and 34.1 cm, respectively in groups A, B, C, and D). Among all women randomised the mean number of women reporting a medical disorder (typically non-specific ailments such as infertility, irregular menses, vomiting in pregnancy, upper respiratory illness) was similar in all four groups (16, 15, 11, and 19% respectively) with no single medical problem giving rise to particular concern.

7% of women who had informative pregnancies stopped taking their capsules before they became pregnant, usually because they lost interest in participating in the trial; among the remaining women, 95.4% took 80% or more of the assigned capsules, 3.8% took 50–79%, and 0.8% took less than 50%, as judged by capsule counts at their quarterly visits. Table VII shows the 10th, 50th, and 90th percentile of serum folate concentrations according to randomisation group. The samples were taken at the visit immediately before they became pregnant (median interval between this visit and the first day of the last menstrual period was 7 days). The concentrations were substantially higher in the women allocated to folic acid than in those who were not (even at the 10th centile) while those in the groups without

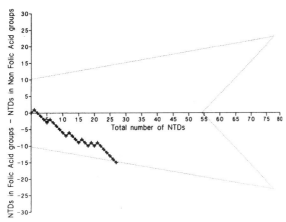

Sequential analysis, showing cumulative difference between number of neural tube defects (NTDs) in the folic acid and non-folic-acid groups plotted against total number of NTDs.

The boundaries of the diagram define the stopping points of the study. Upper and lower boundaries of the figure were constructed by use of approximation that number of events in the folic acid groups minus number in the groups without folic acid follows a gaussian distribution with mean N(1 − r)/(1 + r) and variance N, where r is the relative risk and N is the total number of neural tube defects in the study [22] By taking the parameters of this gaussian distribution, equations given by Armitage [23] can be used to specify the upper and lower boundaries of the figure.

folic acid were not materially different from the baseline concentrations at the time of randomisation. The red cell folate results were similar. Compliance, therefore, was good.

DISCUSSION

Our results show that folic acid supplementation can prevent neural tube defects. The relative risk estimate for the women allocated to take folic acid was 0.28 compared with the control groups — that is, 72% of neural tube defects were prevented (95% CI 29% to 88%). The result is unlikely to be due to chance and the randomised double-blind design excludes bias as an explanation. The results also demonstrate that it is folic acid, rather than any of the other vitamins, that is responsible for the preventive effect.

We can be confident about the reliability of the diagnoses of neural tube defects in the trial. In the 27 cases recorded, 23 of the women had a termination of pregnancy and 4 had live births. Of these 4, in 2 cases the mothers were known to have declined termination and in 2 the reason was not known; 2 of the 4 survived. 18 of the 25 dead cases were confirmed by necropsy reports and in the remaining 7 descriptions confirmed the diagnosis. The diagnosis was unbiased with respect to randomisation group, since this was not known to local participants.

6 women allocated to folic acid had neural tube defect pregnancies. Their serum folic acid concentrations (22, 36, 38, 118, 186, 194 ng/ml) were not unusually low for supplemented women. Lack of compliance with the regimen, or failure of folic acid absorption, is unlikely to be an explanation for these failures of prevention.

Table VII

Serum folic acid concentrations at last visit before beconing pregnant according to randomisation group among women with informative pregnancies

Randomisation			Serum folic acid (ng/ml)		
Folic acid	Other vitamins	No*	10th centile	50th centile	90th centile
A +	−	277 } 538	21 } 23	44 } 44	187 } 194
B +	+	261	25	46	204
C −	−	267 } 541	3 } 3	5 } 5	10 } 9
D −	+	274	3	5	9

*Number tested was less than number of informative pregnancies because women became pregnant before the first three-monthly visit (64) or because a blood sample was not taken at the last visit before becoming pregnant (52).

Results have been reported from two other randomised trials — the South Wales trial [14] referred to earlier, and more recently an interim analysis from a study performed in Budapest in which a multivitamin capsule containing 0.8 mg of folic acid was given daily to unselected women instead of women with a previous neural tube defect pregnancy.[8] In the first the recurrence rate was 2/60 in the folic acid group compared with 4/51 in the controls, and in the second the occurrence rates were 0/599 and 3/703, respectively. Both results suggested an effect but were inconclusive. Six observational studies of dietary folate or the use of folic acid and other vitamin supplements and neural tube defects have been published [9–14] and one recent non-randomised folic acid supplementation study.[15] All but one showed an association but all may have suffered from the selection bias outlined above, and none could specifically identify folic acid as the responsible vitamin.

The non-randomised intervention study reported by Smithells and his colleagues yielded a sevenfold ratio in risk between supplemented and unsupplemented women,[3,16] compared with our threefold ratio. A likely explanation for this difference is that the result from the non-randomised study reflects a combination of vitamin prophylaxis and selection bias, while our randomised trial reflects the prophylactic effect alone. However, the size of the studies is too small to exclude chance as a possible explanation.

Our trial was conducted among women who had had one or more neural tube defect pregnancies because of their higher risk of a recurrence, about ten times the general risk. There is, however, no reason to believe that the preventive effect of folic acid is restricted to this group. If additional folic acid can prevent a second neural tube defect pregnancy it is also likely to prevent a first one. It is implausible that serial occurrences of the same event have separate causes. Each woman who has had a recurrent neural tube defect pregnancy must have had a first; it is extremely unlikely that a method of preventing the second will not also tend to prevent the first, though the quantitative effect may be different in women having recurrences from that in women in general. If women who have already had an affected infant were genetically more susceptible to having affected pregnancies than women in general, the relative effect of an environmental cause such as a lack of folic acid would, in expectation, be the same in causing first cases as in causing subsequent ones if the effects of the environmental and genetic factors combine as the product of the two alone. It would be an underestimate if they combined additively. Insofar as the former is the more likely model, our result will be an unbiased estimate of the effect in the general population; if it were the latter, it would be conservative. If the genetic factor relied exclusively on a relative lack of folic acid to express the defect but otherwise folic acid had no role in the causation of neural tube defects, the effect would be greater in preventing recurrences than in preventing first cases. It is, however, a less likely model and one that does not explain the results of observational studies of folic acid intake and neural tube defects among women in the general population.[10,11,13,14] Prophylaxis may, in practice, be lower in general because a smaller proportion of women who have not had an affected pregnancy may take folic acid supplements than women seeking to avoid a recurrence.

Women at high risk, having already experienced an affected pregnancy, have more to gain from supplementation than women at low risk, so a risk of toxicity that is acceptable in the former may be less acceptable in the latter. We recognise that a trial such as our own that has sufficient statistical power to demonstrate efficacy usually has insufficient power to answer the question of safety for public health purposes. A judgment on safety needs to be taken on wider grounds. Folic acid is water soluble and readily excreted, and is not known to be toxic. Over 95% of pregnancies with neural tube defects occur in women without a previous affected pregnancy and this, taken with the fact that there is now a proven benefit, argues for increasing the intake of folic acid among all women who wish to become pregnant, not only those at high risk.

There remains the question of the dose of folic acid. If a 4 mg per day supplement is effective, a lower dose (for example, 0.36 mg per day as used by Smithells and his colleagues [3]) is also likely to be effective, though possibly less so. A very large trial would be needed to estimate the relative efficacy of the two doses.

One reason for questioning the view that a relative lack of folic acid is a major cause of neural tube defects has been the observation that the United Kingdom has had one of the highest rates of neural tube defects in the world but was unlikely to be unusually deficient in folic acid. Either the UK does, in fact, have a lower folic acid intake than other countries, perhaps partly through losses in cooking, or the conjugates of folic acid in foods typically eaten in the UK may be relatively poorly absorbed, or there are other dietary factors that interfere with its absorption or metabolism, or there is an interaction with a genetically controlled disturbance of folic acid metabolism.

Another reason to question the efficacy of folic acid is the fact that individual studies have not shown a significant difference in the serum folic acid concentrations of women with affected and unaffected pregnancies; differences in red cell folate levels have been found but they have not been very large.[17-21] It is possible that the range of values of blood folic acid levels among women in most populations is too narrow for such differences (if present) to be readily demonstrable. The position would then be analogous to examining the mean difference in number of cigarettes between lung cancer cases and controls in a study of smoking and lung cancer among individuals who all smoke between 15 and 20 cigarettes a day. The mean difference would be extremely small, and not discernible except in very large studies. The lack of a clear association between serum folate levels and neural tube defects and only a modest difference in red cell folate levels is not, therefore, inconsistent with the protective effect of folic acid supplementation.

Folic acid supplementation can now be recommended for all women who have had a previously affected pregnancy, and public health measures should be taken to ensure that all women of childbearing age receive adequate dietary folic acid. The demonstration that folic acid is the effective agent avoids the need to use a mixture of vitamins with the associated extra costs and concern over possible toxicity (eg, from vitamin A). It is less clear whether all women planning a pregnancy should take folic acid supplements. The case rests upon questions of safety and cost. In any event, community-wide prevention may be difficult to achieve by providing supplements to everyone and consideration should be given to extending the fortification of staple foods with folic acid.

This study has established the specific role of folic acid in the prevention of neural tube defects. It has produced a clear answer to an important medical question on which opinion and practice have been divided. The trial has resolved the uncertainty and has provided a basis for concerted preventive practice.

Steering committee
John Burn, Malcolm Ferguson-Smith, Edmund Hey, Paul Polani, Charles Rodeck, Geoffrey Rose (chairman), Nicholas Wald (study coordinator and principal investigator), and J. Modle and M. Hennigan (departments of health observers).

Data monitoring committee
Eva Alberman, Peter Armitage (chairman), and Geoffrey Chamberlain.

Trial office
Administration: Joan Sneddon, Karen Fordham (formerly Alison Bickmore and Patricia Collins). Computing: James Densem. Statistics: Chris Frost. Laboratory analysis: Rossana Stone, Stephanie Collishaw (formerly Robert Barlow and Christine Jones).

Participating centres

Representatives in the United Kingdom were: M Hall, D Campbell, and P Terry (Aberdeen); W Goldthorp (Ashton-under-Lyne); B Hibbard, K M Laurence, E M Williams, E Jones, and C Morgan (Cardiff); D Taylor (Dundee); M Hulten and B Baverstock (East Birmingham); J A Raeburn and A Lowie (Edinburgh); M Connor, M A Ferguson-Smith, S Malcolm Macnaughton, and M White (Glasgow); C R Stewart (Leicester); J G Grudzinskas and R Hamer (The London Hospital); J Burn, A Hill, and D Gibson (Newcastle-upon-Tyne); the late Sir Alec Turnbull, D Barlow, N Wald, and Nancy Wald (Oxford); C Rodeck and L Abramsky (Queen Charlotte's Hospital, London); I D Cooke, R B Fraser, and H King (Sheffield); J F Miller (Southampton); T Chard, N Wald, and R Hamer (St Bartholomew's Hospital, London). M Pearce (St George's Hospital, London); and M Lucas and H Ward (University College Hospital, London).

Representatives outside the UK were: E F Robertson (Adelaide, Australia); B Field (Sydney, Australia); L Sheffield and T Colgan (Melbourne, Australia); E Winsor and C Veinot (Halifax, Canada); RG, Davidson, S Epstein, D Whelan, and S Steele (Hamilton, Canada); JG Hall and B Keena (Vancouver, Canada); S Guibaud and E Robert (Lyon, France); A Czeizel and L Timar (Budapest, Hungary); Z Papp and O Torok (Debrecen, Hungary); S Gardo and K Bajnoczky (Gyor, Hungary H Kovacs, A Harsanyi and M Garvai (Mskolc, Hungary); B Pejtsik (Pecs, Hungary); G Szemere (Szeged, Hungary); L Szabo (Szombathely, Hungary); G Barkai and J Shmueli (Israel); and E Lillyn and Gerasimova (Moscow, USSR).

We thank all the women who participated in the study; Sir James Gowans, past Secretary of the Medical Research Council, for his personal involvement in judging the need for the trial and his commitment to it once the case of need was clear; and Prof John Davis, chairman of the steering committee for the first year of the study and Prof Ian Cooke, member of the steering committee until 1989. The capsules used in this trial were provided free of charge by the Boots Company plc and we are indebted to the Medical Director of the company, Dr Mervyn Busson, and his colleagues for their help and unstinting support during the course of this trial. We thank Hoffmann La Roche, and in particular Dr Richard Salkeld and Dr RE Wacheberger, for carrying out independent quality control checks on the potency of the capsule constituents without charge; Margaretha White-van Mourik for her contribution to recruitment of women into the trial in Scotland; the Association for Spina Bifida and Hydrocephalus, particularly its past Executive Director, Moyna Gilbertson, for its continuing assistance and cooperation, the staff of the Clinical Trials Service Unit in Oxford for providing the randomisation service, Malcolm Law and Leo Kinlen for their helpful criticisms and comments; and Jan Clarke for typing the manuscript. The trial was supported financially by the Medical Research Council.

References

[1] Hibbard BM. The role of folic acid in pregnancy with particular reference to anaemia, abruption and abortion. *J Obstet Gynaecol Br Commonw* 1964;**71**:529–42.

[2] Hibbard ED, Smithells RW. Folic acid metabolism and human embryopathy. *Lancet* 1965; **i**: 1254.

[3] Smithells RW, Shephard S, Schorah CJ, et al. Possible prevention of neural-tube defects by periconceptional vitamin supplementation. *Lancet* 1980; **i**: 339–40.

[4] Laurence KM, James N, Miller MH, Tennant GB, Campbell H, Double-blind randomised controlled trial of folate treatment before conception to prevent recurrence of neural-tube defects. *Br Med J* 1981; **282**: 1509–11.

[5] Wald NJ, Polani PE. Neural-tube defects and vitamins: the need for randomized clinical trial. *Br J Obstet Gynaecol* 1984; **91**: 516–23.

[6] Longo D, Herbert V. Radioassay for serum and red cell folate. *Lab Clin Med* 1976; **87**: 138–51.

[7] Whitehead J, Brunier H. Planning and evaluation of sequential trials. Manual to software package PEST 2.0, University of Reading, 1989.

[8] Czeizel A, Fritz G. Ethics of a randomized trial of periconceptual vitamins. *JAMA* 1989; **262**; 1633–34.

[9] Laurence KM, James N, Miller MH, Tennant GB, Campbell H. Increased risk of recurrence of pregnancies complicated by fetal neural tube defects in mothers receiving poor diets, and possible benefit in dietary counselling. *Br Med J* 1980; **281**: 1592–94.

[10] Winship KA, Cahal DA, Weber JCP, Griffin JP. Maternal drug histories and central nervous system anomalies. *Arch Dis Child* 1984; **59**: 1052–60.

[11] Mulinare J, Cordero JF, Erickson D, Berry RJ. Periconceptional use of multivitamins and the occurrence of neural tube defects. *JAMA* 1998; **260**: 3141–45.

[12] Mills JL, Rhoads GG, Simpson JL, et al. The National Institute of Child Health and Human Development Neural Tube Defect Study Group. The absence of a relation between the periconceptional use of vitamins and neural-tube defects. *N Engl J Med* 1989; **321**: 430–35.

[13] Bower C, Stanley FJ. Dietary folate as a risk factor for neural-tube defects: evidence from a case-control study in Western Australia. *Med J Aust* 1989; **150**: 613–18.

[14] Milunsky A, Jick H, Jick SS, et al. Multivitamin/folic acid supplementation in early pregnancy reduces the prevalence of neural tube defects. *JAMA* 1989, **262**: 2847–52.

[15] Vergel RG, Sanchez LR, Heredero BL, Rodriguez PL, Martinez AJ. Primary prevention of neural tube defects with folic acid supplementation: Cuban experience. *Prenat Diagn* 1990; **10**: 149–52.

[16] Smithells RW, Seller MJ, Harris R, et al. Further experience of vitamin supplementation for prevention of neural tube defect recurrences. *Lancet* 1983; **1**: 1027–31.

[17] Emery AEH, Timson J, Watson-Williams EJ. Pathogenesis of spina bifida. *Lancet* 1969; **ii**: 909–10.

[18] Smithells RW, Sheppard S, Schorah CJ. Vitamin deficiencies and neural tube defects. *Arch Dis Child* 1976; **51**: 944–49.

[19] Hall MH. Folates and the fetus. *Lancet* 1977; **i**: 648–49.

[20] Molloy AM, Kirke P, Hillary I, Weir DG, Scott JM. Maternal serum folate and vitamin B_{12} concentrations in pregnancies associated with neural tube defects. *Arch Dis Child* 1985; **60**: 660–65.

[21] Yates JRW, Ferguson-Smith MA, Shenkin A, Guzman-Rodriguez R, White M, Clark BJ. Is disordered folate metabolism the basis for the genetic predisposition to neural tube defects? *Clin Genet* 1987; **31**: 279–87.

[22] Whitehead J. The design and analysis of sequential clinical trials. Chichester: Ellis Horwood, 1983.

[23] Armitage P. Restricted sequential procedures. *Biometrika* 1957; **44**: 9–26.

This article was first published in the BMJ and is reproduced by permission of the BMJ

SECONDARY PREVENTION CLINICS FOR CORONARY HEART DISEASE: RANDOMISED TRIAL OF EFFECT ON HEALTH

Neil C Campbell, Joan Thain, H George Deans, Lewis D Ritchie, John M Rawles, Janet L Squair

Neil C Campbell, *clinical research fellow*; H George Deans, *clinical senior lecturer*; Lewis D Ritchie, *Mackenzie professor of general practice* – Department of General Practice and Primary Care, Foresterhill Health Centre, Aberdeen AB25 2AY

Joan Thain, *health visitor* – Denburn Health Centre, Aberdeen AB25 1QB

John M Rawles, *honorary senior lecturer* – Medicines Assessment Research Unit, Medical School, Foresterhill, Aberdeen AB25 2ZD

Janet L Squair, *research fellow*, Department of Public Health Medical School, Foresterhill, Aberdeen AB25 2ZD

Correspondence to: Dr Campbell n.campbell@abdn.ac.uk

BMJ 1998;**316**:1434-7

ABSTRACT

Objective: To evaluate the effects of secondary prevention clinics run by nurses in general practice on the health of patients with coronary heart disease.

Design: Randomised controlled trial of clinics over one year with assessment by self completed postal questionnaires and audit of medical records at the start and end of the trial.

Setting: Random sample of 19 general practices in northeast Scotland.

Subjects: 1173 patients (685 men and 488 women) under 80 years with working diagnoses of coronary heart disease who did not have terminal illness or dementia and were not housebound.

Intervention: Clinic staff promoted medical and lifestyle aspects of secondary prevention and offered regular follow up.

Main outcome measures: Health status measured by the SF-36 questionnaire, chest pain by the angina type specification, and anxiety and depression by the hospital anxiety and depression scale. Use of health services before and during the study.

Results: There were significant improvements in six of eight health status domains (all functioning scales, pain, and general health) among patients attending the clinic. Role limitations attributed to physical problems improved most (adjusted difference 8.52, 95% confidence interval 4.16 to 12.9). Fewer patients reported worsening chest pain (odds ratio 0.59, 95% confidence interval 0.37 to 0.94). There were no significant effects on anxiety or depression. Fewer intervention group patients required hospital admissions (0.64, 0.48 to 0.86), but general practitioner consultation rates did not alter.

Conclusions: Within their first year secondary prevention clinics improved patients' health and reduced hospital admissions.

INTRODUCTION

General practitioners have been encouraged to target patients with manifest coronary heart disease for secondary prevention.[1] Strong evidence exists to support this strategy; reductions in cardiovascular events and mortality can be achieved by, for example, taking aspirin,[2] control of blood pressure,[3] lowering lipid concentrations,[4,5] exercise,[6] healthy diets,[7] and stopping smoking.[8]

A comprehensive package of secondary prevention is, however, a considerable undertaking for patients, many of whom are elderly and may have other health priorities.[1] There are risks that health may worsen with polypharmacy, drug side effects, and patient discordance. Weighed against the risks, however, are possible benefits: patients may appreciate extra support, uncontrolled symptoms may be identified earlier, and health promotion to patients with angina can improve symptoms.[9] We conducted a randomised trial of secondary prevention clinics run by nurses in general practice to assess their effects on uptake of secondary prevention. In this paper we report the effect on patients' symptoms and health.

SUBJECTS AND METHODS

Of 28 general practices selected randomly in northeast Scotland (formerly Grampian region), 19 agreed to participate in the study.[10] Patients with diagnoses of coronary heart disease in their general practice records who did not have a terminal illness or dementia and were not housebound were eligible: 1343 (71%) of a random sample of 1890 completed baseline questionnaires and agreed to participate.[10]

We used random numbers tables to centrally randomise patients (by individual after stratification for age, sex, and practice) to intervention or control groups. Patients assigned to the intervention group were invited to attend secondary prevention clinics

3

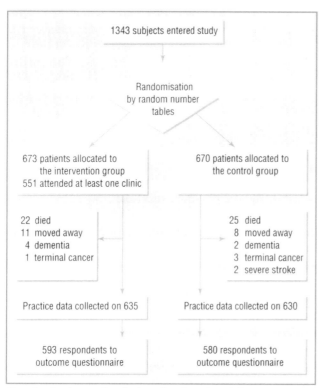

Randomisation and exclusion of patients in trial

during which their symptoms were reviewed; treatment was reviewed and use of aspirin promoted; blood pressure and lipid management were reviewed; and lifestyle factors were assessed and, if appropriate, behavioural change negotiated. The clinics ran for one year. Patients were invited for a first appointment during the first three months and were followed up depending on clinical circumstances (usually two to six monthly). Patients in the control group received usual care by their general practitioner.

We collected data on health and symptoms by postal questionnaire before intervention and at one year using the following instruments:

SF-36 health survey questionnaire—This is a general outcome measure that uses eight scales to assess three aspects of health: functional status (physical functioning, social functioning, role limitations attributed to physical problems, role limitations attributable to emotional problems), wellbeing (mental health, energy and fatigue, pain), and general health perception.[11] It has been validated for use in the United Kingdom.[12]

Angina type specification—This is designed for use with the SF-36 questionnaire to assess several aspects of chest pain.[13] Its measurements of presence, frequency, and course of chest pain have been found to predict future cardiovascular events.[14]

Hospital anxiety and depression scale—A well validated and widely used instrument to assess mental state.[15] We collected data about attendance at general practice by, audit of general practice records. Data about hospital admissions were obtained from patients' responses to the angina type specification.

A sample size of 1300 at baseline was projected to give 808 responders at outcome, which was sufficient to detect five point "clinically and socially relevant" differences in all SF-36 domains.[11] We analysed data with standard statistical techniques on an intention to treat basis using SPSS for Windows version 6.1.3. Binary, outcomes were analysed by logistic regression and continuous scales by analysis of covariance, with adjustment where appropriate for age, sex, practice, and baseline performance. Frequency of chest pain, length of hospital stay, and numbers of general practitioner consultations were analysed with the Mann-Whitney U test.

The study was effectively open because practice staff who ran the clinics knew which patients were in the intervention group. Questionnaire data were entered blind to group allocation, but masking of data collection about general practitioner consultations was impracticable because indicators were often present in medical records. The study was approved by the Grampian Health Board and University of Aberdeen joint ethics committee.

RESULTS

The figure shows the randomisation of subjects and follow up. Table 1 shows the baseline characteristics of patients in the intervention and control groups. There were no large differences, but the intervention group scored slightly better for "energy" than the control group.

Table 2 shows the mean changes in SF-36 scores that occurred between baseline and one year. Before the analysis of covariance we analysed variables that were thought to be potential confounders (age, sex, practice, and baseline performance) for their effect on outcome

Table 1

Characteristics of control and intervention group at bas

	No of subjects (intervention/ control)	Intervention group	Control gr
No (%) of men	593/580	346 (58)	339 (5
No (%) with angina at baseline*	554/544	273 (49)	279 (5
No (%) admitted to hospital in previous year	540/518	132 (24)	137 (2
No (%) with myocardial infarction	593/580	273 (46)	255 (4
Median (interquartile range) years since myocardial infarction	271/254	5 (8)	6 (
Mean (SD) age	593/580	65.9 (7.9)	66.3 (8.
Mean (SD) SF-36 scores:			
Physical	573/555	58.6 (25.7)	57.1 (25.
Social	592/579	77.3 (26.4)	76.1 (25.
Role physical	550/532	49.7 (43.6)	47.9 (42.
Role emotional	545/529	67.2 (41.4)	67.3 (41.
Mental	575/563	75.7 (17.6)	73.9 (17.
Energy	577/563	54.2 (22.3)	51.3 (21.
Pain	590/576	64.8 (26.4)	62.9 (25.
General	552/539	56.5 (22.7)	54.7 (21.

*Number of subjects with chest pain in the past week.

Table 2

Mean changes in SF-36 scores between baseline and one year in intervention and control groups

Domain	No of subjects (intervention/ control)	Mean change in score		Adjusted difference (95% CI)*	P value
		Intervention group	Control group		
Physical	554/541	2.28	−1.58	4.33 (2.12 to 6.54)	<0.001
Social	590/577	0.20	−2.79	3.51 (0.94 to 6.08)	0.007
Role physical	511/497	4.71	−3.04	8.52 (4.16 to 12.88)	<0.001
Role emotional	493/491	2.08	−2.42	4.66 (0.11 to 9.21)	0.045
Mental	556/532	0.32	−0.13	1.05 (−0.50 to 2.61)	0.185
Energy	559/545	1.52	0.71	1.58 (−0.17 to 3.33)	0.077
Pain	583/569	1.45	−0.33	2.50 (0.18 to 4.83)	0.035
General	514/496	1.06	−0.82	2.34 (0.50 to 4.19)	0.013

*Adjusted for age and baseline performance.

scores. No significant difference in mean change in score between practices was found in any domain with analysis of variance, and the independent samples t test showed no significant differences between sexes. Baseline performance and age, however, were found to correlate significantly with changes in scores, and we therefore adjusted for these in subsequent analyses.

Of 508 patients in the intervention group, 257 (51%) reported chest pain during the past week at baseline and 232 (46%) at one year. The corresponding figures for 498 control patients were 258 (52%) and 250 (50%). After age, sex, practice, and baseline performance were adjusted for, the odds ratio for chest pain in the intervention group was 0.81 (95% confidence interval 0.61 to 1.08, P = 0.143).

Fifty one of 519 (10%) patients in the intervention group reported that the course of their chest pain was worsening ("getting a little worse" or "getting much worse") at baseline and 37 (71%) at one year. The figures for 500 control patients were 47 (91%) and 54 (11%). After age, sex, practice, and baseline performance were adjusted for, the odds ratio was 0.59 (0.37 to 0.94, P = 0.025).

Among patients reporting chest pain, the median frequency during the past week for intervention and control groups at baseline was three (P = 0.110). There was no change at one year (P = 0.722).

Table 3 shows the hospital anxiety and depression scores. Patients from rural practices and men were significantly less anxious, and age and baseline performance significantly correlated with anxiety and depression. These confounders were included in analysis of covariance, which confirmed that there were no significant effects from intervention (adjusted difference −0.10 (−0.42 to 0.23, P = 0.560) for anxiety and −0.16 (−0.44 to 0.13, P = 0.281) for depression in the intervention group).

Of 540 patients in the intervention group, 132 (241%) were admitted to hospital during the year before the study and 106 (20%) during the study year. The corresponding figures for 518 control patients were 137 (26%) and 145 (28%). After age, sex, general practice,

and baseline performance were adjusted for the odds ratio of requiring admission to hospital for the intervention group was 0.64 (0.48 to 0.86, P = 0.003). The difference was explained only partly by "cardiac" admissions: there were 36 (7%) in the intervention group and 49 (9%) in the control group during the study year. It was not due to differences in non-fatal Myocardial infarctions: 13 (2%) in the intervention group, 12 (2%) in the control group.

At baseline the median length of stay in hospital was seven days in the intervention group and six in the control group (P = 0.435). The median stay at one year was six days in both groups (P = 0.408). The median number of general practitioner consultations in three months for intervention and control groups at baseline was one (P = 0.107). There was no change at one year (P = 0.488).

DISCUSSION

We assessed the effects of secondary prevention clinics on the health of patients with established coronary heart disease in typical general practices and found that patients receive important early benefits. The effect of clinics on uptake of secondary prevention will be reported later.

Table 3

Hospital anxiety and depression scores at baseline and one year for intervention and control groups

	No of subjects	Mean scores		Difference (95% CI)	P value*
		Baseline	1 year		
Anxiety:					
Intervention	556	5.78	5.77	0.01 (−0.24 to 0.26)	0.932
Control	552	6.14	6.19	−0.05 (−0.27 to 0.17)	0.660
Depression:					
Intervention	568	4.50	4.38	0.11 (−0.09 to 0.32)	0.281
Control	556	4.63	4.60	0.03 (−0.18 to 0.23)	0.794

*Paired samples t test.

Against a background of overall deterioration among the control group, the general health of patients who were invited to attend the clinics improved. There were significant differences in most domains of the SF-36 questionnaire, but the largest improvements were in functional status. It was in these aspects of health that this population scored most poorly at baseline compared with a general population,[12] and where, therefore, improvement might be most welcome. The lowest baseline and greatest benefit were in role limitations attributed to physical problems, and the size of this effect would be expected to be clinically and socially relevant.[11]

Although not directly comparable, our findings are similar to those of a study in Belfast of health promotion in patients with angina.[16] The Belfast study had important differences: all its subjects had angina; the intervention did not include medical aspects of secondary prevention; numbers of patients were smaller; and the Nottingham Health Profile was used to evaluate effects on perceived health. However, significant improvements in physical mobility and trends towards improvement in most other scales were reported. Our study provides stronger evidence of benefit to all patients with coronary heart disease in more areas of health but confirms that most benefit occurs in physical aspects.

Chest pain

Fewer patients in the intervention group suffered chest pain at one year, but this difference was not significant and there were no differences in the frequencies of pain among those who reported it. Significantly fewer subjects, however, reported that their chest pain was deteriorating; such patients have been found previously to have poorer prognoses.[14] Overall, therefore, the intervention caused a small but important improvement in chest pain. Once again, these findings are in line with those of the Belfast study, where health promotion was found to reduce angina.[9]

Anxiety and depression

Intervention produced no significant improvement in hospital anxiety and depression scores or in the mental health domain of the SF-36. However, at baseline only 14% of subjects were anxious and 6% depressed (hospital anxiety and depression score > 10). These estimates and the baseline mental health scores were similar to those expected in the general population,[12,17,18] so it was unsurprising that there were no psychological benefits from intervention.

Most previous studies of anxiety and depression in coronary heart disease have been conducted on patients soon after myocardial infarction, when their psychological distress peaks.[19] Among patients with coronary heart disease in general practice, however, recent myocardial infarction is uncommon.[10] Our results suggest that anxiety and depression do not warrant additional attention in patients with stable coronary

> **Key messages**
> - Nurse led clinics in general practice were used to promote secondary prevention to patients with coronary heart disease
> - Within the first year the health of patients invited to the clinics improved
> - Most benefit was in functional status, but chest pain improved too
> - There was no effects on anxiety or depression
> - There were significant reductions in hospital admissions in the first year

heart disease. It was reassuring, however, that the pursuit of comprehensive secondary prevention did not lead to increased psychological distress.

Use of health services

To assess the wider impact of improved general health on patients we studied their use of health services. These patients were high users: a quarter of subjects required hospital admissions in the year before the study. During the study year, however, there was a significant reduction in the numbers of patients in the intervention group requiring hospital admissions. We would not expect the increased secondary prevention to have such an immediate effect, and, indeed, there were no significant reductions in deaths or non-fatal myocardial infarctions. Neither did the fall in other "cardiac" admissions fully account for the difference. It is possible, however, that improved general health and closer monitoring helped to avoid other hospital admissions.

Relevance and limitations

Our study relied on self completed questionnaires to measure health, but we used instruments that have been validated and used extensively.[11–15] Recruitment rates of general practices and patients were good, and differences between respondents and non-respondents were modest.[10] There were few exclusions and response rates were good, so the sample was reasonably representative of northeast Scotland. Local factors may affect results of clinics in other regions or countries, but the concordance between our results and those of the most similar previous study (in Belfast)[9,16] suggests that our results will be widely relevant A follow up of one year is relatively short, but improvements in secondary prevention should lead to medium and long term reductions in cardiovascular events and deaths. Longer term follow up is planned to study this.

CONCLUSIONS

Overall, secondary prevention clinics improved patients' health. Most benefit was in functional status, but there were also improvements in chest pain and less need for hospital admissions. Targeting secondary prevention in a general practice population can achieve significant and important benefits to patients' health within the first year.

We thank Sandra Skilling and Janis Bryant for help with data collection and Jeremy Grimshaw for help with the study design. The clinics were run by the following health visitors, practice nurses and district nurses: June Anderson, Liz Brown, Mary Brown, Linda Bruce, Jas Burnett, Liz Clouston, Ann Darnley, Mary Duguid, Sheena Durno, Sandra Farquharson, Cath Gilbert, Gillian Grant, Linda Harper, Fiona Leitch, Heather MacAskill, Susan MeSheffrey, Kirsten Masson, Pat Murray, Lynn Phillips, Hilary Plenderleith, Shiela Rattray, Marjorie Smith, Beth Struthers, Margo Stuart, Lynette Sykes, Fiona Travis, Ann Williams, Jean Wood.

The following general practices provided patients and assisted administratively: Danestone Medical Practice, Elmbank Group, Dr Grieve and partners, Kincorth Medical Practice, King Street Medical Practice, Old Machar Medical Practice, Rubislaw Medical Group, Spa-Well Medical Group, and Victoria Street Medical Group in Aberdeen; Aboyne Medical Practice, Kemnay Medical Practice, Drs Mackie and Kay, Skene Medical Practice, and Turriff Medical Practice in Aberdeenshire; Benreay Practice, Dr Crowley, The Laich Medical Practice, Dr MacFarquhar and partners, and Seafield Medical Practice in Moray.

Contributors: NCC participated in the study protocol, intervention design, and training, collected and analysed the data, and drafted the paper. JT participated in the study proposal, intervention design and training, assisted with data collection, and edited the paper. HGD participated in the study proposal, intervention design and training, discussed core ideas, and edited the paper. LDR and JMR participated in the study proposal, discussed core ideas, and edited the paper. JLS supervised data analysis and edited the paper. NCC and LDR are guarantors.

Funding: Health Services and Public Health Research Committee of the Chief Scientist Office at the Scottish Office and Grampian Healthcare Trust. Accommodation and nurse time for the clinics were provided by the contributing primary care teams.

1   Moher M, Schofield T, Weston S, Fullard E. Managing established coronary heart disease. *BMJ* 1997;**314**:69–70.
2   Antiplatelet Trialists' Collaboration. Collaborative overview of randomised trials of antiplatelet therapy. 1. Prevention of death, myocardial infarction, and stroke by prolonged antiplatelet therapy in various categories of patients. *BMJ* 1994;**308**:81–106.
3   Browner WS, Hulley SB. Clinical trials of hypertension treatment: implications for subgroups. *Hypertension* 1989; **13**(suppl. 1):151–6.
4   Scandinavian Simvastatin Survival Study Group. Randomised trial of cholesterol lowering in 4444 patients with coronary heart disease: the Scandinavian simvastatin survival study (4S). *Lancet* 1994;**344**:1383–9.
5   Sacks FM, Pfeffer MA, Moye LA, Rouleau JL, Rutherford JD, Cole TG, et al. The effect of pravastatin on coronary events after myocardial infarction in patients with average cholesterol levels. *N Engl J Med* 1996;**335**:1001–9).
6   O'Connor GT, Buring JE, Yusuf S, Goldhaber SZ, Olmstead EM. An overview of randomised trials of rehabilitation with exercise after myocardial infarction. *Circulation* 1989;**80**:234–44.
7   Moher M. *Evidence of effectiveness of interventions for secondary prevention and treatment of coronary heart disease in primary care.* Oxford: Anglia and Oxford Regional Health Authority, 1995.
8   Daly LE. Long term effect on mortality of stopping smoking after unstable angina and myocardial infarction. *BMJ* 1983;**287**:324–6.
9   Cupples ME, McKnight A. Randomised controlled trial of health promotion in general practice for patients at high cardiovascular risk. *BMJ* 1994;**309**:993–6.
10 Campbell NC, Thain J, Deans HG, Ritchie LD, Rawles JM. Secondary prevention in coronary heart disease: a baseline survey of provision and possibility in general practice. *BMJ* 1998;**316**:1430–4.
11 Ware JE. *SF-36 health survey-manual and interpretation guide.* Boston: Nimrod Press, 1993.
12 Garratt AM, Ruta DA, Abdalla MI, Buckingham JK, Russell IT. The SF 36 health survey questionnaire: an outcome measure suitable for routine use within the NHS? *BMJ* 1993;**306**:1440–4.
13 Pryor DB. *User's manual: Angina type specification.* Bloomington: Health Outcomes Institute, 1993.
14 Pryor DB, Shaw L, McCants CB, Lee KL, Mark DB, Harrell FE Jr, et al. Value of the history and physical in identifying patients at increased risk for coronary artery disease. *Ann Intern Med* 1993;**118**:81–90.
15 Zigmond AS, Snaith RP. The hospital anxiety and depression scale. *Acta Psychiatr Scand* 1983;**67**:361–70.
16 Cupples ME, McKnight A, O'Neill C, Normand C. The effect of personal health education on quality of life of patients with angina in general practice. *Health Educ J* 1996;**55**:75–83.
17 Hale AS. ABC of mental health: anxiety. *BMJ* 1997;**314**:1886–9.
18 Hale AS. ABC of mental health: depression. *BMJ* 1997;**315**:43–6.
19 Mayou R. Rehabilitation after heart attack. *BMJ* 1996;**313**:1498–9.

(Accepted 23 February 1998)

4

This article was first published in Family Practice and is reproduced by permission of Oxford University Press

PATIENTS' EXPERIENCE OF EPILEPSY AND HEALTH CARE

Nicola Mills, Max Bachmann, Ian Harvey, Mervyn McGowana[a] and Iain Hinea[a]

Family Practice 1997; **14**: 117–123
Received 10 October 1996; Accepted 5 November 1996.

Department of Social Medicine, University of Bristol. Bristol BS8 2PR and
[a]North Western Bristol General Practice Locality Group, Bristol, UK.

Objective. The aim of this study was to assess the severity of epilepsy and its effect on patients' lives, and to describe patients' use of and attitudes to health care.
Method. A questionnaire was sent to 595 people with epilepsy identified from 14 general practices in north-west Bristol. All patients aged 16 years and over receiving anti-epileptic medication for their epilepsy were included in the study. Areas investigated included severity of epilepsy and its effect on quality of life, anti-epileptic medication and its perceived effect, health care utilization and preferences for health care.
Results. Seizure frequency was strongly associated with adverse effects of epilepsy. Attacks of epilepsy were experienced at least monthly by 20.4% (95% confidence intervals (CI) 17.0–23.7%) of patients, 29.4% (25.4–33.4%) took more than one anti-epileptic drug, 56.1 % (50.1–62.2%) reported drug side effects, 74.1 % (70.3–77.8%) would prefer to receive all or most of their epilepsy care in a general practice setting, and 69.8% (63.5–76.2%) would like contact with a primary care-based epilepsy specialist nurse. During the previous year 42.4% (35.9–48.8%) of patients had not seen a doctor about their epilepsy. Of patients who had attended the general practice only 13.4% (9.6–17.2%) had regular arrangements to see their GP about epilepsy. Patients receiving both primary and secondary care had the greatest needs and wants for improved care.
Conclusions. Structured care, including regular appointments, co-ordination of primary and secondary care, and increased monitoring and discussion, may improve the quality of life of people with epilepsy, but requires evaluation.
Keywords. Epilepsy, health care, patients' perspective, quality of life.

INTRODUCTION

Epilepsy is one of the most common chronic diseases and its potential adverse effects include physical morbidity, social stigma, the inconvenience of frequent health care use and, more generally, impaired quality of life.[1,2] In recent years, efforts to improve the quality of care for chronic diseases have elicited innovative variations in service and staff mix based on attempts to make expertise more accessible to primary care teams and hence to patients. Successes with structured and shared diabetes care have led to suggestions that epilepsy care should be similarly organized, with particular emphasis on the role of specialist nurses.[3]

A recent review summarized the main problems with epilepsy care as: lack of systematic follow-up, inappropriate poly-pharmacy, non-compliance with medication, communication failure and poor patient knowledge.[1] Population needs for epilepsy care have been outlined [4] but these have not formally considered patients' preferences and have not been based on quantitative assessments of current problems and health care coverage. Ridsdale *et al.* [5] confirmed many of the above problems, taking into account patients' views, and showed that many patients with epilepsy preferred to receive care in general practice. This study goes further, to examine several different influences on patients' quality of life and health care preferences, and compares these factors between hospital and general practice patients.

This study arose when 14 Bristol general practices, comprising the North West Locality Group, obtained health commission funding for a pilot project. One epilepsy specialist nurse was employed to work part time, based in one practice but consulting with patients in all practices, aiming to provide individual counselling, education to primary care teams, and liaison between components of the health service. This paper reports on a survey of people with epilepsy in the locality which served as a baseline for evaluating the intervention. The aims of the survey were to assess the severity of epilepsy and its effect on patients' lives, to describe patients' use of and attitudes to health care, and to investigate factors influencing quality of life and desire for the new service.

METHOD

The study was cross-sectional, providing baseline information for the planned intervention study. The follow-up study will compare changes over time in seven practices serviced by the epilepsy specialist nurse with seven control practices. Control practices will receive the new service in the second but not the first year of the project.

The study population comprised 595 people with epilepsy aged 16 years and over from 14 general practices based in the north-west of Bristol. This corresponds to an estimated 0.93% (595/63772) prevalence of all patients in this category receiving medication for epilepsy. The population was defined as all patients currently on anti-epileptic drugs and designated as having epilepsy by their GP. No patients were excluded for reasons such as learning disabilities or psychological disorders since carers were invited to fill in the form on their behalf. This population was the same as that which the epilepsy specialist nurse intended to serve. Patients were identified by practices from drug record data, and GPs removed patients using anti-epileptic drugs for reasons other than epilepsy. Local Research Ethics Committee approval was obtained.

Self-completion questionnaires were posted to all patients. Questionnaires were accompanied by a covering letter from the patients' GPs informing them of the purpose of the study. Those who did not respond to the first mailing were sent a second copy of the questionnaire 7 weeks later. The questionnaires were based upon the Living with Epilepsy survey instrument developed by Jacoby and colleagues [6] and used previously in several British surveys.[2,5,6] The areas investigated were: frequency of epilepsy attacks and severity; drug treatment and its perceived effect; use of, attitudes to, and preferences for primary- and secondary-based epilepsy care; perceived effect of epilepsy and its treatment on everyday life.

Most questions had multiple choice answers. Patients indicated 'how you feel about your life as a whole' on a seven-point analogue scale with smiling, neutral or sad faces. This scale has been used for other chronic diseases' and appears to have fair reliability, validity [8,9] and responsiveness to change.[10] For analysis, responses scoring 1 or 2 were defined as 'happy' while those scoring 3 or more were defined as 'not happy'. Data were analysed on SAS. For the main prevalence estimates, 95 % confidence intervals were adjusted for possible cluster effects due to inter-practice variation.[11] Proportions were compared with Pearson's c^2 test and c^2 test for linear trend. To examine the independent influences of personal characteristics and different aspects of epilepsy on well being and desire for the proposed service, multiple logistic regression was used.

RESULTS

The study population comprised 595 patients aged 16 years or over and receiving medication for epilepsy, 394 of whom completed the questionnaire (response rate of 66.2%; 327 (83.0%) replying to the first mailing and 67 (17.0%) to the second). This is similar to the response rate found in a previous similar study.[2] Because some respondents did not answer some questions, the relevant denominator is provided for respective questions. The mean age of the 394 patients was 52.0 years (standard deviation (SD) 17.3, range 16–94 years), and 52.7 % were male. Long-term health problems in addition to epilepsy

were reported by 47.0% (95% CI 42.9–51.2 %), and 5.3 % of all patients belonged to the British Epilepsy Association or the National Society for Epilepsy.

Epilepsy severity and its effect on quality of life

During the previous year, 58.1% (52.8–63.4%) of 363 patients had not had a single epilepsy attack, 21.5 % (17.2–25.7 %) had fewer than one attack per month and 20.4 % (17.0–23.7 %) had one or more attacks a month: 36.2 % of patients had never had a period of 2 years or more free of epileptic attacks. Of those who answered questions on injuries resulting from an epilepsy attack, 4.3 % (8/184) reported a dental injury, 5.9 % (11/185) reported a fracture (excluding to the head), 7.3 % (14/193) reported having an attack while bathing or swimming, 7.6 % (14/184) reported a burn or scald and 22.5 % (43/191) reported a head injury in the previous year. The proportions reporting that epilepsy and its treatment adversely affected different aspects of their daily lives increased significantly with increased frequency of epilepsy attacks (Table 1). Perceived stigma due to epilepsy was also positively associated with attack frequency (Table 1).

Of 343 patients, 52.2 % indicated they were 'happy' about their lives as a whole on the faces scale (scores 1–2). Factors independently associated with a response of 'not happy' (scores 3–7) in a logistic regression model were: epilepsy attack in the previous year (odds ratio (OR) 2.81, 95 % CI 1.66–4.23), feeling as if they were treated 'like an inferior person' by some people (OR 2.13, 1.05–4.32), other long-term health problem (OR 2.06, 1.22–3.48) and male gender (OR 2.11, 1.25–3.55).

Anti-epileptic medication

Of 391 patients, 65.7 % were on monotherapy, 24.5 % were on two drugs, 4.1 % were on three drugs and 0. 8 % were on four drugs; in total 29.4 % (95 % CI 25.4–33.4%) were receiving polypharmacy. The remaining 4.9 % stated they were not currently taking any anti-epileptic medication. The number of drugs taken was positively associated with frequency of epilepsy attacks: 33.9 % of patients on monotherapy, 62.5 % on two drugs and 72.2 % on three or more drugs had one or more attacks in the previous year (x^2 for linear trend = 26.4; df = 1; $P < 0.00001$). Drug side effects, especially sedation, concentration and memory problems, were reported by 56.1% (50.1–62.2 %), and were more common with multiple drug therapy than monotherapy (72.9% versus 48.8%; x^2 = 17.6; df = 1; $P < 0. 001$).

Of 364 patients, 94.2 % considered their epilepsy to be very or fairly well controlled by drugs. Reported good control was inversely associated with number of anti-epileptic drugs used (x^2 for linear trend = 14.2; df = 1; $P = 0.00017$). Of 72 patients who had epilepsy attacks at least monthly, 75.0 % reported very or fairly good control; 78.7% (73.7–83.7%) reported never missing their medication, 16.4 % (11.5–21.3 %) missed medication but less than once monthly, and 4.9% (2.9–6.9%) missed their medication at least monthly.

4

Table 1

Perceived effect of frequency of epilepsy attacks on everyday life and perceived stigma in the previous year (number (%) who report either 'a lot' or 'some' effect)

A lot/some effect on:	Epilepsy attack frequency (no. (%) of patients)				x^2 for linear trend	
	None	< 1 /month	≥ 1 /month	Total[a]	x^2	P
Relationship with partner[b]	19 (10.1)	9 (12.7)	22 (32.8)	57 (16.3)	17.2	0.00003
Relationship with family	24 (12.5)	15 (20.8)	25 (37.3)	74 (20.8)	19.1	0.00001
Relationship with friends	16 (8.5)	16 (21.9)	28 (40.0)	70 (19.7)	34.9	< 0.00001
Social life/activities	31 (16.1)	28 (38.9)	38 (55.1)	106 (29.8)	41.4	< 0.00001
Ability to do paid employment	33 (19.9)	20 (30.8)	24 (38.7)	80 (25.8)	9.1	0.0026
Kind of paid work[c]	35 (18.9)	17 (23.6)	16 (24.6)	69 (20.1)	1.2	0.28
Overall health	33 (17.6)	26 (35.6)	49 (72.5)	119 (33.7)	66.3	< 0.00001
Feelings about yourself	36 (18.8)	29 (40.3)	41 (62.1)	117 (33.0)	45.0	< 0.00001
Future plans/ambitions	27 (14.3)	28 (40.0)	44 (66.7)	105 (30.3)	67.0	< 0.00001
Standard of living	20 (10.5)	27 (38.0)	40 (58.8)	93 (26.3)	65.8	< 0.00001
'Because of my epilepsy I feel that some people:						
Are uncomfortable with me'	33 (17.9)	19 (27.5)	30 (47.6)	88 (26.2)	20.9	< 0.00001
Treat me like an inferior person'	27 (15.3)	13 (19.1)	13 (24.1)	58 (18.3)	2.2	0.13
Would prefer to avoid me'	22 (12.5)	12 (18.2)	15 (27.8)	52 (16.5)	7.0	0.0082

[a] Includes patients who did not report on frequency of attacks.
[b] 112 (32.0%) patients not applicable.
[c] 185 (53.9%) patients not applicable.

Use of health services

During the previous year many patients had seen neither GP nor hospital doctor about their epilepsy, and patients receiving both hospital and GP care had the poorest control of epilepsy attacks (Table 2; consultations with the GP not concerning epilepsy were excluded). Of 339 patients, 71.7 % had consultations with the GP for any purpose in the previous year, with a mean of 3.5 (SD 4.8) visits per patient; the mean number of visits specifically for epilepsy was 1.6 (SD 2.7). In comparison the mean number of hospital visits for epilepsy, mainly to a local general neurology or neuropsychiatric clinic, was 0.6 (SD 1.3). Of those who attended the general practice, only 13.4% (9.6–17.2 %) had a regular appointment to see a GP for their epilepsy. The likelihood of having a regular arrangement increased slightly, but not significantly, with frequency of epilepsy attacks (x^2 for linear trend = 2.3; df = 1; P = 0.129).

During the previous year 9.6% had been admitted to a hospital as an inpatient, 9.7% attended an accident and emergency department and 11. 1% had an electroencephalogram for their epilepsy. The likelihood of each of these events increased with frequency of epilepsy attacks (x^2 for linear trend = 14.7, 29.7, 15.2; df = 1; P = 0.00013, < 0.00001, 0.0001 respectively). Blood levels of anti-epileptic drugs had been measured in the previous year in 47.4% of patients, and in 66.7 % of those who had one or more epilepsy attacks a month.

The mean time taken to see the GP or hospital doctor (including travelling and waiting) was 46.7 (SD 30.0) minutes and 131.0 (SD 78.8) minutes respectively. The mean distance to the GP was 1.2 (SD 2.4) miles: the last time patients visited 59.0% walked and 23.3% travelled by car. By comparison the mean distance to the hospital was 5.7 (SD 12.6) miles and only 8.5% walked while 46.9% travelled by car. Two-thirds of the people who attended the hospital took somebody else with them compared with only one-third who attended the general practice.

Table 2

Sources of epilepsy care and percentage of patients in each care category who had one or more epilepsy attacks in the previous year

	Sources of epilepsy care in previous year			
	None	GP only	Hospital only	GP and hospital
n (%)	111 (42.4)	84 (32.0)	18 (6.9)	49 (18.7)
95% confidence intervals (%)	35.9–48.8	26.0–38.1	4.2–9.6	14.0–23.4
n (%) ≥ 1 attack in previous year [a,b]	20 (19.1)	49 (63.6)	7 (38.9)	36 (78.3)

[a] Not all patients who stated source of care gave information on attacks.
[b] Pearson's x^2 test = 60.1; df = 3; P < 0.001.

Table 3

Perceived main source of care against preferred main source of care

Preferred main source of care	Perceived main source of care (% of patients)				
	GP (n = 220)	GP and hospital equally (n = 51)	Hospital (n = 30)	Neither (n = 14)	Total (n = 320)[a]
GP	65.0	21.6	16.7	35.7	51.9
General practice-based epilepsy clinic	18.2	27.4	43.3	14.3	22.2
Hospital	0.9	15.7	26.7	7.1	6.2
Indifferent	15.9	35.3	13.3	42.9	19.7
Total	100.0	100.0	100.0	100.0	100.0

[a] Includes five patients who did not report on perceived main source of care.

Patients' perceptions of and preferences for care

Of 368 patients, 69.6% perceived their epilepsy care to be provided by the GP in the main, 9.8 % by a hospital doctor, 16.0 % equally shared between GP and hospital, and 4.6 % by neither. Table 3 shows that all categories of patients expressed a preference for mainly receiving care in a primary setting, this was expressed most strongly by patients who perceived the GP as providing their main epilepsy care. Patients who felt the hospital provided the main care were most likely to favour a general practice-based epilepsy clinic (Table 3). The main reasons for preferring care from the GP, general practice-based epilepsy clinic or hospital were given as: "the doctor knows more about me and my history", "the care is more personal" and "the doctor knows more about epilepsy", respectively.

Previous discussion of several topics related to epilepsy was most likely in shared GP and hospital patients and least likely in patients who had not received epilepsy care in the past year (Table 4). Of patients who had not discussed these topics those who received shared care and hospital only care were most in favour of discussion (Table 4). Patients who had had an epilepsy attack in the past year were more likely to want discussion, significantly so for hospital attenders (76.2% versus 46.8%; x^2 10.0; df = 1; $P = 0.002$), but not for GP attenders (71.7% versus 61.6%; $x^2 = 2.6$; df = 1; $P= 0.109$). However, perceived adequacy of information provided and perceived adequacy of staff knowledge in hospitals and general practices were similar (58.2% versus 62.5% and 87.3% versus 77.5%, respectively). The proportions who reported it very or fairly easy to talk to staff about

Table 4

Proportions (%) of patients who had ever discussed topics relating to epilepsy with GPs and/or hospital staff and those that would have liked discussion

Topic discussed	Sources of epilepsy care in previous year (% of patients)					x^2	P	No. with complete information
	None (n = 111)	GP only (n = 84)	Hospital only (n = 18)	GP and hospital (n = 49)[a]	Total (n = 262)			
Possible causes of epilepsy	35.8	42.2	44.4	49.0	40.9	2.7	0.448	259
Type of epilepsy	38.5	46.1	35.3	65.3	45.8	10.6	0.014	253
Would like to discuss above	*42.1*	*58.2*	*68.8*	*69.8*	*54.7*	*11.2*	*0.011*	*214*
Possible side effects of drugs	38.9	43.2	47.1	70.8	46.9	14.3	0.003	254
Interactions with other drugs	42.5	50.5	38.9	67.4	49.4	9.2	0.027	255
Effect of alcohol and drugs	43.7	40.7	47.1	69.4	48.0	11.5	0.009	250
Contraception/pregnancy	30.0	11.8	20.0	33.3	24.6	4.9	0.179	118
Would like to discuss above	*38.6*	*47.0*	*71.4*	*58.1*	*47.4*	*8.0*	*0.047*	*211*
Laws about driving	41.0	48.8	61.1	55.1	47.6	4.3	0.228	252
Effect of work/study	16.8	23.4	29.4	36.7	23.6	7.7	0.052	250
Effect of family life	13.1	20.0	17.7	30.6	19.0	6.8	0.078	253
Effect of social life/activities	13.0	17.3	29.4	30.6	18.8	8.3	0.041	255
Self-help epilepsy groups	5.6	13.6	17.7	16.3	11.0	6.0	0.111	255
Would like to discuss above	*32.0*	*44.0*	*53.3*	*62.5*	*43.2*	*13.2*	*0.004*	*241*

[a] Discussed with either GP or hospital doctor.

problems or worries because of their epilepsy were 71.6% for hospital attenders and 85.4% for GP attenders.

Of 348 patients, 69.8 % (95% CI 63.5–76.2 %) stated that they would like to make contact with an epilepsy specialist nurse in the general practice; this was most likely (91.8 %) among those who had used both hospital and GP in the previous year. In a multiple logistic regression model, desire to see the epilepsy specialist nurse was greater for those who had had an epilepsy attack in the previous year (OR 2.04, 95 % CI 1.36–4.23), or were 'not happy' on the faces scale (OR 2.57, 1.48–4.45), but was not associated with other long-term health problems or gender.

DISCUSSION

The study quantified, for a geographically defined population, problems with epilepsy care that have been identified previously in other settings:[1] lack of systematic follow-up, inappropriate polypharmacy, noncompliance with medication and communication failure. The study is original both in its assessment of the accessibility of primary and secondary care, and in its comparison of the health care experiences and preferences of patients using primary and/or secondary care. Experiences and preferences of patients in Bristol can be compared with those reported from Liverpool[6] and south-east England.[5] Many patients did not receive any epilepsy care over the period of a year but most of those who received care did so in a primary setting, which would have been preferred by many hospital patients. It also suggested that patients using both primary and secondary care had the greatest unmet needs concerning: control of epilepsy attacks, discussion of issues and desire for contact with the specialist nurse.

Although the majority of patients were not affected by their epilepsy, one-fifth reported epilepsy attacks at least monthly, and epilepsy adversely affected several aspects of many patients' lives, with effects strongly associated with the frequency of attacks. The finding that frequency of attacks was associated with adverse psychosocial effects and with perceived stigma supports the results of other studies [6,12] that used the same methods.

The finding that three-quarters of those having one or more epilepsy attacks a month felt very or fairly well controlled by medication supports the claim by Betts and Smith that "many patients and their medical advisors still accept a level of control which is far from the ideal (i.e. no seizures, a normal quality of life, free from side effects of medication)".[13] There is clearly scope for more intensive counselling and monitoring to reduce attack frequency and to help patients cope with the psychosocial effects of epilepsy. Around half of the patients wished to discuss certain issues surrounding epilepsy but had never done so, supporting Ridsdale et al.[5] who reported that 35% of patients in their study stated they had not received enough information about their epilepsy.

Two-thirds of patients were on monotherapy, which is slightly less than the proposed 70–80% that it has been stated could be controlled on one drug.[1] It is of concern, however, that over half of all patients reported drug side effects which might be improved by tailoring drug choices and doses. The finding that nearly 79% of patients reported never missing taking their tablets suggests better compliance than the 50–70% reported elsewhere,[1] but the positive association between compliance and control of epilepsy attacks indicates that benefits could be gained from still better compliance rates.

The lack of structured care is illustrated by the finding that only one in seven GP patients had arrangements regularly to see their GP about epilepsy. This is similar to the 17% reported by Ridsdale et al.[5] using the same method. The study shows the greater accessibility of primary than secondary care, in terms of distance, time and transport costs, which partly explains the preference of hospital patients for a specialist service based in primary care. Accessibility is arguably the main advantage of a shift of specialist skills to primary care.

The findings of Ridsdale et al.[5] on patients' preferences for source of care confirm our findings that patients generally preferred to receive epilepsy care in the primary care setting. Unlike Ridsdale et al., this study allowed patients to consider the option of a specialist nurse based in the general practice. The district epilepsy service of Taylor et al.,[14] with community-based specialist liaison nurses, appears to be a workable model for improving epilepsy care, and has been shown to have a positive impact on epilepsy management. Decentralizing specialist services by means of epilepsy specialist nurses, and structured care with annual or 6-monthly consultations [5] may, however, be costly, and costs need to be estimated. Although more frequent and structured epilepsy care may be effective, this has not yet been unequivocally demonstrated in rigorous evaluation studies.

The methodological issues that require comments are: sampling frame completeness, response rate and validity of patients' responses. Drug record data are an imperfect method of identifying all patients with epilepsy, but were most appropriate as the new service used the same data to define its target population. Non-responders are likely to have been systematically different from responders, and it is plausible that the former included patients whose learning disabilities prevented them or their carers from completing the questionnaire. Other studies [5,6] have excluded this category of patients which may have contributed to their higher response rates but limited their generalizability. Some patients may not have been motivated to respond because their lack of epilepsy-related problems made them uninterested in service development. However, Jacoby et al.[6] found little difference in the level of current seizure activity between responders and non-responders to their questionnaire, upon which ours is based. Patients' questionnaire responses may have been inaccurate, but they were preferable to medical records, which have been shown often to be incomplete.[5] They provided current information on patients who had not received epilepsy care for some time and they allowed patients' experiences of and preferences for health care to be elicited. The investigators propose to use qualitative methods to examine more deeply patients' and health professionals' perceptions and preferences regarding epilepsy and its health care.

In future years it is likely that primary care for epilepsy in Britain will be developed to address the problems shown in this study, following the example of diabetes care. This may however, require considerable resources and organization. Priorities for population needs assessments in future include patients' own views and evaluation of innovations in structured epilepsy care.

ACKNOWLEDGEMENTS

We thank all patients for their information and the partners and practice staff of participating general practices for their support and for allowing access to their patients. Thanks to Dr Ann Jacoby, Professor David Chadwick, and Dr Gus Baker for the use of their questionnaire. Finally, thanks to Ann Fokke, epilepsy nurse specialist, for her comments on earlier drafts. Funding was obtained from Avon Health Authority.

There was no conflict of interest.

References

1 Thapar AK. Care of patients with epilepsy in the community: will new initiatives address old problems? *Br J Gen Pract* 1996; **46**: 37–42.

2 Jacoby A. Quality of life and care in epilepsy. In Chadwick DW, Baker GA, Jacoby A (eds). *Quality of Life and Quality of Care in Epilepsy.* Royal Society of Medicine Round Table Series Number 31. London: Royal Society of Medicine Services, 1993: 66–78.

3 Ridsdale L. Matching the needs with skills in epilepsy care. *Br Med J* 1995; **310**: 1219–1220.

4 Brown SM, Betts T, Chadwick DW, Hall B, Shorvon SD, Wallace S. An epilepsy needs document. *Seizure* 1993; **2**: 91–103.

5 Ridsdale L, Jeffery S, Robins D, McGee L, Fitzgerald A, Epilepsy Care Evaluation Group. Epilepsy monitoring and advice recorded: general practitioners' views, current practice and patients' preferences. *Br J Gen Pract* 1996; **46**: 11–14.

6 Jacoby A, Baker GA, Steen N, Potts P, Chadwick DW. The clinical course of epilepsy and its psychosocial correlates: findings from a UK community study. *Epilepsia* 1996; **37**: 148–161.

7 Anderson R. The quality of life of stroke patients and their carers. In Anderson R, Bury M (eds). *Living with Chronic Illness: The Experience of Patients and Their Families.* London: Unwin Hyman, 1988: 14–42.

8 Bowling A. *Measuring Health: A Review of Quality of Life Measurement Scales.* Milton Keynes: Open University Press, 1991.

9 Wilkin D, Hallam L, Doggett M-A. *Measures of Need and Outcome for Primary Health Care.* Oxford: Oxford University Press, 1992.

10 Kinnersley P, Peters T, Stott N. Measuring functional health status in primary care using the COOP-WONCA charts: acceptability, range of scores, construct validity, reliability and sensitivity to change. *Br J Gen Pract* 1994; **44**: 545–549.

11 Bennett S, Woods T, Liyanage WM, Smith DL. A simplified general method for cluster-sample surveys of health in developing countries. *World Health Statistics Q* 1991; **44**: 98–106.

12 Ridsdale L, Robins D, Fitzgerald A, Jeffery S, McGee L, Epilepsy Care Evaluation Group. Epilepsy in general practice: patients' psychological symptoms and their perception of stigma. *Br J Gen Pract* 1996; **46**: 365–366.

13 Betts T, Smith K. New departures in epilepsy care: an epilepsy liaison service. *Seizure* 1994; **3**: 301–308.

14 Taylor MP, Readman S, Hague B, Boulter V, Hughes L, Howell S. A district epilepsy service, with community-based specialist liaison nurses and guidelines for shared care. *Seizure* 1994; **3**: 121–127.

4

This article was first published in the BMJ and is reproduced by permission of the BMJ

A RANDOMISED CONTROLLED TRIAL OF GENERAL PRACTITIONER SAFETY ADVICE FOR FAMILIES WITH CHILDREN UNDER 5 YEARS

Margaret Clamp, Denise Kendrick

Margaret Clamp, *general practitioner*, Colwick Vale Surgery, Colwick, Nottingham NG4 2DU,
Denise Kendrick, *senior lecturer*, Division of General Practice, University of Nottingham Medical School, Queen's Medical Centre, Nottingham NG7 2UH

Correspondence to: Dr Kendrick Denise.Kendrick@nottingham.ac.uk

BMJ 1998; **316**: 1576-9

ABSTRACT

Objective: To assess effectiveness of general practitioner advice about child safety, and provision of low cost safety equipment to low income families, on use of safety equipment and safe practices at home.

Design: Randomised, unblinded, controlled trial with initial assessment and six week follow up by telephone survey. Twenty families from intervention and control groups were randomly selected for a home visit to assess validity of responses to second survey.

Setting: A general practice in Nottingham.

Subjects: 98% (165/169) of families with children aged under 5 years registered with the practice.

Interventions: General practitioner safety advice plus, for families receiving means tested state benefits, access to safety equipment at low cost. Control families received usual care.

Main outcome measures: Possession and use of safety equipment and safe practices at home.

Results: Before intervention, the two groups differed only in possession of fireguards. After intervention, significantly more families in intervention group used fireguards (relative risk 1.89, 95% confidence interval 1.18 to 2.94), smoke alarms (1.14, 1.04 to 1.25), socket covers (1.27, 1.10 to 1.48), locks on cupboards for storing cleaning materials (1.38, 1.02 to 1.88), and door slam devices (3.60, 2.17 to 5.97). Also, significantly more families in intervention group showed very safe practice in storage of sharp objects (1.98, 1.38 to 2.83), storage of medicines (1.15, 1.03 to 1.28), window safety (1.30, 1.06 to 1.58), fireplace safety (1.84, 1.34 to 2.54), socket safety (1.77, 1.37 to 2.28), smoke alarm safety (1.11, 1.01 to 1.22), and door slam safety (7.00, 3.15 to 15.6). Stratifying results by receipt of state benefits showed that intervention was at least as effective in families receiving benefits as others.

Conclusions: General practitioner advice, coupled with access to low cost equipment for low income families, increased use of safety equipment and other safe practices. These findings are encouraging for provision of injury prevention in primary care.

INTRODUCTION

The *Health of the Nation* suggests that primary healthcare teams should provide safety advice to parents during child health surveillance programmes, advise on and provide access to safety equipment, check and advise on hazards in the home, provide advice on first aid, and advise the community on safety.[1] Studies have suggested that a lack of time and expertise are often quoted as factors that limit the provision of injury prevention in primary care.[2-10] Hence, it has been suggested that any initiative to be introduced into general practice must be quick and easy to carry out.[11]

Studies in the United States have shown that counselling by physicians improved safety behaviour and reduced hazards,[12-15] and one small study showed a reduction in falls in infants.[16] In addition, increasing access to safety equipment increased the installation of smoke alarms[17] and socket covers but not cupboard locks, which were more difficult to install. [18,19]

However, differences between the healthcare systems of the United Kingdom and the United States may limit the generalisability of these studies to UK settings. We therefore undertook this study to assess the effectiveness of counselling on injury prevention by a general practitioner in conjunction with access to low cost safety equipment for families on a low income in the United Kingdom. The study received approval from the ethics committee of Queen's Medical Centre.

SUBJECTS AND METHODS

Subjects

The study population comprised the 169 families with children aged ≤ 5 years that were registered with a single handed general practice in an urban area of Nottingham. The 165 (98%) families that responded to a questionnaire on child safety practices were numbered from 1 to 165, and we used random number tables to allocate them, by number, to an intervention or a control group. We calculated that 73 families were required in each group, based on $\beta=0.1$, $\alpha=0.05$, a baseline possession of safety equipment of 60%,[20] and a difference of 25% in possession of safety equipment. The figure shows the flow of families through the trial.

Questionnaire

We used a questionnaire to obtain information on families' use of safety equipment; storage of sharp objects, cleaning products, and medicines; risk factors for unintentional injury; and sociodemographic factors.

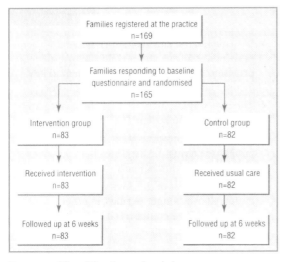

Progress of families through trial

The questions on risk and sociodemographic factors had previously been validated.[21] The questionnaire was designed to be administered by telephone or postal survey. It was piloted in another general practice with a similar patient population, with 30 questionnaires administered by each method. No major changes were made to the questionnaire based on the pilot study.

The questionnaire was pre-coded. Each safety practice was assigned a category combining several aspects of safety. For example, for the storage of sharp objects, safe storage was defined as all sharp objects stored above adult eye level or always kept in cupboards or drawers that were always locked. Moderately safe storage was defined as some sharp objects stored below adult eye level in cupboards or drawers that were only sometimes locked or only some of which had locks. Unsafe storage was defined as some or all sharp objects always stored below adult eye level in cupboards or drawers that were not locked.

The questionnaire was administered at baseline and at follow up, six weeks after intervention, by telephone by the general practitioner (MC) or sent by post to those families without a telephone. Non-responders to the postal questionnaire were sent a reminder three weeks later.

The validity of the responses was assessed by home visits to a random sample of 10 families in each of the intervention and control groups two weeks after the second questionnaire. MC, who was blind to the responses on the questionnaire, made the home visits.

Intervention

The intervention consisted of standardised advice and safety leaflets concerning smoke alarms, stair gates, fireguards, cupboard locks, covers for electric sockets, door slam devices, safe storage of medicines, sharp objects, and cleaning materials. Families receiving means tested state benefits were offered a smoke alarm for 50p and two window locks, three cupboard locks, six socket covers, or a door slam device for 20p, all available from the surgery at the time of the consultation. Stair gates and fireguards were offered at £5 per item via the health district's low cost scheme, which was available to families receiving benefits across Nottingham Health District (including control families) and was accessed via health visitors, with equipment being delivered to a local health centre for collection by parents.

The intervention took place during child health surveillance consultations or opportunistically during other consultations, or the family was asked to make an appointment specifically for the intervention. The control group received routine child health surveillance and routine consultations, but without the intervention. The mean length of consultation for safety advice was 20 minutes.

Statistical analysis

We analysed the data, on an intention to treat basis, using SPSS for Windows.[22] The results are presented as relative risks (95% confidence intervals) of using safety equipment and behaving safely, and the number needed to treat to facilitate one family to use safety equipment or behave safely. We assessed the consistency between the responses to the questionnaire and observed safety practices by means of κ coefficients.[23]

RESULTS

The consistency of responses to the questionnaire and at the home visit was high: 21 questions showed complete agreement, with κ coefficients of 1; for five questions $\kappa=0.75$-0.99; for six questions $\kappa=0.59$-0.74; and for four questions $\kappa<0.60$. Two questions had almost complete agreement (95% in each case), but the κ coefficient was low because all but one of the responses were positive on the first questionnaire.[24] The two remaining questions with low κ coefficients concerned the level at which sharp objects were stored in the kitchen ($\kappa=0.49$) and the use of socket covers on unused sockets ($\kappa=0.33$).

Table 1 shows the baseline characteristics of the study population. Thirty three per cent of the families in the intervention group and 35% of those in the control group reported that at least one of their children had

Table 1

Sociodemographic characteristics of study population.
Values are numbers of families

Sociodemographic characteristics	Intervention group (n=83)	Control group (n=82)
Single parent family	7	10
Not owner occupiers	20	15
Receiving means tested state benefits	30	23
Without access to car	15	11
Jarman score:		
<0	5	9
0.1-22.9	64	59
>23	14	14
Overcrowded*	12	8
Not in paid employment:		
Respondent	42	38
Partner of respondent	11	6
Ethnic minority group	1	1

* Defined as >1 person per room, excluding kitchens <2 m wide and bathrooms.

Table 2

Use of safety equipment by families after safety intervention

Safety equipment used	No of families		Relative risk (95% CI)	Number needed to treat*
	Intervention group (n=83)	Control group (n=82)		
Fireguard[†]	36/65	19/60	1.89 (1.18 to 2.94)	4
Stair gate[††]	51/82	40/78	1.26 (0.95 to 1.67)	9
Smoke alarm	82	71	1.14 (1.04 to 1.25)	8
Socket covers	76	59	1.27 (1.10 to 1.48)	5
Window catches	80	72 1.	1.10 (1.00 to 1.20)	12
Cupboard locks:				
To lock away sharp objects	23	29	0.78 (0.50 to 1.23)	–
To lock away cleaning materials	49	35	1.38 (1.02 to 1.88)	6
To lock away medicines	15	15	0.99 (0.52 to 1.89)	–
Door slam devices	51	14	3.60 (2.17 to 5.97)	2

* Number needed to treat to facilitate one family using safety equipment (not calculated when relative risk <1).
† Families without open, gas, or electric fires excluded from analysis.
†† Families without stairs excluded from analysis.

had more than one attendance at the general practice or accident and emergency department for an injury.

After the intervention, families in the intervention group were more likely to use a range of items of safety equipment than were control families (table 2). A higher proportion of families in the intervention group were categorised as safe for their storage of sharp objects and medicines and for safety of windows, fireplaces, electric sockets, smoke alarms, and door slams (table 3), suggesting that even when these families did not obtain items of safety equipment, such as cupboard locks and window catches, they did change their safety behaviour.

After stratifying the results by receipt of means tested benefits, we found that, among those receiving benefits, a significantly higher proportion of families in the intervention group than controls were categorised as safe for five of the nine safety practices. Among those not receiving benefits, significantly more families in the intervention group were categorised as safe for three of the nine safety practices. This suggests that the intervention was equally, if not more, effective in the families receiving benefits.

DISCUSSION

The high response rate to the baseline questionnaire suggests the results of this study are generalisable to the practice population. The similarity of the study population to that of Nottingham in terms of sociodemographic factors[25] suggests these results may be applicable to a wider population, although the lower proportion of families belonging to an ethnic minority in the study means that caution must be exercised in extrapolating the results of this study to minority groups.

Table 3

Proportion of families categorised as behaving very safely on range of practices after safety intervention

Safety practice	Intervention group (n=83)	Control group (n=82)	Relative risk (95% CI)	Number needed to treat*
Fireplace safety[†]	56	30	1.84 (1.34 to 2.54)	3
Stairway safety[††]	53	50	1.05 (0.83 to 1.33)	11
Smoke alarm safety	80	71	1.11 (1.01 to 1.22)	10
Socket cover safety	68	38	1.77 (1.37 to 2.28)	3
Window safety	67	51	1.30 (1.06 to 1.58)	5
Storage of sharp objects	52	26	1.98 (1.38 to 2.83)	3
Storage of cleaning materials	59	49	1.19 (0.95 to 1.49)	9
Storage of medicines	79	68	1.15 (1.03 to 1.28)	8
Door slam safety	42	6	7.00 (3.15 to 15.6)	2

* Number needed to treat to facilitate one family behaving very safely.
† Families without open, gas, or electric fires categorised as behaving very safely.
†† Families without stairs categorised as behaving very safely.

Key messages

- We assessed the effectiveness of general practitioner advice about child safety, and provision of low cost safety equipment to low income families, on safe practices at home

- The intervention increased safe behaviour and use of safety equipment

- The intervention was equally effective in families receiving means tested benefits as in those not receiving benefits

- The effectiveness of this intervention should be evaluated over longer periods, in other practices, and when delivered by other members of the primary healthcare team

As safety practices were self reported, it is possible that families receiving the intervention overreported safety practices to a greater degree than did control families, so overestimating the effect of the intervention.[26] However, the high degree of consistency of responses to questionnaire and the safety practices observed on the home visit suggest that overreporting did not occur to any great degree and did not occur differentially in the intervention group.

The results from this small study suggest that general practitioners can increase safety practices through giving routine safety advice and providing low cost safety equipment. The short follow up period means we cannot draw conclusions about the long term effectiveness of such an intervention, and further studies are needed. Further evaluation is needed in other practices to see if our findings can be replicated elsewhere. Furthermore, the effectiveness and cost effectiveness of other members of the primary care team undertaking the same intervention programme requires evaluation. The short time scale and small sample size of this study precluded any assessment of reductions in frequency or severity of injury, but such evaluations are needed before new interventions are introduced into routine primary care.

Our finding that the intervention was at least equally effective in families receiving benefits is important as there is debate about the relative effectiveness of population versus targeted approaches to injury prevention in primary care. [21 27 28] This study used a population approach, with tailoring of the interventions to specific groups in order that families relying on state benefits were not disproportionately disadvantaged by taking part in the interventions. This is the first UK study to suggest that a population approach would be equally effective in different socioeconomic groups. It has been argued that the population approach would lead to widening inequalities in health, as interventions may be less effective in those most at risk.[27] This study suggests this is not the case, but further work, with a larger sample from a larger number of practices, is needed to confirm this finding.

ACKNOWLEDGMENTS

The safety leaflets used in this study included *Play it Safe* (Health Education Authority, 1996), *Your Baby's Safety At Home and At Play* (Mothercare, 1994), and *Home Safety Checklist* (Child Accident Prevention Trust, 1996).

DK coordinated the formulation of the primary study hypothesis, discussed core ideas, designed the protocol and questionnaire, and participated in data analysis and writing of the paper. MC initiated the idea for the study; discussed core ideas; carried out the literature search and pilot studies; modified the questionnaire; administered the questionnaire, intervention, and validation studies; entered and verified the data; and participated in data analysis and writing of the paper.

Funding: Nottingham Health Authority provided a grant of £500 for the purchase of safety equipment. This research was undertaken as part of a Masters Degree in Medical Science in Primary Health Care, in the Division of General Practice at Nottingham University.

Conflict of interest: None.

References

1 Department of Health. *The health of the nation. Key area handbook: accidents.* London: DoH, 1993.
2 Carter YH, Bannon MJ, Jones PW. Health visitors and child accident prevention. *Health Visitor* 1992; **65**: 115-117.
3 Carter YH, Jones PW. General practitioners' beliefs about their role in the prevention and treatment of accidents involving children. *Br J Gen Pract* 1993; **43**: 463-465.
4 Greig T. The GP's role in child accident prevention. *Practitioner* 1987; **231**: 1612-1616.
5 Kendrick D. The role of the primary health care team in preventing accidents to children. *Br J Gen Pract* 1994; **44**: 372-375.
6 Levene S. Accident prevention: the health visitor's role. *Health Visitor* 1992; **62**: 340-341.
7 Kendrick D, Marsh P, Williams EI. General practitioners: child accident prevention and "The Health of the Nation." *Health Educ Res* 1995; **10**: 345-353.
8 Kendrick D, Marsh P, Williams EI. How do practice nurses see their role in childhood injury prevention? *Injury Prev* 1995; **1**: 159-163.
9 Marsh P, Kendrick D, Williams EI. Health visitors' knowledge, attitudes and practices in childhood accident prevention. *J Public Health Med* 1995; **17**: 193-199.
10 Laidman P. *Health visitors and preventing accidents to children. Research report 12.* London: Health Education Authority, 1987.
11 Phalp A. Child accidents: common, serious and preventable. *Practitioner* 1994; **238**: 766-769.
12 Bass JL, Mehta KA, Ostrovsky M, Halperin SF. Educating parents about injury prevention. *Pediatr Clin North Am* 1985; **32**: 233-272.
13 Kelly B, Sein C, McCarthy PL. Safety education in a pediatric primary care setting. *Pediatrics* 1987; **79**: 818-824.
14 Katcher ML, Landry GL, Shapiro MM. Liquid-crystal thermometer use in paediatricians' office counselling about tap water burn prevention. *Pediatrics* 1989; **83**: 766-771.

15 Thomas KA, Hassanein RS, Christopherson ER. Evaluation of group well-child care for improving burn prevention practices in the home. *Pediatrics* 1984; **74**: 879-881.

16 Kravitz H. Prevention of accidental falls in infancy by counselling mothers. *Illinois Med J* 1973; **144**: 570-573.

17 Miller RE, Reisinger KS, Blatter MM, Wucher F. Pediatric counselling and subsequent use of smoke detectors. *Am J Public Health* 1982; **72**: 392-393.

18 Dershewitz RA. Will mothers use free household safety devices? *Am J Dis Child* 1979; **133**: 61-64.

19 Dershewitz RA, Williamson JW. Prevention of childhood household injuries: a controlled clinical trial. *Am J Public Health* 1977; **67**: 1148-1153.

20 Kendrick D. Children's safety in the home: parents' possession and perceptions of the importance of safety equipment. *Public Health* 1994; **108**: 21-25.

21 Kendrick D, Marsh P. Injury prevention programmes in primary care: a high risk group or a whole population approach? *Injury Prev* 1997; **3**: 170-175.

22 SPSS. *Statistical package for social sciences for windows.* Release 6.1.3. Chicago IL: SPSS, 1995.

23 Landis JR, Koch GG. The measurement of observer agreement for categorical data. *Biometrics* 1977; **33**: 159-174.

24 Streiner DL, Norman GR. *Health measurement scales: a practical guide to their development and use.* Oxford: Oxford University Press, 1995.

25 Office of Population Censuses and Surveys. *1991 Census. Report for England. Regional Health Authorities parts 1 and 2.* London: HMSO , 1993.

26 Scott I. You can't believe all that you're told: the issue of unvalidated questionnaires. *Injury Prev* 1997; **3**: 5-6.

27 Moller J. Population strategies for injury prevention? If only it were that simple. *Injury Prev* 1997; **3**: 162-164.

28 Ward H. Should injury prevention programmes be targeted? *Injury Prev* 1997; **3**: 160-162.

5

(Accepted 22 April 1998)

This article was first published in Occupational Medicine and is reproduced by permission of Occupational Medicine

COMMUNICATION BETWEEN AN OCCUPATIONAL PHYSICIAN AND OTHER MEDICAL PRACTITIONERS — AN AUDIT

A M de Bono

Occupational Health Department, Leicester General Hospital, Gwendolen Road, Leicester, UK
Occup. Med. Vol. 47, 349–356, 1997

Four hundred and seventy-two consecutive referral episodes relating to 386 patients attending the Occupational Health Department of a general teaching hospital were analyzed to evaluate the frequency, content and effect on management of communications between the occupational physician and other doctors. In all, 250 episodes (53%) were associated with such a communication. The likelihood of a communication was strongly influenced by reason for referral, particularly in respect of long or short term sickness absence; univariate odds ratios (OR) = 10.58, 95% CI = 8.13–27.08) and 2.65, 95% CI = 1.55–4.60) respectively; a medical diagnosis of psychiatric illness (OR = 3.17, 95% CI = 1.69–5.97)); and by number of consultations. Communication was also more likely when the occupational outcome was ill health retirement, rehabilitation in work or modified work. Ninety-eight per cent of specific requests for information or an opinion elicited a reply. Information received from other doctors influenced the occupational health physician's management in 52 referral episodes (20%). Specific action by GPs as a result of communication was documented in 54 and by specialists in 37 episodes. The importance of communication between occupational health physician and other doctors in the occupational health process is confirmed.
Key words: Audit; communication: occupational health consultation.

Received 19 December 1996; accepted in final form 8 May 1997.

Correspondence and reprint requests to: A. M. de Bono, Occupational Health Department, Leicester General Hospital, Gwendolen Road, Leicester, UK. Tel: (+44) 116 2584930; Fax: (+44) 116 2875792; email: 106110.3106@compuserve.com

INTRODUCTION

The work of an occupational physician includes medical consultations in many respects identical to those of other physicians with their patients. The strict definition of a patient is 'one receiving or registered to receive treatment' (OED): many occupational health 'clients' would not fall into this category.[1,2] A second factor which distinguishes consultations between occupational physicians and their patients or clients is that the latter are usually already in a therapeutic relationship with other physicians, who are seldom primarily involved in seeking the occupational medicine consultation.

The tensions inherit in this situation have been recognized and codes of ethics for communication between occupational physicians and other doctors proposed by the Faculty of Occupational Medicine and the British Medical Association.[3,4] The importance of such communication was emphasized recently in the NHS Executive guidelines on occupational health services for NHS staff.[5]

There have been few formal investigations of the role of communication between occupational physicians and other doctors in contributing to the effective management of the occupational health problem or the long-term health and well-being of the patient. The transfer of information between general practitioners and hospital specialists has previously been studied, but only in the context of the interface between primary and secondary medical care.[6,7] A survey of 400 general practitioners and 300 occupational physicians showed a striking difference in their perception of the frequency with which communication occurred between them.[8,9] Seventy per cent of the occupational physicians felt that occupational health services communicated frequently, with general practitioners about their patients whereas only eight per cent of general practitioners thought this to be true.

There appears to be no previous systematic study of the nature and recorded purpose of communication between occupational physicians and general practitioners. Seaton [10] has argued strongly for an active role of the occupational physician in offering to assist the general practitioner in the management of his patient. Apart from Parker's finding [9] that the majority of a sample of 400 general practitioners thought that occupational health services had a useful role in helping the disabled, and that occupational health services should not refer patients to NHS consultants without obtaining express permission from the patients general practitioner, there is little information about the general practitioner's view of the role of occupational physicians in the management of their patients.

The object of this study was to examine the nature and purpose of communication between the occupational physician and other doctors arising from the occupational medicine consultation, in the setting of an occupational health service in an NHS teaching hospital.

METHODS

Study population

The study population comprised members of NHS staff working on site who had been referred by a third party or self referred for occupational medical assessment to the occupational physician in the Occupational Health Department at Leicester General Hospital over a 3-year period from November 1991. Casual referrals or emergency presentations including acute illness or accident in the workplace were excluded. Leicester General Hospital is an NHS Trust University Teaching hospital employing approximately 2,700 staff (21% male, 79% female). During the study period an on-site occupational health service was provided by two nurses and a part-time occupational physician (the author).

Data collection

From November 1991 all consultations were logged on a database written in EPI-Info version 5.00 maintained on a laptop portable computer with appropriate backup, and clinical notes recorded in the staff member's occupational health record folder. Of 390 patients logged, records were traced and retrieved for 386 (98.9%). A code number was allocated to each patient and a structured questionnaire was used to collect information about each identified referral episode from the computer database and the clinical notes. Some referrals to the occupational physician generated follow up consultations; the term 'referral episode' was applied to the consultation or series of consultations which related to a specific occupational health problem. For the purposes of this study, a referral episode terminated when a final opinion was given to the referrer. Where more than one referral of an individual to the occupational physician was made during the study period, each episode was analyzed separately in chronological order and the number of previous referrals noted.

All staff were classified into one of eight occupational groups; the source of referral was recorded and the reason for referral classified into one of nine groups. Clinical diagnoses were recorded on the computer database at the time of each consultation. For the purposes of this study the diagnoses were grouped into five categories according to the principal clinical problem identified during the referral episode. The occupational outcome at the termination of each referral episode was recorded, classified into one of nine categories. Any documented evidence of modification to the patient's working hours or duties on the recommendation of the occupational physician was separately recorded.

Communication between the occupational physician and other medical practitioners was analyzed according to a standard proforma developed for the purpose of this study and included in the questionnaire. The contents of letters and documented telephone conversations were assessed by the author and coded according to whether occupational or clinical information was given and whether information or an opinion was specifically requested. The same criteria were applied to all referral episodes. The criteria for communicating with a general practitioner or specialist were (i) that the occupational physician believed information she possessed would assist the other practitioner in their management of the patient or (ii) that the occupational physician believed that the other practitioner could contribute useful information concerning the patient. All letters to general practitioners and specialists were personalized for specific patients and problems. Standardized letters such as 'routine' pre-employment enquiries were not used.

The existence of a recorded reply to the occupational physician's communication was noted and its contents assessed for the provision of new information and for a recorded agreement or disagreement with the assessment offered to the other doctor by the occupational physician. Any invoices sent by outside practitioners in connection with reports on their patients were recorded.

Records were scrutinized by the author for any evidence of action taken by a general practitioner or hospital specialist following receipt of a letter or telephone communication from the occupational physician. A judgement was made as to whether the occupational physician's subsequent management of the patient was altered by information provided by the general practitioner or hospital consultant in their replies.

REVIEW PANEL

A randomized subset of anonymized case histories and verbatim anonymized letters relating to 10% of referral episodes in which written communication occurred between the occupational physician and other doctors was presented to a panel of three independent occupational physicians for validation. The panel included a fellow and two associates of the Faculty, all with more than five years occupational medicine experience. One of the physicians works in the NHS, two in other industries. They were asked to analyze the communications using the standard proforma.

Statistical methods

Results of univariate analyses are presented as odds ratios (odds of a communication resulting in a population identified by a specified variable compared with the odds of a communication in the population without that variable) with 95% confidence intervals based on a Poisson distribution.[11] Two x two contingency tables were tested for significance using the Chi-squared test with Yates' correction[12] Multiple logistic regression analysis was used in an attempt to identify independent predictor variables.[13] Analysis was carried out using MINITAB 7.2, Minitab Inc., Philadelphia USA, 1989, and SPSS for Windows) Release 6.0, 1993.

A random selection of case records for panel verification was made using a computer-generated random numbers list. Consistency of the panel's agreement (or otherwise) with the authors' assessment of the content and outcome of communications was measured using the Kappa score, which is the proportion of the observed distribution of answers not accounted for by a hypothetical random distribution of answers.

RESULTS

There were 472 referrals relating to 386 patients, 112 referrals (23%) relating to male and 360 (77%) to female patients. Mean age was 41 years (range 19–72) and the age distribution is shown in Figure 1. Occupational groups from which the patients came, sources of referral and reasons for referral are shown in Table 1. Three hundred and fourteen patients were seen for a single referral, 60 for two referral episodes, 10 for three and two for four episodes.

The number of consultations per episode and the distribution of clinical diagnoses and occupational outcomes are also shown in Table 1. For the purposes of the study respiratory, cardiovascular and other medical conditions were grouped together, partly because numbers within each group were small, and partly because communication patterns were broadly similar. Modified work was defined as short or long term alteration of hours or conditions of working on the advice of the occupational physician. It was possible for patients to have more than one diagnosis.

An analysis of the frequency, mode and reason for communication between occupational physician and general practitioner or specialist is shown in Table 2. About half of all referral episodes (53%) resulted in a communication with general practitioner or specialist, and about a quarter (23%) in a communication with a specialist. Nearly all the communications with general practitioners sought to convey both occupational (98%) and clinical (94%) information, as did most of the communications with specialists (81% and 70% respectively). Communications with specialists were more likely to request factual information (47% *vs.* 20%, Chi square 24.3, *p* < 0.001) or to request an opinion (84% *vs.* 12%, Chi square 166, *p* < 0.001) than communication with general practitioners.

Table 1

Characteristics of patient population in 472 referral episodes

	No.	%
Categories of staff		
Nurse	140	30
Ancillary	134	28
Nursing auxiliary	83	17
Other professional	32	8
Clerical	31	7
Medical	23	5
Management	11	2
Other	18	3
Sources of referral		
Management	236	50
Occupational health nurse	178	37
Self	45	9
Other	13	3
Reasons for referral[a]		
Sickness absence > 3 months	54	11
Sickness absence < 3 months	72	15
Recurrent sickness absence	100	21
Work related ill-health	34	7
Fitness for work	74	16
Pre-employment	13	3
Medical opinion	53	11
Vaccination related	68	14
Ill-health retirement	4	1
No. of consultations per episode		
1	242	51
2	124	26
3	52	11
4	30	7
5	8	2
>5	16	4
Clinical diagnoses[b]		
Musculoskeletal	152	32
Psychiatric	58	12
Vaccination related[b]	75	16
Other medical	140	30
Sickness absence behaviour	32	7
No clinical diagnosis	28	6
Occupational outcome[c]		
Continued present post	300	64
Rehabilitated in work	39	8
Ill-health retirement	35	7
Returned to work	28	6
Contract terminated	26	5
Continued sick leave	16	3
Fit for employment	12	3
Resigned from post	8	2
Transferred to alternative post	8	2

[a] Definitions: Long term sickness absence > 3 months, short term < 3 months, recurrent: multiple episodes in preceding year. Work related ill-health: where possible workplace aetiology was queried by referrer. Fitness for work: not related to sickness absence but where the person's fitness to do their job was questioned by referrer. Vaccination related: administration of vaccine, assessment of or advice about immune status.
[b] *n* = 485 because there were 13 patients with two diagnoses. In seven patients the clinical diagnosis was 'vaccination related' although the patient had initially been referred for another reason. 'Other medical' includes respiratory (37), cardiovascular (21), metabolic (17), urogenital & gynaecological (13), neurological (12), abdominal (12), skin (9), ENT & eyes (8).
[c] Modified work (short or long term alteration of hours or conditions of working on the recommendation of the occupational physician) was arranged for 62 patients (13%).

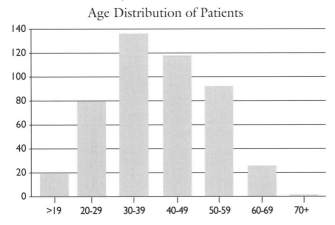

Figure 1. *Age distribution of 386 patients in 472 referral episodes.*

Table 2

Analysis of numbers and reasons for communication with GP or specialist (total number of referral episodes = 472)

	Referral episodes	
	No.	% of total episodes
Any communication	250	53
Communication with GP	225	48
Communication with specialist	108	23
Communication with GP and specialist	83	18
Communication to elicit information	124	26
Communication to impart information	250	53
Communication to elicit and impart information	124	26

Communications with general practitioners	*Letter*	*'Phone*	*Either*[a,b]
To request factual information	36	12	46 (20%)
To request an opinion	18	8	26 (12%)
To convey occupational information	200	43	222 (98%)
To convey clinical information	190	40	211 (94%)

Communications with specialists	*Letter*	*'Phone*	*Either*[a,c]
To request factual information	47	5	51 (47%)
To request an opinion	82	12	91 (84%)
To convey occupational information	92	14	87 (81%)
To convey clinical information	81	13	75 (70%)

[a] Either indicates *any* communication during the episode; in some episodes communication was made by letter and telephone.
[b] Figures in brackets are % of all communications with GPs ($n = 225$).
[c] Figures in brackets are % of all communications with specialists ($n = 108$).

Communication patterns were further analyzed according to the reason for original referral, medical diagnosis, number of consultations, and occupational outcome (Table 3). There were marked differences in communication pattern according to reason for referral, with long or short term sickness absence or (to a lesser extent) assessment of fitness for work being the most likely to result in a communication, whereas a request for a medical opinion, consultation for work-related ill-health, pre-employment assessment or vaccination-related problems were less likely to result in a communication.

Patients with a psychiatric diagnosis were more likely to be seen in a consultation generating a communication (OR = 3.17, 95% CI = 1.69–5.97 and interestingly this applied both to communications imparting (OR = 3.19, 95% CI = 1.49–6.23) and eliciting (OR = 2.96, 95% CI = 1.40–5.26) information. Conversely vaccination related or sickness absence behaviour related episodes were less likely to lead to communication. The 'occupational outcomes' of rehabilitation at work, modified work and ill-health retirement were significantly more likely to be associated with communication, with both general practitioner and specialist. In patients referred for assessment of long term sickness absence, there was no difference in communication pattern between those who returned to work and those who did not.

There was no significant time-related change in communication pattern when the three years of the study were analyzed individually (data not shown).

It is clear that many of the variables which correlate with particular communication patterns are interrelated: for example a single referral may involve a patient with a psychiatric illness seen because of long-term sickness absence and requiring multiple consultations. Multiple logistic regression analysis was used in an attempt to identify independent predictor variables (significant at $p < 0.05$ level). Potential predictor variables chosen were those listed in Table 3, entered stepwise in order of their univariate odds ratios. Occupational outcomes were not included, since these would not be known 'a priori'. Additional variables examined were age, source of referral and occupation.

Number of consultations were classified as 'multiple consultations' (i.e., > 1) or 'no consultations'. Independent predictors identified were *multiple consultations* (adjusted OR = 3.5, 95% CI = 2.7–4.5, $p = 0.001$), a *psychiatric diagnosis* (adjusted OR = 1.8, 95% CI = 1.5–2.4, $p = 0.02$), and *long-term (> 3 months) sickness absence* (adjusted OR = 1.7, 95% CI = 1.4–2.3, p -0.02). The predictive value (cumulative R) of the best model was 17%.

The response of general practitioners and specialists to requests for information or an opinion about their patients is shown in Table 4. The response rate to

Table 3

Likelihood of 'any communication' analyzed by reason for referral, diagnosis, number of consultations and occupational outcome

	% referrals leading to communication	Univariate odds ratio and 95% CI
Reason for referral		
Sickness absence < 3 mo.	72	2.65 (1.55–4.60)
Sickness absence > 3 mo.	91	10.58 (4.13–27.08)
Sickness absence recurrent	51	0.92 (0.60–1.45)
Fitness for work	65	1.80 (1.07–3.00)
Medical opinion	21	0.20 (0.10–0.39)
Pre-employment	0	
Work related ill-health	32	0.42 (0.20–0.90)
Vaccination related	37	0.51 (0.30–0.87)
Diagnosis		
Musculoskeletal	58	1.40 (0.94–2.06)
Psychiatric	75	3.17 (1.69–5.97)
Other medical	60	1.49 (0.99–2.24)
Sickness absence behaviour	38	0.50 (0.30–0.83)
No. of consultations		
1	30	0.13 (0.08–0.20)
2	65	2.00 (1.30–3.05)
>2	90	13.2 (6.67–26.18)
Outcome		
Rehabilitation in work	80	3.44 (1.55–1.74)
Modified work	80	3.35 (1.76–6.33)
Ill-health retirement	100	99[a]

[a] All episodes resulting in ill-health retirement were associated with a communication: under these circumstances the odds ratio is very large and cannot be calculated accurately

requests for factual information or an opinion was high — 98% for both general practitioners and hospital consultants. Letters from the occupational physician assessed as seeking to impart information only were followed by replies from general practitioners in 25% of cases. There were two 'unsolicited' letters from specialists.

Replies from consultants were more likely to be assessed as providing new information (72% *vs.* 46%, Chi square 12.75. $p < 0.001$) than those from general practitioners. The proportion of replies from specialists and general practitioners which recorded agreement with the occupational physician was similar (50% *vs.* 43%, Chi square 0.51, $p = 0.6$). Recorded disagreement with the occupational physician occurred in three cases, in a fourth case a patient continued to receive sick certification from a doctor in the general practice despite recorded agreement with the occupational physician's assessment of fitness to return to work from both the patient's own general practitioner and hospital consultant.

Requests for payment accompanied eight of the 91 replies from general practitioners, four in the first year of the study, three in the second and one in the third. Twenty-one anonymized case histories and verbatim

anonymized letters were independently assessed by the review panel. Their answers to 14 questions were recorded and the consistency of their agreement with the author is shown in Table 5. The Chi-square statistic showed that agreement was greater than would be expected by random chance for all the questions. The Kappa scores, which measure the proportion of agreement which could not be accounted for by random chance, show better agreement where the question asked was basically a factual one, for example whether the communication provided occupational or clinical information than when a subjective opinion was requested, for example whether the reply provided new information. A possible anomaly may have occurred with the question 'Did the letter request an opinion?' as the wording may have been open to subjective interpretation.

Scrutiny of the occupational health records identified specific actions taken by other doctors following communication from the occupational physician. Actions by general practitioners followed 24% of communications (in 54/225 referral episodes) and specialist actions followed 21% of communications (in 33/108 referral episodes). A broad classification of those actions is shown in Table 6.

One hundred and eight-nine replies were recorded from general practitioners (91) and hospital consultants (98) of which 30% (52/189) were judged to have altered the subsequent management of the patient by the occupational physician (Table 7). Reports from specialists were more likely to do so than those from general practitioners (38% *vs.* 21%, Chi square = 5.75, $p = 0.05$).

DISCUSSION

This study describes the work of a single occupational health physician, in what could arguably be described as a specialized workplace environment. There are few published data on the workload and case mix of occupational health physicians in an NHS setting, and these are likely to vary from unit to unit. A pattern which clearly emerges is that the need for and intensity

Table 4

The response of general practitioners and specialists to requests for information or an opinion

Communication from occupational physician	No. sent	Reply received	%
To GP to request information or opinion	48	47	98
To GP to impart information	177	44	25
To specialist to request information or opinion	91	89	98
To specialist to impart information	8	7	87

Table 5

Panel assessment of communication content

	n	Kappa	Chi-square	p
Letters from OHP to GP				
Did letter convey occupational information?	21	89%	131	< 0.001
Did letter convey clinical information?	21	76%	103	< 0.001
Did letter request factual information?	21	65%	78.3	< 0.001
Did letter request an opinion?	21	55%	58.3	< 0.001
Replies from GP to OHP				
Did reply provide new information?	6	69%	42.0	< 0.001
Did reply express agreement?	6	50%	27.8	< 0.001
Did reply express disagreement?	6	33%	17.1	< 0.01
Letters from OHP to specialist				
Did letter convey occupational information?	12	76%	68.9	< 0.001
Did letter convey clinical information?	12	61%	44.8	< 0.001
Did letter request factual information?	12	32%	17.8	< 0.001
Did letter request an opinion?	12	17%	9.3	< 0.03
Replies from specialist to OHP				
Did reply provide new information?	12	40%	22.0	< 0.001
Did reply express agreement?	12	48%	32.4	< 0.001
Did reply express disagreement?	12	86%	84.0	< 0.001

6

of communication is crucially affected by case mix. Letters and telephone communications were more likely to be exchanged when there was a need to unravel a medical problem. This occurs particularly in relation to long or short term sickness absence. Staff referred because of current sickness absence will almost always be in possession of a 'sick certificate' at the time of consultation and communication with the doctor who has provided that certificate would seem appropriate. Relatively uncomplicated patients, those not absent

Table 6

Actions by other doctors following communication from occupational physician

Action	No.
Action by general practitioners[a]	
Certification	25
Specialist referral	15
Initiation or review of treatment	10
Surgery consultation	3
Initiation of further liaison with OP	4
Action by specialists[b]	
Arrange or expedite consultation	14
Specialist investigation	9
Initiation or review of treatment	10
Initiation of further liaison with OP	4

[a] Total 57 actions relating to 54 referral episodes involving 54 patients.
[b] Total 37 actions relating to 33 referral episodes involving 31 patients.

from work at the time of consultation, and staff referred in relation to immunization or possible work related ill-health were less likely to be the subjects of communication between doctors. Assessment of the contribution of workplace factors to ill-health or of the need for infection control measures depend upon the workplace knowledge of the occupational physician, assisted when appropriate by the specialist opinion of others, for example dermatologists if patch testing were required. This may explain the pattern of communication observed in these groups, in which communication with general practitioners was entirely to convey information. The large number of vaccination-related referrals, mainly relating to hepatitis B status, is specific to the NHS context.

An audit of 225 medical consultations selected at random from the occupational health services of three Scottish health boards between 1989 and 1991[14] found a significant difference in the frequency with which 'career' occupational physicians recorded communications to general practitioners: 73% of consultations compared with 46% of consultations for their 'non-career' colleagues (usually sessional doctors, often themselves general practitioners). No distinction was reported between communications to elicit or convey information. It was suggested that the difference might reflect the use of alternative methods of communication, for example by non-recorded telephone calls, or a difference in attitude between the two groups with 'career' occupational physicians feeling that they had contributed a professional 'added value' worthy of

Table 7

Alterations in management by occupational physician following communication from other doctors

Action by OP	Following reply from specialist	Following reply from GP
Decision on fitness for work	19	10
Recommendation for modified work	6	0
Long-term occupational advice	3	0
Advice in relation to workplace hazard	5	0
Treatment*	4	2
Referral for further specialist assessment	0	7
Totals	37	19

* These actions relate to 52 referral episodes

imparting to the employee's general practitioner. It is difficult to compare these results with the present study without a more detailed knowledge of case mix — for example 'career' occupational physicians (consultants, senior registrars and lecturers) may have seen more complicated cases including a higher proportion of sickness absence or ill-health retirement cases or patients with psychiatric illness. Communication with specialists is not reported in the Scottish audit.

Certain clinical diagnoses were also more likely to be associated with a greater density of communication, particularly psychiatric ill-health. The Clothier Inquiry following the Allitt case, in which a nurse administered lethal drug overdoses to patients under her care, highlighted the need for communication between occupational health services and general practitioners as a safeguard against the employment of psychiatrically unfit health care staff.[15] Although the present study did not investigate this point, there is a strong impression that psychiatric morbidity among health care personnel has been much more intensively investigated since the report's publication. A recent report has also emphasized the important contribution of psychiatric ill-health to early retirement.[16]

Communication was also more likely to be involved in referral episodes which involved multiple consultations, presumably because these reflected more complex or difficult problems: the odds ratio for any communication in a referral episode involving more than two consultations compared with all referral episodes was 13.20 (95% CI = 6.67–26.18).

In the present study, a high proportion of communications from the occupational physician were assessed as conveying occupational (98% of communication to general practitioners, 81% to specialists) and clinical (94% to general practitioners, 70% to specialist) information. In addition, 20% of communications to general practitioners and 47% of those to hospital specialists requested factual information, and 12% of communications to general practitioners and 84% of those to specialists requested an opinion. Virtually all (98%) of specific requests for information or an opinion elicited a reply. In addition, 25% of letters sent to general practitioners to 'convey information' only elicited a reply.

The response rate to communications from the occupational physician is high in this study. In addition the number of instances where a general practitioner communicated useful information even when not specifically asked to do so is significant and would support a policy of communication with general practitioners on matters relating to the health of their patients. It is possible that the practice of conveying clinical and occupational information (with the patient's consent) at the same time as requesting facts or an opinion may have encouraged participation in a 'clinical partnership' conducive to sharing information. This might also explain why requests for payment from general practitioners were minimal. Another explanation is that very few requests were made for information of a routine or unfocused nature which could have been elicited directly from the patient. A possible reason for the impression among general practitioners that occupational physicians seldom write to them may simply be that these communications form only a small proportion of the total number they receive.[9]

A higher percentage of replies from hospital specialists (72%) were assessed as providing new information than those from general practitioners (46%), not a surprising finding since consultants' letters are likely to contain results of hospital investigations or specialist assessments based on their particular expertise. Stated disagreement with the occupational physician's assessment by either general practitioner or specialist was unusual, occurring in only three cases, and there was only one instance of discordant certification.

Actions taken by general practitioner, specialist and occupational physician as a result of communication encompassed a wide variety of activities ranging from simple recertification to arranging specialist referrals and altering patient management. A general picture which emerges is of therapeutic co-operation, with specialists in different disciplines collaborating to ensure the best medical and occupational outcome for the patient. It was not possible from the present study to deduce whether the long-term outcome of the referral was influenced by communication between the occupational physician and other doctors. It could be argued that the only way to do so would be deliberately to randomize patients prospectively at referral to communication or non-communication policies and compare the outcomes in the two groups. The ethics of doing this would be questionable.

The relevance of the present study to occupational health services in other industries will depend on the extent to which these deal with a comparable casemix, and to some extent on the model of occupational health care delivery which is used. Pilling has emphasized the importance of a consensus view on the appropriateness or

6

otherwise of ill-health retirement from all the medical practitioners involved with a particular patient, and this view could be extended to other outcomes.[17] Assessments regarding continuing fitness to work or sickness absence have been shown to be the most common clinical activities for all occupational physicians.[18]

Agius and colleagues[14] in their audit of occupational medicine consultation records identify seven stages in the process of problem solving in occupational medicine. Communication with other doctors' is not identified as a specific stage but may be assumed to be a possible component of all their identified stages, particularly collecting information and reliably processing that information, formulating a conclusion and communicating the advice appropriately. New technologies, and in particular the use of electronic mailing, present important opportunities for conveying and requesting information, and their appropriate incorporation into occupational health services needs to be planned and implemented. At the same time, the challenges of confidentiality, format and relevance of information need to be met.

Acknowledgements

I should like to thank Drs Yvonne Bladon, Margaret Leverment and Douglas Scarisbrick for forming the review panel, Dr David McBride for helpful advice, and colleagues in the Department of Medicine and Therapeutics, University of Leicester, for statistical assistance.

References

1. British Medical Association. *The Handbook of Medical Ethics*. London, UK: BMA, 1984: 11.
2. Lee WR. Medical ethics in industry. In: Howard JK, Tyrer FH, eds. *Textbook of Occupational Medicine*. Edinburgh, UK: Churchill Livingstone, 1987: 82–86.
3. Faculty of Occupational Medicine. *Guidance on Ethics for Occupational Physicians, Fourth Edition*. London, UK: Royal College of Physicians, 1993; 4.5, 7.2–7.5.
4. British Medical Association. *The Occupational Physician*. London, UK: BMA, 1994:16–17.
5. NHS Executive. Occupational Health Services for NHS Staff. NHS Executive, 1994; NHS Executive Publ. No. HSG (94) 51; 29.
6. Westerman RF, Hull FM, Bezemer PD, Gort G. A study of communication between general practitioners and specialists. *Br J Gen Practice* 1990; **40**: 445–449.
7. Tudor Hart J, Treasure T. The hospital letter. *Br J Hosp Med* 1989; **441**: 175–177.
8. Parker G. Attitudes of general practitioners to occupational health services. *J Soc Occup Med* 1991; **41**: 34–36.
9. Parker G. The relationship between occupational health and primary care. An investigation into attitudes and experiences. Dissertation MFOM, 1992.
10. Seaton A. Occupational medicine — let's keep our white coats and stethoscopes. *Occup Med* 1993; **43**: 63–64.
11. Morris JA, Gardner MJ. Calculating confidence intervals for relative risks (odds ratios) and standardized ratios and rates. *Br Med J* 1988; **296**: 1213–1216.
12. Campbell MJ, Machin D. *Medical Statistics: A Commonsense Approach, Second Edition*. Chichester, UK: John Wiley & Sons, 1993: 78–82.
13. Campbell MJ, Machin D. *Medical Statistics: A Commonsense Approach, Second Edition*. John Wiley & Sons, 1993: 100–103.
14. Agius RM, Lee RJ, Symington IS, Riddle HFV, Seaton A. An audit of occupational medicine consultation records. *Occup Med* 1994; **44**: 151–157.
15. Report of the independent inquiry relating to deaths and injuries on the children's ward at Grantham and Kesteven General Hospital during the period February to April 1991 ('The Allitt Inquiry'). HMSO 199X.
16. Poole CJM. Retirement on grounds of ill health: cross sectional survey in six organisations in the United Kingdom. *Br Med J* 1997; **3314**: 929–932.
17. Pilling KJ. Ill health retirement guidance. In: Cox RAF, Edwards FC, McCallum RI, eds. *Fitness for Work, the Medical Aspects, Second Edition*. Oxford, UK: Oxford University Press, 1995: 500–503.
18. Agius RM, Lee RJ, Murdoch RM, Symington IS, Riddle HFV, Seaton A. Occupational physicians and their work: prospects for audit. *Occup Med* 1993; **43**: 159–163.

This article was first published in the BMJ and is reproduced by permission of the BMJ

DO CLINICAL GUIDELINES INTRODUCED WITH PRACTICE BASED EDUCATION IMPROVE CARE OF ASTHMATIC AND DIABETIC PATIENTS? A RANDOMISED CONTROLLED TRIAL IN GENERAL PRACTICES IN EAST LONDON

Gene Feder, Chris Griffiths, Clare Highton, Sandra Eldridge, Matthew Spence, Lesley Southgate

Gene Feder, *senior lecturer*; Chris Griffiths, *senior lecturer*; Clare Highton, *research associate*;
Matthew Spence, *research assistant*; Lesley Southgate, *professor*
Department of General Practice and Primary Care,
St Bartholomew's and Royal London Hospital Medical College, London EC1M 6BQ

Sandra Eldridge, *statistician*
Department of Epidemiology and Medical Statistics, Queen Mary and Westfield College, University of London, London.
Correspondence to: Dr Feder

BMJ 1995; **311**: 1473-8

ABSTRACT

Objective—To determine whether locally developed guidelines on asthma and diabetes disseminated through practice based education improve quality of care in non-training, inner city general practices.
Design—Randomised controlled trial with each practice receiving one set of guidelines but providing data on the management of both conditions.
Subjects—24 inner city, non-training general practices.
Setting—East London.
Main outcome measures—Recording of key variables in patient records (asthma: peak flow rate, review of inhaler technique, review of asthma symptoms, prophylaxis, occupation, and smoking habit; diabetes: blood glucose concentration, glycaemic control, funduscopy, feet examination, weight, and smoking habit); size of practice disease registers; prescribing in asthma; and use of structured consultation "prompts."
Results—In practices receiving diabetes guidelines, significant improvements in recording were seen for all seven diabetes variables. Both groups of practices showed improved recording of review of inhaler technique, smoking habit, and review of asthma symptoms. In practices receiving asthma guidelines, further improvement was seen only in recording of review of inhaler technique and quality of prescribing in asthma. Sizes of disease registers were unchanged. The use of structured prompts was associated with improved recording of four of seven variables on diabetes and all six variables on asthma.
Conclusions—Local guidelines disseminated via practice based education improve the management of diabetes and possibly of asthma in inner city, nontraining practices. The use of simple prompts may enhance this improvement.

INTRODUCTION

Clinical guidelines pervade primary and secondary care. It is now recognised that the development of guidelines based on research evidence must be complemented by dissemination and implementation strategies that encourage clinicians to use guidelines in practice.[1,2] In a systematic review of 91 studies Grimshaw and Russell concluded that guidelines had the greatest chance of chance of changing clinical behaviour when they were developed by the clinicians for whom they were intended, disseminated through a specific educational programme and implemented via patient-specific reminders during consultations.[3] Only six of the studies reviewed were from British general practice. The largest study, in 62 English training practices [4] was disappointing: those receiving "external" guidelines improved neither process nor outcome of care for children with common acute disorders. How can we make guidelines effective in general practice?

The Hackney collaborative clinical guidelines project was a local initiative started in 1991 in east London that developed primary care guidelines and tested methods of dissemination and implementation. The project was based in the local academic department of general practice and supported by the Hackney General Practice Forum.[5] The East London and City Health Authority has the highest Jarman underprivileged area index in England [6] and a highly mobile population reflected in a 30% average annual turnover of patients on practice lists.[7] During our study most practices in the area were single handed or two handed and based in poor quality premises.

Morbidity from asthma in Hackney is high: admission rates in east London are between 80% and 100% above the national average for all age groups.[8] For patients with diabetes admission rates in east London are high for both amputation and ketoacidosis.[9] We aimed principally to determine whether guidelines on asthma and diabetes disseminated via an educational package to non-training inner city practices affected the quality of care.

Our hypotheses were that practices receiving guidelines for either asthma or diabetes (*a*) improved their recording of key data, reflecting good quality care; (*b*) increased the size of the register for the relevant disease; and (*c*) improved their pattern of prescribing (asthma guidelines only). We also examined the effect of "prompts" (structured records) derived from the guidelines on the quality of care and the effect of the guidelines on consultation rates.

Our dissemination method was practice based, multidisciplinary educational outreach (or "academic detailing"). Studies of educational outreach have been confined to North America, and the measurable effect on prescribing and preventive care by clinicians has been small.[10]

SUBJECTS AND METHODS

Guideline development

The guidelines were developed by local general practitioners working through informal consensus with local hospital specialists and relevant professionals and were not explicitly evidence based.[11] The guidelines on asthma were based on the British Thoracic Society's first national guidelines [12] and the diabetes guidelines on the St Vincents' declaration.[13]

Practice recruitment and diagnostic criteria

In autumn 1992 we invited all 49 non-training practices in Hackney to join the study. Twenty seven (55%) practices agreed; only seven of these practices had disease registers before the start of the study. Participating practices were visited by general practitioner members of the research team who proposed uniform diagnostic criteria for asthma and diabetes [14,15] and prompted creation or updating of disease registers for these conditions. These disease registers were the source of our samples of patients. The diagnostic criteria were derived from the guidelines (both simple summaries and "complex" documents were disseminated). More details of our intervention package are available on request.

In two practices, only one of two partners agreed to participate. These practices essentially ran personal lists with little interaction between partners and were entered as singlehanded practices. One singlehanded general practitioner withdrew owing to illness, one two partner practice was excluded as it could not adequately develop disease registers, and a further two partner practice served as a pilot for data collection and educational intervention, leaving 24 practices comprising 39 principals for analysis (table 1).

After the initial recruitment session described above, practices were stratified by partnership size, list size per general practitioner, employment of a practice nurse,

Table 1

Randomisation of 24 participating practices by five stratifying variables and distribution of other relevant practice variables. Values are numbers of practices unless stated otherwise

Variable	Practices given guidelines on diabetes (n = 12)	Practices given guidelines on asthma (n = 12)
Stratifying variables		
Partnership size:		
1 Partner	7	8
2 Partners	4	3
≥3 Partners	1	1
Employment of nurse	8	6
Median (range) deprivation score*	6.05 (5.48–7.22)	6.07 (5.24–6.97)
Median (range) list size/general practitioner	2038 (1138–4407)	1969 (970–4032)
Existing asthma and diabetes clinics	5	4
Other relevant practice variables		
Employment of practice manager	5	7
Possession of computer	7	7
Existing disease registers at baseline	5	2
≥ General practitioner vocationally trained†	6	8
≥ 1 General practitioner with membership of Royal College of General Practitioners†	2	2
≥ 1 General practitioner with higher exams†‡	4	6
Median (range) age of general practitioners§	50 (33–63)	50 (35–65)
Median (range) No of years experience of general practitioners as principals§	12 (3–25)	7 (1–12)
Median (range) No of years since general practitioner's GMC registration§	18 (6.5–33)	16 (9–37)
Premises quality score‖	3 (2–4)	4 (2–4)

* Derived for each practice from Jarman indices by dividing each practice's total deprivation payment by its list size for a single quarter at start of study.

† Or more than half of general practitioners in the cases of the two practices with [[=]] 3 partners.

‡ For example, (Member of the Royal College of Physicians; Fellow of the Royal College of Surgeons; Member of the Royal College of General Practitioners.

§ Mean values used in practices with ≥ 2 partners.

‖ Rated by family health services authority's adviser on scale 1 to 4 (1 = excellent, 4 = wholly inadequate).

Date:	Asthma review:

	Day	Night	Exercise

Symptoms:

Days unable to work/off school

β Agonist use per day:

Smoking? Yes/no	Occupation:
Peak flow rate Actual: Expected/best: Home range:	Inhaler technique: Good/mod/poor Peak flow meter? Yes/no
Prophylaxis? Increase/decrease Start/stop	Self management plan? Yes/no

Plan:

Fig 1—*Stamp issued to participating doctors for reviewing their asthmatic patients*

deprivation, and prior existence of asthma and diabetes clinics. They were then randomised to two groups to receive the guidelines either for asthma or for diabetes. A postal questionnaire on other practice characteristics was completed by all practices (table 1). Three months after recruitment, practices were revisited and introduced to their respective guidelines. The rolling programme of practice sessions ran from January to June 1993.

Every practice provided data from the notes of both patients with asthma and those with diabetes, but they only received guidelines for one condition, acting as a control for the other condition. "Asthma practices" refers to those receiving the guidelines on asthma and "diabetes practices" refers to those receiving the guidelines on diabetes.

Dissemination of guidelines via practice outreach
Our educational intervention consisted of three lunchtime sessions—approved for the postgraduate education allowance—to which all relevant members of the practice team were invited. The four educators (GF, CG, CH, and a specialist nurse) worked in pairs and visited equal numbers of asthma and diabetes practices.

They standardised the content and delivery of sessions. The first session introduced the allocated guidelines and discussed how the practice's current management could be developed into a practice protocol in line with the recommendations in the guidelines, with an emphasis on patient recall for annual review. Each clinician was given a stamp for reviewing asthmatic patients (fig 1) and a stamp or booklet for reviewing diabetic patients. These "prompts" reflected the content of an annual review consultation for patients with asthma or diabetes as recommended in the guidelines. The session concluded with a practical discussion of home urine monitoring or peak flow measurement. The second session reviewed the practice's organisational decisions and then focused on the clinical content of the guidelines. It concluded with a demonstration of measuring visual acuity or inhaler technique. The third session took place about six months later and focused on audit data from the notes of patients with diabetes or asthma. We also reviewed how the practice was coping with implementing the guidelines. All contacts with practices were logged on a database to estimate the costs of our educational intervention.

Quality of care variables
Quality of care variables are based on data which the guidelines recommended that clinicians should collect in annual review consultations for both conditions. The variables correspond with evidence based audit standards.[16,17]

Prescribing costs
Prescribing costs for drugs for asthma were obtained from Pactline (the Prescription Pricing Authority's online service) for the year preceding the study and the year after the guidelines were introduced. Costs were derived from the *British National Formulary* and expressed as cost per prescribing unit per year. The ratio of the prescribing costs of prophylaxis to bronchodilators was calculated for each practice for the year before and year after intervention. This prescribing index has been validated as a marker of the quality of prescribing in asthma in east London practices.[18] A measure of changes in quality of prescribing during the study, was derived for each practice

Table 2

Median (interquartile range) sizes of disease registers as percentage of list size before and after introduction of guidelines and median (interquartile range) ratio of these two values

	Asthma register			Diabetes register		
	Size before	Size after	Ratio (size after/ size before)	Size before	Size after	Ratio (size after/ size before)
Practices receiving guidelines on asthma	1.3 (1.0, 2.1)	2.6 (1.4, 4.3)	1.7 (1.2, 2.4)	1.6 (0.9, 1.8)	2.0 (1.2, 2.7)	1.1 (1.0, 2.3)
Practices receiving guidelines on diabetes	1.6 (1.1, 3.0)	2.4 (1.6, 3.8)	1.2 (1.0, 1.8)	1.8 (1.4, 2.8)	2.2 (1.6, 2.4)	1.1 (0.9, 1.5)

by dividing the index before intervention by the index after intervention.

Size of disease registers is a measure of case finding by practices. All the asthma registers of the practices in our study (table 2) were smaller at baseline than even conservative estimates of adult asthma in cast London, whereas the diabetes registers were close to expected prevalence in east London (1.7% (95% confidence interval 1.1 to 2.6) (I Jones, personal communication)). Changes in size of disease register were calculated as the ratio of the size after the introduction of guidelines to that before.

Collection of process and prescribing data

Sample size was based on practice audits in Hackney: peak flow and blood glucose concentrations had been recorded within the previous year in about 40% of the notes of asthmatic and diabetic patients respectively. Detection of a 50% relative increase in the recording of these two variables (from 40% to 60%) with a power of 95% at a significance level of 5% required a total sample of 310 patients. A sample size of 390 patients (10 patients per principal) was sufficient to detect a clinically relevant difference even with a trend towards increased recording in "control" practices and reduction of power when the practice rather than the patient was taken as unit of analysis.

Data were gathered from the clinical records of 10 patients with asthma and 10 with diabetes per general practitioner principal, selected from disease registers by a method using random numbers. Only permanently registered NHS patients aged 16 and over were included. "Ghost" patients (those who had had no contact with the surgery for the past two years)[19] and patients whose asthma or diabetes had been diagnosed less than 12 months previously were excluded and replacement patients randomly selected. For baseline

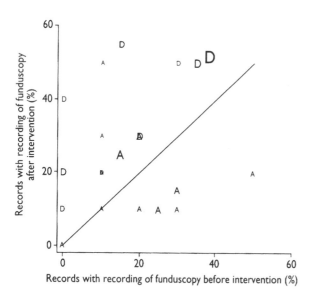

Fig 2—*Percentages of records of diabetic patients with recording of funduscopy at baseline and one year later in practices receiving guidelines on asthma (A) and on diabetes (D). (Size of letter A or D corresponds to size of practice in terms of number of general practitioner principals)*

data, these records were scrutinised for all entries relating to asthma and diabetes made during the 12 months up to recruitment of the practice—except for occupation, which was searched for in the three years up to recruitment. Data collection was repeated one year after the introduction of the guidelines, with a new random sample from the disease registers. For notes scrutinised one year after intervention, two further variables were gathered: the number of patients in whom the "prompt" stamp or booklet was used and the number of consultations for the relevant condition during the year before and the year after intervention.

The sources of patient data were written patient records, computerised patient recordings, test results, and hospital letters. The most recent general practice record of any data was entered directly onto a database. If there was no record in the general practice notes within the past year the medical record was searched for letters from hospital clinics or discharge letters within the past year that contained this information.

The accuracy of the gathering and coding of data was validated at baseline by an independent comparison of recording accuracy with the notes of 10 patients with asthma and 10 with diabetes; 96% of the coding was accurate. The consistency of data extraction was assessed by examining coding before the guidelines and one year later using the same 10 sets of notes for asthma and for diabetes. For all but four variables there was perfect agreement. For three variables on asthma (smoking habit, symptom review, inhaler technique) there was substantial agreement ($\kappa = 0.7$). The only variable for which there was poor agreement was examination of feet in diabetic patients ($\kappa = 0.4$).

Analysis

To determine the effect of the introduction of guidelines on the quality of care, analysis of covariance was used to model a practice's level of recording after intervention as a function of the level before intervention and intervention, weighted by the number of patients sampled in each practice. To test hypotheses about prescribing in asthma and size of disease registers, non-parametric tests were used as appropriate owing to the noticeably non-normal distributions of some of the variables.

RESULTS

Practices randomised to receive asthma or diabetes guidelines were similar with respect to stratifying variables and practice characteristics (table 1).

Recording of quality of care variables

Recording of these variables varied greatly both at baseline and after intervention—for example, funduscopy (fig 2). Asthma and diabetes practices had similar distributions of variables at baseline, except for the recording of smoking habit, which was significantly greater in the diabetes practices (table 3). Differences at baseline were taken into account in the regression models testing the effect of the guidelines.

Table 3

Average percentage* of patients with variable recorded at baseline and after one year in practices receiving guidelines on asthma or diabetes with estimated difference between level of recording in intervention and non-intervention practices post intervention

Variable	At baseline		After one year		Difference in proportions (95% confidence interval)
	Practices given guidelines on asthma	Practices given guidelines on diabetes	Practices given guidelines on asthma	Practices given guidelines on diabetes	
Diabetes variables:					
Funduscopy	19.4	20.5	20	38.1	17.6 (6.9 to 33.9)
Blood glucose	57.8	56.8	57.8	75.2	20.2 (6.4 to 33.9)
Weight	37.5	40.4	40	68.1	26.5 (7.7 to 45.4)
Blood pressure	66.1	69.0	58.3	79.5	18.1 (2.8 to 33.4)
Smoking habit	23.2	34.8	31.7	62.4	25.5 (8.7 to 42.3)
Feet examination	28.3	31.4	27.2	51.8	24.7 (7.1 to 42.3)
HbA1 recorded	20.6	24.8	30	48.1	13.8 (1.2 to 26.3)
Asthma variables:					
Smoking habit	19.4	30.9	48.9	47.6	5.6 (−17.2 to 28.3)
Inhaler technique checked	3.9	6.2	22.8	10	12.9 (1.9 to 23.9)
Peak flow	36.1	32.9	41.7	39.5	0.7 (−15.2 to 16.7)
Prophylaxis	54.4	43.8	58.3	51.9	2.7 (−14.4 to 19.7)
Occupation	13.9	13.3	28.9	16.7	12.6 (−4.9 to 30.2)
Symptom review	31.7	32.4	57.2	56.2	1.0 (−13.8 to 15.9)

*Weighted by number of patients sampled in practice.

Table 4

Effect of introduction of guidelines and use of stamp or booklet* on recording levels (odds ratios) (95% confidence interval) for both factors controlling for the other

Recording of variable	Guideline but no use of stamp or booklet	Guideline and use of stamp or booklet
Diabetes variables:		
Smoking habit	2.2 (1.2 to 3.9)	3.1 (1.5 to 6.6)
Weight	1.9 (1.1 to 3.5)	11.5 (3.4 to 38.3)
Blood pressure	1.9 (1.0 to 3.6)	5.2 (1.5 to 17.6)
Funduscopy	2.3 (1.2 to 4.7)	1.4 (0.7 to 2.6)
Blood glucose	2.0 (1.1 to 3.7)	2.1 (0.9 to 4.9)
HbA1	1.9 (1.0 to 3.7)	1.3 (0.7 to 2.4)
Feet examination	1.5 (0.8 to 2.8)	4.4 (2.2 to 9.0)
Asthma variables:		
Peak flow	0.8 (0.5 to 1.2)	27.3 (8.1 to 92.1)
Inhaler technique	1.7 (0.9 to 3.0)	41.6 (17.1 to 100.9)
Symptom review	1.4 (1.0 to 2.0)	44.9 (6.1 to 333.5)
Prophylaxis	1.2 (0.8 to 1.7)	4.3 (1.8 to 10.3)
Occupation	1.3 (0.8 to 2.1)	15.3 (6.9 to 34.0)
Smoking habit	1.3 (0.9 to 1.8)	66.7 (9.0 to 465.8)

* In diabetes practices use of stamp or booklet, or both, ranged from 0% to 80% (median 27–5%). In asthma practices use of stamp ranged from 0% to 70% (median 22.5%).

Analysis of covariance showed that diabetes practices significantly improved their recording of all variables. The difference in percentages and 95% confidence intervals shown in table 3 are based on these analyses. Analysis of place of recording showed that recording within practices improved for all variables except funduscopy; improvement in recording of funduscopy was mostly due to this procedure being performed in hospital. In both groups of practices significant improvements over baseline values were found in the recording of three asthma variables: review of inhaler technique, smoking habit, and symptom review. In asthma practices further improvement was detected in the recording of only one of six variables: review of inhaler technique (table 3).

Practices which already had a disease register before intervention had a higher baseline recording of variables on asthma and diabetes. Proportional improvements in recording were similar irrespective of the previous existence of a disease register.

Size and growth of disease register

Before the introduction of the guidelines the median sizes of disease register (as percentage of a practice's total list size) were 1.5% and 1.6% for asthma and diabetes respectively. No significant differences existed in register sizes for each condition between asthma and diabetes practices (Wilcoxon's two sample test: asthma, $z= -0.81$, P>04; diabetes, $z= -1.41$, P>0.1). Although register sizes increased after the guidelines were introduced in most practices, particularly the asthma practices, there was no significantly greater increase in intervention practices.

Drug prescribing in asthma

In the year preceding the study, the median cost per prescribing unit for bronchodilators was £1.51 (interquartile range £1.29, £1.70) and for prophylaxis was £1.40 (£1.04, £2.25), with no significant differences between the asthma and diabetes practices (Wilcoxon's two sample test: bronchodliators, $z= -0.84$, P=0.4; prophylaxis, $z= -1.3$, P=0.26). The variation in prophylaxis costs between practices was striking, with a 10-fold difference separating the prescribers with the lowest and the highest costs.

In the year after intervention costs for bronchodilators rose by a median of 3p (−12p, 16p) in the asthma practices and 15p (8p, 29p) in the diabetes practices. Costs for prophylaxis rose by 57p (23p, 78p) in the asthma practices and 40p (16p, 64p) in the diabetes practices. The ratio of prescribing indices before and after intervention was calculated for each practice. The median value of this ratio for the asthma practices was 1.43 (1.1, 1.55) and for the diabetes practices was 1.06 (0.99, 1.29). The value for the asthma practices was significantly greater than that for the diabetes practices ($z=2.14$, P=0.03).

Effect of "prompt" stamp or booklet on recording

In addition to the significant effect of our intervention on diabetes practices, the use of a structured "prompt" for a quarter of patients in our sample was associated with increased proportional recording of three out of six variables (smoking habit, blood pressure, and blood glucose (table 4)). For the asthma practices, use of the annual review stamp significantly increased the recording of all six variables on asthma. Although the stamp was used with only 41 patients in the asthma practices, the effect was unambiguous.

Consultation rates

Consultation rates in our sample for asthma and diabetes were generally low for all the practices. In the diabetes practices median consultation rates increased for diabetes by 30% (1.6 to 2.1 consultations per patient per year) and for asthma by 22% (1.2 to 1.4). In the asthma practices consultation rates increased for asthma by 50% (1.0 to 1.5) and for diabetes by 23% (1.1 to 1.4).

Cost of educational intervention

Each practice required about 30 minutes for correspondence, 20 minutes on the telephone, and three hours in personal visits. With two doctors visiting each practice, this equates to £144 per practice of general practice time (at a clinical lecturer's salary of £24 500 a year). Postgraduate education allowance costs on average £439 per practice, giving a total cost of £583 per practice. Although this does not take into account the development of the guidelines or the salary costs of other practice team members, it gives an approximate cost of the educational intervention.

DISCUSSION

This study addresses a practical question: how can we effectively disseminate clinical guidelines to primary care? Our intervention improved the recording of key data associated with good care for patients with diabetes. For patients with asthma, the effect was marginal, with improvements in recording rates for one out of six variables and improved prescribing. These improvements were not limited to practices who had already developed some form of structured care but were seen even in practices which at the start of the study did not have a disease register. Furthermore, we detected improvements despite the absence of a control group not receiving any guidelines; our study design controlled for but did not test for a Hawthorne effect (improvements in performance by virtue of participation in a study). Our results contrast with those in the north of England study in which guidelines improved the quality of care only in those practices in which a practitioner contributed to their development.[4]

The education programme through which we disseminated the guidelines aimed to change practitioners' behaviour by small group methods,[20] which are particularly appropriate for primary care teams. We incorporated some of the most important features of educational outreach: focusing on a specific group of clinicians; defining clear educational and behavioural objectives; establishing credibility; stimulating active participation in the educational sessions; using concise graphic educational material; highlighting and repeating essential messages; and providing positive reinforcement in follow up visits.[21] The excellent rate of participation among many underdeveloped practices reflected widespread acceptability of a programme of guidelines led by peers.[20]

Our results reflect the management of patients on practice disease registers. Diagnostic accuracy and completeness of disease register [22] probably varied between practices. We cannot extrapolate our findings to the management of all patients with asthma or diabetes registered with these practices. However, as systematic bias is unlikely, the variation in quality of disease registers does not invalidate their use in a randomised controlled study.

Why did the diabetes practices make greater improvements in the recording of care than the asthma practices when the educational method and format of the guidelines was the same? There are two possible explanations. Firstly, there was a trend towards improved recording of asthma variables in the diabetes practices. While this could be a result of external factors, such as increased publicity about asthma management, it could also reflect differences in the power of the Hawthorne effect in the two groups of practices. Thus, the more complex nature of the diabetes review and the need for a structured recall system is a larger hurdle for the practice and may require a specific educational intervention, whereas the relatively simpler nature of the asthma review means that intervention around another chronic condition—namely, diabetes—will have an indirect effect on asthma care. A study with a control group of practices receiving no guidelines could test this hypothesis.

Secondly, the diabetes practices might have referred more patients for hospital review, resulting in more information being available from clinic letters. However, the improvements in the recording of diabetes variables persisted, with the exception of funduscopy, even when data from hospital letters were excluded. Thus our intervention prompted an appropriate division of labour between primary and secondary care (the latter being more appropriate for retinopathy screening [23]).

Sampling of disease registers

Our resources required us to sample from disease registers. With samples of 10 patients per doctor, irrespective of register size, the practices with smaller registers contributed a greater proportion of the register to the total patient sample. This sampling method avoids overrepresentation of patients from practices with large registers. It also ensured enough patients per practice to feed back meaningful baseline data as part of the educational intervention. The method does not take account of variation in the size of lists or registers. Alternative sampling methods—proportional to register size or total list size—would have made comparison between practices problematic as the practices varied greatly in these features. Although our sampling method means that sampling errors are not simple random but complex errors, any bias to the substantive results is likely to be small.

Recording of asthma and diabetes variables

The recording of variables varied enormously between practices and was generally poor. At the start of the study some practices had no record of funduscopy or peak expiratory flow rate during the past year for any of the patients sampled. Although these results seem poor compared with previous reports of care of asthmatic and diabetic patients, our study did not exclude patients with poor attendance,[24] and we assessed practices whose patient turnover approached 30% annually.[7] Many of the study practices were only beginning to develop chronic disease management and were doing so under difficult conditions.

There are two caveats about our interpretation of these data. Firstly, we set a harsh standard by counting data only recorded within the past year. Secondly, medical records in general practice do not accurately reflect clinical performance, although laboratory investigations and drug treatment are more likely to be noted than history or physical examination.[25] These limitations were addressed by the controlled nature of our study as long as no systematic bias existed in the distribution of diagnostic or recording inaccuracy.

Drug prescribing in asthma

The 10-fold variation in prescribing costs of asthma prophylaxis is unlikely to be fully explained by variations in generic prescribing, list inflation, or case mix. Most practices at the start of our study were spending less than one third as much on prophylaxis as general practitioners with an interest in asthma surveyed in a recent nation-wide study.[26] Our intervention resulted in more appropriate prescribing by practices receiving guidelines on asthma. This is the first demonstration of changes in prescribing resulting from a guidelines programme in British general practice.

Effect of "prompt" stamp or booklet

The use of prompts was associated with improved recording of variables for both conditions. This is further evidence that patient specific prompts may enhance the effect of guidelines on clinicians' behaviour,[27] although—in the absence of randomisation—we cannot be certain that improved recording was due to the effect of the prompt itself rather than more diligent clinicians choosing to use the prompt.

The use of prompts was relatively evenly spread across practices, which suggests an independent effect of prompts, but this requires further investigation. Manual prompts are a particularly appropriate method in an area where few practices use computers in consultations.

Acceptability of external audit method

External audit was acceptable to study practices that joined our study. Some practices expressed concern about confidentiality but were reassured that data would be available to outside bodies only in an anonymised form. Strengths of this method are convenience for practices, consistency, and therefore comparability of results. External audit is a potentially powerful tool for assessing the quality of chronic disease management.[28]

CONCLUSION

Our study shows that local guidelines disseminated with practice based education can improve the management of diabetic patients and probably of asthma patients in inner city, non-training practices. The use of simple recording prompts enhances this improvement. This form of dissemination was acceptable to a wide range of practices, many of which were underdeveloped. Our crude estimation of costs suggests that a modest investment can have a meaningful effect on chronic disease management. In a one year project we could not judge whether these improvements persist with time. Even if they do, our educational method of guidelines dissemination still needs to be tested against other methods of quality improvement and in relation to patient outcomes.[29]

Key messages

- Clinical guidelines can improve the quality of management of diabetes and possibly asthma in general practice if disseminated via a practice based educational programme

- The use of structured consultation prompts for the recording of clinical information recommended by the guidelines improves implementation of the guidelines in practice

- Relatively underdeveloped inner city practices can respond positively to this form of dissemination of guidelines and external audit

We thank all the participating practices; Moira Spence for inspiration and managerial advice; Jeremy Grimshaw for advice on design; Jon Deeks and Stephen Evans for statistical advice; Judith Duddle for participation in the practice education sessions; Jeanette Murphy for help with design of the educational intervention; and Joanne Turner, Katie Featherstone, Sarah Mott, and Michelle Ricken for support.

Funding: The North East Thames Regional Health Authority and the Department of Health.

Conflict of interest: None.

References

1   Delamothe T. Wanted: guidelines that doctors will follow. *BMJ* 1993;**307**: 218.
2   Haines A, Feder G. Guidance on guidelines. *BMJ* 1992;**305**:785–6.
3   Implementing clinical practice guidelines: can guidelines be used to improve clinical practice? *Effective Health Care* 1994;**8**:1–12.
4   North of England Study of Standards and Performance in General Practice. Medical audit in general practice: effects on doctors' clinical behaviour and the health of patients with common childhood conditions. *BMJ* 1992;**304**:1480–8.
5   Graffy, J, Willams J. Purchasing for all: an alternative to fundholding. *BMJ* 1994;**38**:391–4.
6   Jarman B. Underprivileged areas: validation and distribution of scores. *BMJ* 1984;**289**:1587–92.
7   Inkley-Leitch G, Arnold L. *A collaborative development plan for primary health care in City and East London*. London: City and East London Family Health Services, 1993.
8   East London and the City Health Authority. *Health in the East End. Annual public health report 1994/95.* London: ELCHA, 1995.
9   North Thames Regional Health Authority. Population outcome indicators: diabetes. London: NTRHA, 1994.
10 Oxman AD. *No magic bullets: a systematic review of 102 trials of interventions to help health care professionals deliver services more effectively or efficiently.* London: North East Thames Regional Health Authority, 1994.
11 Royal College of General Practitioners. *The development and implementation of clinical guidelines.* London: RCGP, 1995. (Report from general practice No 26.)
12 Statement by the British Thoracic Society, Research Unit of the Royal College of Physicians of London, King Fund's Centre, National Asthma Campaign. Guidelines for the management of asthma in adults: 1–chronic persistent asthma. *BMJ* 1990;**301**:651–3.
13 Krans HM, Porta M, Keen H, eds. *Diabetes care and research in Europe: the St Vincent Declaration action program.* Copenhagen: Copenhagen World Health Organisation Regional Office for Europe, 1992.
14 *Hackney asthma guide.* London: Department of General Practice, Medical College of St Bartholomew's and the Royal London Hospitals, 1991.
15 Harris M, Hadden WC, Knowles WC, Bennett PH. International criteria for the diagnosis of diabetes and impaired glucose tolerance. *Diabetes Care* 1985;**8**:562–4.
16 Eli Lilley National Clinical Audit Centre. *Monitoring asthma.* Leicester: University of Leicester, 1994.
17 Eli Lilley National Clinical Audit Centre. *Monitoring diabetes.* Leicester: University of Leicester, 1993.
18 Naish J, Sturdy P, Toon P. Appropriate prescribing in asthma and its related costs in east London. *BMJ* 1995;**310**:97–100.
19 Warren R. *List discrepancy and morbidity project.* London: Limehouse Practice 1992.
20 Mitman BS, Tonesk X, Jacobson PD. Implementing clinical guidelines: social influence strategies and practitioner behaviour change. *Quality Review Bulletin,* 1992,**18**:413–22.
21 Soumerai SB, Avorn J. Principles of educational outreach ("academic detailing") to improve clinical decision making. *JAMA* 1985;**263**:549–56.
22 Patchelt P, Roberts D. Diabetic patients who do not have diabetes: investigation of a register of diabetic patients in general practice. *BMJ* 1994;**308**:1225–6.
23 Finlay R, Griffiths J, Jackson G, Law D. Can general practitioners screen their own patients for diabetic retinopathy *Health Trends* 1991,**23**,104–5.
24 Parnell SJ, Zalin AM, Clarke CWF. Care of diabetic patients in hospital clinics and general practice clinics: a study in Dudley. *Br J Gen Pract* 1993;**43**:65–9.
25 Rethans J-J, Martin E, Metsemakers J. To what extent do clinical notes by general practitioners reflect actual medical performance? A study using simulated patients. *Br J Gen Pract* 1994;**44**:153–6.
26 Jones K. Impact of an interest in asthma on prescribing costs in general practice. *Quality in Health Care* 1992;**1**:110–3.
27 Grimshaw JM, Russell IT. Achieving health gain through clinical guidelines. II. Ensuring guidelines change practice. *Quality in Health Care* 1994,**3**:45–52.
28 Benett J, Lambert C, Hunds, Kirion C. Standards for diabetes care from a city-wide primary care audit. *Diabet Med* 1994,**11**:489–92.
29 Pringle M. Outcomes and general practice. In: Delamothe T, ed. *Outcomes into clinical practice.* London: BMJ Publishing, 1994:135–40.

(Accepted 2 November 1995)

This article was first published in the British Journal of General Practice and is reproduced by permission of the Royal College of General Practitioners

EVALUATION OF AN EDUCATIONAL PROGRAMME TO IMPROVE THE RECOGNITION OF PSYCHOLOGICAL ILLNESS BY GENERAL PRACTITIONERS

Philip C Hannaford, Chris Thompson, Morag Simpson

Philip C Hannaford MD MRCGP and Morag Simpson PhD
Royal College of General Practitioners' Manchester Research Unit.
Chris Thompson BSc MPhil FRCPsych professor,
Faculty of Medicine, Southampton, Royal South Hants Hospital, Southampton.

Submitted: 15 March 1995; accepted: 20 December 1995

BJGP 1996, **46**, 333–337

SUMMARY

Background. Take Care is a commercially sponsored educational package for the detection and management of depression by all members of the primary health-care team.

Aim. This study was designed to evaluate whether the educational package affects the recognition of psychological illness by general practitioners.

Method. General practitioners working in 13 practices in North West England or Trent Regional Health Authorities took part the evaluation. Patients who scored more than eight on the depression or anxiety component of the Hospital Anxiety and Depression (HAD) scales, and who were thought by their general practitioner to have a totally physical problem or no illness, were deemed to have a psychological illness that had been 'missed' by the doctor. Changes in the proportion of missed cases before and after exposure to Take Care were estimated.

Results. When all practices were considered together, the general practitioners missed a depressive illness in 24.1% of patients before Take Care, and 17.1 % afterwards; absolute decrease 7.0% [95% confidence interval (CI) -2.0 to -12.0%]. An improvement was seen in most practices (Wilcoxon matched-pair test P < 0.05). The programme was also associated with a small reduction in the overall proportion of episodes of anxiety missed by the doctor (absolute decrease 4.5%; 95% CI -1.0 to -8.0%) a reduction was found in most practices (Wilcoxon matched-pair test P < 0.05). There was no material difference in the diagnostic false-positive rate of the doctors before and after the introduction of the programme.

Conclusion. Exposure to an educational package for depression was associated with improved recognition of psychological illness by general practitioners.

Keywords: depression; education; recognition of psychological illness.

INTRODUCTION

Current estimates suggest that about one in 20 adults in the general population suffer from a depressive illness at any one time.[1] Many episodes are likely to go undetected and untreated.[1] In order to raise the level of awareness of the disorder within the health profession, the Royal College of Psychiatrists and the Royal College of General Practitioners launched the Defeat Depression campaign in January, 1992.[2] The Government has also recognised the importance of depression by identifying deaths from suicide as a key area for improvement in its *Health for the Nation* strategy for England.[3]

Take Care complements these important initiatives by providing an educational package about the recognition and management of depression by all members of the primary health care team. The programme includes a handbook on depression, an *aide-mèmoire* for assessing patients with depression, some Hospital Anxiety and Depression (HAD) scales, patients information leaflets and videos, and a poster to display in the practice. The handbook has a modular design, and contains four main sections on the detection and diagnosis of depression, its initial and continuing management, and the value of a multidisciplinary approach to the problem. More recent modules include protocol development, audit and problem solving. Another key component of Take Care is access to a regionally based depressive care advisor who is an experienced registered mental health nurse. These advisors visit each practice regularly in order to help develop its preferred way of managing patients with depression. Practices are free to work through the programme at their own pace, concentrating on the elements that they feel most appropriately address their needs.

The programme has been produced under the guidance of a steering committee of general practitioners, psychiatrists, practice nurses, academic and health service managers (Appendix). Although sponsored by SmithKline Beecham, great care has been taken to ensure that the programme is non-promotional especially with respect to the role of any particular class or brand of antidepressant treatment.

Take Care was launched in June 1993, when 100 practices in eight regional health authorities in England (North East, North West, North East Thames, North West Thames, South West Thames, Trent, West Midlands and Yorkshire), South Wales and Scotland were offered the opportunity to participate. Each practice had four or more partners and employed a practice nurse. By May 1994, 1040 practices had expressed interest in participating in the programme, and 520 had completed the original four modules. This paper examines whether the programme has affected the recognition of psychological illness by general practitioners.

METHOD

Selection of practices for the evaluation

In May 1993, the 200 practices in the North West England and Trent regional health authorities who were going to be invited to enrol for Take Care were approached by the Royal College of General Practitioners' Manchester Research Unit asking for their help in the programme's evaluation. The practices were given brief details of Take Care and the evaluation exercise. Eighteen practices, agreed to help; 13 in the North West England region and five in Trent. Full details of the evaluation procedure were then provided, either at an evening meeting or during a visit to the practice. The research staff involved in the evaluation had no direct involvement in the running of the Take Care programme itself. After the preliminary visit, communication between the collaborating practices and the Manchester Research Unit was deliberately minimized to reduce the effects that this might have on the results. However, we were requested by several ethics committees to supply the practices with the study numbers of patients who may have had a missed episode of depression after each part of the evaluation.

Baseline assessment before exposure to Take Care

The baseline assessment was conducted between May and July 1993, before the practices had received any written educational material or been visited by the nurse advisor. Each practice was asked to distribute the HAD scales to 300 consecutive surgery attendees aged 16 years and above. Patients who were unable or unwilling to complete the questionnaire were excluded from the evaluation. The HAD scales consist of 14 questions about anxiety and depression and can be used as a self-reporting screening of questionnaire to identify individuals who have a high probability of suffering from anxiety or depression. Although the scale was originally designed for the hospital setting,[4] it has been validated in general practice.[5]

The patients completed the HAD scale in the waiting room, and returned it to the person distributing the questionnaires before seeing the general practitioner.

'Blind' to its result. the doctor conducted a normal consultation before indicating on a separate assessment sheet which category most accurately described the nature of the patient's illness: totally, physical. predominately physical. predominately psychological, totally, psychological or no illness present. Most, if not all, of the partners in each practice completed the assessment exercise. Trainees were allowed to be included, but only if they were going to be present for both assessments.

The completed HAD scales and assessment sheets were returned to the RCGP Manchester Research Unit for data processing but only the general practitioners were able to identify individual patients.

Follow-up assessment after exposure to Take Care

The second assessment was conducted approximately 3 months after the practice had completed the recognition of depression module of the programme. The practices took a varying length of time to complete this first module, and therefore the follow-up assessment was performed over a 5-month period between November 1993 and March 1994. The practices were asked to distribute another 300 HAD scales to consecutive surgery attendees. In order to obtain approximately comparable groups in both parts of the evaluation, the practices were provided with the initials and surgery times of the doctors who completed the baseline assessment so that the new set of questionnaires could be distributed in roughly the same pattern. Five practices were unable to complete the follow-up assessment, mainly because of workload pressures. These practices were scattered throughout the regions without any obvious clustering.

'Missed' psychological illness

Patients who scored more than eight on the depression scale and who were thought by the doctor to have a totally physical problem or no illness were deemed to have a depressive illness that had been 'missed' by the general practitioner. The threshold of eight was chosen because previous work in general practice has shown this value to be the best compromise between sensitivity and the false-positive rate.[5] The probability of a patient with a HAD score of more than eight being diagnosed as having depression during a psychiatric research interview (positive predictive value) is 81%.[5] A threshold of eight on the anxiety scale was similarly used to identify patients with a missed case of anxiety.

The 95% confidence intervals (CI) for the difference in the overall proportion of missed cases of depression and anxiety before and after exposure to Take Care were calculated using the confidence interval analysis program.[6] In addition, because there was evidence of variation in the detection of psychological illness between practices, the non-parametric Wilcoxon matched-pairs test [7] was used to test whether the 'average' level of missed cases decreased across most practices.

Table 1

Number and characteristics of patients included in the assessments before and after participating in Take Care.

	Before	After
Total number of HAD scales returned	4107	3582
Total number of complete HAD scales	3863	3395
Total number of patients aged 16 + years with complete HAD scales and GP assessment	3390	2973
Males	1161 (34.2%)	993 (33.4%)
Females	2077 (61.3%)	1851 (62.3%)
Unknown	152 (4.5%)	129 (4.3%)
Mean age:		
males	48.0 years	48.7 years
females	44.3 years	44.6 years
Patient completed HAD scales:		
high* for depression only	72 (2.1%)	70 (2.4%)
high* for anxiety only	1027 (30.3%)	861 (29.0%)
high* for both depression and anxiety	443 (13.1%)	405 (13.6%)
low* for both depression and anxiety	1848 (54.5%)	1637 (55.1%)

* Low ≤ 8; high > 8.

Power of the study

Previous research has found that about one-third of patients consulting their general practitioner have an anxiety and/or depressive state. [5] On this basis, it was estimated that each practice would have to assess 255 patients before and after exposure to Take Care in order to detect an improvement in the recognition of psychological illness from 50 to 75% (5% significance, 90% power, two-sided test).

RESULTS

The 13 practices which participated in both parts of the evaluation provided 3390 sets of fully completed HAD scales and doctor assessments before exposure to Take Care, and 2973 sets (Table 1). The age and sex of the patients in both parts of the exercise was very similar, as were the results of the HAD scales, suggesting that the matching of clinics in both assessments was good. Approximately 2% of patients had high scores on the depression scale alone, 30% on the anxiety scale alone and 13% on both scales. Thus, about 15% of patients had scores on the depression scale in the morbid range, as previously established by Zigmond &-Snaith. [4] This is similar to another study based in primary care. [5]

Tables 2 and 3 detail the distribution of the results of the HAD scales and doctor's assessment before and after exposure to Take Care. On both occasions, patients who had high scores on both the anxiety and depression scales were more likely to be assessed by their general practitioner as having a psychological problem than those with high scores on the anxiety or depression scales alone. When all practices were considered together, the general practitioners missed a depressive illness in 24.1 % (124/515) of patients before Take Care, and 17.1 %

Table 2

Distribution of patient completed had scales by the general practitioner's assessment of the nature of the illness, before participating in take care.

General practitioner assessment of nature of the Illness	HAD scales				
	High* for depression and anxiety	High* for depression only	High* for anxiety only	Low* for depression and anxiety	Total
	Number (%)	Number (%)	Number (%)	Number (%)	Number (%)
Totally psychological	111 (25.1)	1 (1.4)	115 (11.2)	43 (2.3)	270 (8.0)
Predominantly psychological	120 (27.1)	11 (15.3)	183 (17.8)	140 (7.6)	454 (13.4)
Predominantly physical	118 (26.6)	30 (41.7)	318 (31.0)	570 (30.8)	1036 (30.6)
Totally physical	84 (19.0)	28 (38.9)	380 (37.0)	980 (53.0)	1472 (43.4)
No illness	10 (2.3)	2 (2.8)	31 (3.0)	115 (6.2)	158 (4.7)
Total	443 (100.0)	72 (100.0)	1027 (100.0)	1848 (100.0)	3390 (100.0)

* Low ≤ 8; high > 8.

Table 3

Distribution of patient completed HAD scales by the general practitioner's assessment of the nature of the illness, after participating in take care.

General practitioner assessment of nature of the Illness	HAD scales								Total	
	High* for depression and anxiety		High* for depression only		High* for anxiety only		Low* for depression and anxiety			
	Number	(%)	Number	(%)	Number	(%)	Number	(%)	Number	(%)
Totally psychological	115	(28.4)	2	(2.9)	69	(8.0)	29	(1.8)	215	(7.2)
Predominantly psychological	99	(24.4)	16	(22.9)	172	(20.0)	147	(9.0)	434	(14.6)
Predominantly physical	127	(31.4)	35	(50.0)	306	(35.5)	602	(36.8)	1070	(36.0)
Totally physical	60	(14.8)	17	(24.3)	292	(33.9)	793	(48.4)	1162	(39.1)
No illness	4	(1.0)	0		22	(2.6)	66	(4.0)	92	(3.1)
Total	405	(100.0)	70	(100.0)	861	(100.0)	1637	(100.0)	2973	(100.0)

* Low ≤ 8; high > 8.

(81/475) afterwards; absolute decrease 7% (95% CI -2.0 to -12.0%). The Wilcoxon matched-pairs test was statistically significant ($P < 0.05$), reflecting the fact that, individually, most practices (nine) showed an improvement in the recognition of depression (Table 4).

The Take Care programme does not include much information about the detection and management of anxiety and so a change in the detection of this problem was not expected. However, using a threshold of eight on the anxiety scale as indicative of such a problem, overall 34.4% (505/1470) of cases of anxiety were missed before exposure to Take Care and 29.9% (378/1266) afterwards; absolute decrease 4.5% (95% CI −1.0 to −8.0%). Again, most practices (10) showed an improvement (Wilcoxon matched-pairs test $P < 0.05$) (data not shown).

Table 4

Number of HAD scales returned by each practice, percentage of missed cases of depression before and after exposure to take care, and difference.

Practice	Number of HAD scales returned*		Missed cases of depression		Difference (%)
	Before Take Care	After Take Care	Before Take Care (%)	After Take Care (%)	
A	321	327	47.3	26.4	−20.9
B	222	181	35.6	14.9	−20.7
C	159	109	22.7	8.0	−14.7
D	274	126	27.9	18.2	−9.7
E	329	263	17.0	8.6	−8.4
F	245	218	27.8	20.5	−7.3
G	243	308	11.8	5.3	−6.5
H	316	240	25.4	23.8	−1.6
I	161	199	32.1	31.8	−0.3
J	245	200	20.7	21.2	+0.5
K	241	162	16.1	18.9	+2.8
L	283	289	10.7	13.9	+3.2
M	350	349	7.8	11.5	+3.7
N	260		19.1	-	-
O	235		27.9	-	-
P	286		31.4	-	-
Q	85		36.4	-	-
R	295		44.0	-	-

* Not all of the HAD scales could be used because the scale was incomplete, there was no accompanying general practitioner assessment or the patient was younger than 16 years.

The improvements in the recognition of depression and anxiety did not occur at the expense of an increase in the false positive rate of the general practitioner's diagnosis. Before Take Care, 9.9% of patients had low scores on both the anxiety and depression scales but were thought by their general practitioner to have a totally or predominantly psychological problem (Table 2). The corresponding figure after exposure to Take Care was 10.8% (Table 3) (absolute difference 0.9%; 95% CI −2.9 to 1.2%).

The patients from the five practices that completed only the first part of the evaluation were similar, in terms of age, sex and HAD scores, to those from the 13 practices that completed both parts of the exercise (data not shown). The practices that dropped out did not appear to have a particularly high (or low) proportion of missed cases of depression at the baseline assessment, compared with the other practices (Table 4).

DISCUSSION

An important limitation of this evaluation was the absence of a comparison group of practices who had not been exposed to Take Care. Therefore, the improvement in the detection of depression could be the result of other influences such as the Defeat Depression campaign. The participating doctors were asked in a questionnaire sent after the evaluation whether they had been aware of any other initiatives about depression during the study period. One doctor stated that he knew of a local audit of suicide and parasuicide, and another was conducting his own research into depression. There was also some knowledge of the Defeat Depression campaign (mentioned by seven doctors), drug promotions for specific preparations (two) and awareness of the Health of the Nation target for suicide reduction (one). In most cases, the doctors were usually aware of the general publicity surrounding these initiatives rather than specific local activities. Therefore, it seems unlikely, that other initiatives will have contributed materially to the observed effects.

It is possible that the apparent beneficial effects of the programme occurred because of the requirement imposed by several local ethics committees to inform the practices, after each assessment, of patients who may have had a depressive illness missed by the general practitioner. Little is known about whether such feedback affects subsequent detection rates by general practitioners. A study of hospital physicians providing primary care services to residents of Baltimore, Maryland, USA, found a slightly higher proportion of patients with a documented episode of psychiatric illness after a randomized trial of the feedback of the results of another screening instrument for depression, the General Health Questionnaire (21% after, compared with 16% before).[8] However, the authors were unable to tell whether the difference was the result of changes in the recording of illness and/or an increased sensitivity to psychiatric problems. Any effects of feedback would have to be long lasting if they were to influence our results, since the interval between baseline and follow-up assessment was at least 4 months.

The study assessed only the patient's illness on the day of surgery attendance. Some patients may have been known to have depression but consulted for another problem on the day of the assessment. For example, a depressed woman may have seen her doctor for oral contraception. In this instance, the woman will had a high HAD scale score but the general practitioner would have assessed her as not having an illness as the cause of that particular consultation, and consequently, will have been deemed to have 'missed' her depression. The number of occasions in which these circumstances arose were probably small. Furthermore, provided that the doctors completed the assessment sheets in an identical manner in both parts of the evaluation before and after comparisons remain valid.

The general practitioners in the study were all volunteers. Although this means that the results do not necessarily reflect the effect of Take Care on other practitioners, it does not invalidate the internal 'before and after' comparisons. Arguably, the volunteer doctors were more likely to be interested in psychiatric illness, and more able to recognize such problems before Take Care. The effect of such volunteer bias would have been to underestimate the true effect of the educational programme. We were unable to collect any information about the patients who did not participate in the study. Some may have refused because of language difficulties, problems which could also affect the presentation and recognition of depression. However, it is unlikely that the proportion of patients with such difficulties will have been large. Furthermore, the same problems should have affected the baseline and follow-up assessments, so internal comparisons remain valid.

General practitioners were chosen for this evaluation because they are the members of the primary health-care team most likely to have received some training in the recognition and management of depression. The results do not necessarily represent the experience of other members of the team. Greater benefits may be observed among other members of the team, especially practice nurses. It is noteworthy that practice nurses appear to be more responsive to the Take Care programme than general practitioners (Jo Newton, SmithKline Beecham, personal communication).

This evaluation looked only at the short-term effects of the Take Care programme. Further work is needed in order to determine whether the benefit appears to persist and to identify, which aspect of the programme (such as the provision of the nurse advisor) is responsive for the change.

With the increasing demand for continuing professional development and training, more educational programmes like Take Care are likely to be produced. As with any intervention in medicine, these initiatives should be evaluated. We have shown that this can be done, provided that the methodology is kept simple and does not impose unreasonable work on participants clinicians.

Appendix

Members of the Steering Committee were: Professor Chris Thompson (Chairman), Dr David Baldwin, Dr Stuart Bootle, Dr Ralph Burton, Jan Cox, Brian Edwards, Dr Simon Fradd, Atie Fox, Dr Philip Hannaford, Dr Simon Holmes, Mark Jones, Dr Chris Manning, Professor Roy McClelland and Dr Robert Peveler.

References

1. Paykel ES, Priest RG. Recognition and management of depression in general practice: consensus statement. *BMJ* 1992: **305**: 1198–202.
2. Priest RG. A new initiative on depression. *Br J Gen Pract* 1991; **41**: 487.
3. Secretary of State for Health. *The health of the nation: a strategy for health in England (CM 1986)*. London: HMSO, 1992.
4. Zigmond AS, Snaith RG. The hospital anxiety and depression scale. *Acta Psychiatr Scand* 1983, **67**: 361–370.
5. Wilkinson MJB, Barczak P. Psychiatric screening in general practice: comparison of the general health questionnaire and the hospital anxiety depression scale. *J Roy Coll Gen Pract* 1988; **38**: 311–13.
6. Confidence Interval Analysis. London: British Medical Journal, 1991.
7. Altman DG. *Practical statistics for medical research*, pp. 203–205. London: Chapman and Hall, 1991.
8. Shapiro S, German PS, Skinner EA, VonKorff M, Turner RW, Klein LE, *et al.* An experiment to change detection and management of mental morbidity in primary care. *Med Care* 1987; **25**: 327–339.

Acknowledgements

We thank the practices of Drs Addis, Calland, Couper, Dowrick, Ellwood, Fraser, Gibbons, Graves, Hibbert, Hudson, Lecky, Loudensack, Meredith, Redmond, Shah, Stokell, Summerscales and Turner, their patients, and SmithKline Beecham who provided a research grant to the Royal College of General Practitioners' Manchester Research Unit for the evaluation.

Address for correspondence

Dr PC Hannaford, Royal College of General Practitioners' Manchester Research Unit, Parkway House, Palatine Road, Manchester M22 4DB.

8

This article was first published in the Journal of Medical Screening and is reproduced by permission of the BMJ Publishing Group

CAN POSTAL PROMPTS FROM GENERAL PRACTITIONERS IMPROVE THE UPTAKE OF BREAST SCREENING? A RANDOMISED CONTROLLED TRIAL IN ONE EAST LONDON GENERAL PRACTICE

Alison M O'Connor, Chris J Griffiths, Martin R Underwood, Sandra Eldridge

AM O'Connor, *registrar*, Lower Clapton Health Centre, Hackney, E5 0PD, UK
CJ Griffiths, *senior lecturer*; MR Underwood, *senior lecturer*; S Eldridge, *lecturer in medical statistics*, Department of General Practice and Primary Care, St Bartholomew's and the Royal London School of Medicine and Dentistry, Medical Sciences Building Queen Mary and Westfield College, Mile End Road, London E1 4NS, UK
Correspondence to: Dr AM O'Connor at St Bartholomew's

Accepted for publication 8 December 1997

(*J Med Screen* 1998;**5**:49–52)

ABSTRACT

Objective – To determine the effect on the uptake of breast screening of a personalised letter from the general practitioner recommending mammography, sent to coincide with an invitation from the NHS breast screening programme.
Design – Randomised control trial with stratification of prognostic variables.
Setting – A group practice in Hackney, east London.
Subjects – 473 women invited for breast screening by the City and East London Breast Screening Service.
Outcome measure – Attendance for mammography.
Results – All women in the randomised trial were followed up; 134 of 236 (57%) randomly allocated to receive the prompting letter attended for mammography compared with 120 of 234 (51%) controls. This difference was not significant (x^2 =1.43, p=0.23)
Conclusion – Personal recommendation by a letter prompting attendance for mammography from the general practitioner known best to women due to be screened did not improve uptake of breast screening in this east London practice. Other strategies are needed to increase uptake of mammography in inner cities.
Keywords: breast cancer; general practitioners; patient compliance

One in 12 women will develop breast cancer at some stage in their life.[1] In an effort to tackle this major public health problem, the National Health Service breast screening programme (NHSBSP) invites all women aged 50 to 64 for a mammogram every three years. Seventy per cent of women need to accept their invitations if the Health of the Nation target of a 25% reduction in breast cancer mortality by the year 2000 is to be achieved.[2,3] Although nationally 71% of eligible women were screened in 1991–92 [4] a more recent review reports uptake rates of 77% in 1995.[5] Uptake in inner cities has been low and uptake in City and East London Health Authority (Hackney, Tower Hamlets, and Newham) was 45% between 1989 and 1992.[6] A more recent report gives uptake rates as low as 38% in this area.[7]

A systematic review of computer generated reminders for doctors and patients suggested that they probably increase the uptake for cancer screening services.[8] However, few of the studies cited were randomised, and most were based in America, in "academic" rather than community settings. A small retrospective analysis in a Scottish general practice showed that personal knowledge of the general practitioner was positively related to attendance.[9]

Defining simple interventions that can be used by inner city primary health care teams to increase mammography uptake may be crucial to the success of the NHSBSP. We used a randomised controlled trial to test the effect on breast screening uptake rates of a personal letter prompting attendance for mammography from the general practitioner best known to each woman.

METHOD

The trial took place in an inner city training general practice in Hackney, east London, comprising seven principals with a list size of 11 194. The area has one of the highest levels of deprivation in the United Kingdom, and a large Turkish population.[10] In March 1996 the NHSBSP was conducting its third screening round in this practice. We used the prior notification list of the practice patients currently in the breast screening age range from the Central and East London Breast Screening Service to identify the study population. We checked patients' addresses against family health services authority records using general practitioner (GP) links; a computer system enabling immediate transfer and checking of data between the practice computer and the health services authority computer.[11] We examined both paper and computer patient records for the following potential confounding variables:

(1) Previous breast screening attendance

We categorised women as:
- *First call* (those who had just entered the screening age range and had not been invited for mammography before)
- *Previous attender* (those who attended after their most recent screening invitation)
- *Previous non-attender* (those who had failed to attend after their most recent screening invitation).

(2) Previous cervical screening attendance

We categorised women as:
- *Attenders*
- *Non-attenders* (those who had not had a cervical smear for more than five years)
- *Not indicated* (those recorded as virgo intacta or as having had a total hysterectomy).

(3) Ethnicity

As Turkish was the major non-English speaking ethnic minority in the practice population, we categorised women as:
- *Turkish*
- *Other.*

Participant flow and follow-up

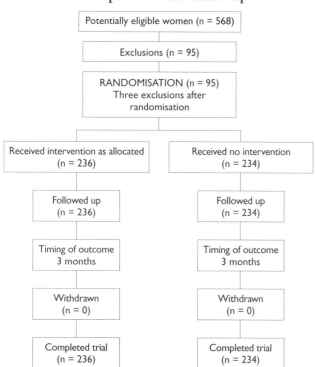

Women excluded for the following reasons:
Mammography in past 3 years (suspended) (n = 37)
Under investigation for breast disease (n = 8)
Terminal illness (n = 6)
Currently living abroad (n = 7)
Left practice area (n = 7)
Ghosts (n = 21)
Cervical smear data unavailable (n = 9)

Three women were excluded from the control group after randomisation: two had been recently screened, the other had moved from the practice area.

Figure 1 Participant flow and follow up.

Table 1

Randomisation of women by the three stratification variables: mammography, cytology, and ethnicity

Stratification variables	Intervention (n=236)	Control (n=234)
Mammography		
First call	53	56
Attended last call	110	106
Did not attend last call	73	72
Cervical smear		
Attended for smears	154	152
Did not attend for smears	36	39
Not indicated	46	43
Ethnicity		
Turkish	12	12
Other	224	222

We obtained ethnicity data from our computer records where available and through our Turkish health advocate, who identified the Turkish speaking women primarily from her personal knowledge of them but also by their surnames.

Selection of general practitioner best known to each woman

We determined the general practitioner best known to each woman by identifying the principal with whom they had consulted most frequently in their past 10 consultations. Consultations with locums or general practitioner registrars were excluded. If fewer than three of the last 10 consultations were with any one principal we recorded the GP best known as the principal with whom they were registered.

Exclusions

We used the following exclusion criteria:
- Mammography within the past 3 years
- Currently under investigation for breast disease
- Terminal illness
- Currently living abroad
- Moved from practice area
- "Ghosts" (no consultations for at least five years)
- "Cervical smear data unavailable" (women for whom smear data were unavailable).

Intervention

We sent women in the intervention group a letter on practice headed notepaper, signed personally by the GP best known to them. The letters were positive, explanatory, reassuring, and encouraging. We included an explanatory leaflet about breast screening and an invitation to attend the surgery to discuss breast screening if desired. We sent Turkish women in the intervention group leaflets and signed copies of the letter in both English and Turkish. We added a reminder to the computer records of all women in the intervention group. We sent letters about two weeks before their expected invitation from the breast screening unit. Both groups were called by the breast screening unit in the usual manner, receiving an invitation with appointment time, date, and an information leaflet with translations in several languages. If the first invitation produced no response the policy of the breast screening unit was to send one further follow up letter.

Outcome measure

The study outcome was attendance for mammography three months after invitation. Attendance results were routinely sent to the practice from the breast screening unit and we gathered any missing data directly from the unit.

Statistical analysis

In an interim audit of 60 women on a fail safe prior notification list (produced every six months to include women who might have been missed off the last official screening round — for example, because they had recently moved into the area), the previous uptake for breast screening in this practice was 36%. We considered a clinically important increase in attendance to be 15%. To detect such a difference at a 5% significance level with a power of 80%, 209 patients in each group were needed. Differences in attendance between intervention and control groups were calculated by the x^2 test. Differences between groups are shown with 95% confidence intervals.

Assignment

We generated the randomisation sequence using a computer minimisation program. This allocated each woman randomly while minimising the differences in the stratification variables between the two groups. The allocation schedule was held on the database and the recommendation letters for the women in the intervention group were produced and signed by the relevant principal.

Blinding

The researchers, the GP principals, and the patients were not blind to the intervention once allocation had occurred. Data entry of results, however, was carried out by a researcher without access to the patient allocation.

RESULTS

Participant flow and follow up

Figure 1 shows the participant flow and follow up; all patients included in the study were accounted for at the end of the study.

The prior notification list contained 568 women between the ages of 50 and 64 who were potentially eligible for breast screening. Ninety five women were excluded before randomisation (fig 1), almost all (86 women) because they were either ineligible for screening or had moved from the practice area. Three women were excluded from the study after randomisation when it was found they were ineligible, one had moved from the practice area, two others had been recently screened. All three were from the control group and were included in a sensitivity analysis as having attended for mammography. Intervention and control groups were well matched after randomisation (table 1).

Seventy five per cent of the women in the study had had four or more of the most recent 10 consultations with a practice principal. No letters were returned undelivered to the practice.

Attendance for mammography

Table 2 shows attendance for mammography subdivided according to previous breast screening attendance. There was no significant difference in attendance between women who were sent a recommendation letter and those who were not. We carried out a sensitivity analysis which assumed that the three worner, excluded from the control group after randomisation had attended for mammography (x^2= 1.14, p=0.28).

	Table 2			
Attendance for mammography subdivided by previous mammography attendance between intervention and control				
Previous mammography attendance	Intervention No (%)	Control No (%)	Difference (%)	95% Confidence interval
First call	29/53 (55)	22/56 (39)	15.4	–3.1 to 34.0
Previously attended	81/110 (74)	74/106 (70)	3.8	–8.1 to 15.8
Previously not attended	24/73 (33)	24/72 (33)	0	–15.8 to 14.9
Total	134/236 (57)	120/234 (51)	5.5	–3.5 to 14.5

x^2=1.43, p=0.23.

Discussion

Our results show that a personal recommendation from the GP known best to women due to be screened, sent to coincide with the invitation from the NHSBSP, did not improve attendance for mammography in this east London practice. Despite previous work suggesting its potential,[12,13] this simple and cheap intervention, sent to all women invited for screening, is unlikely to help improve low mammography uptake rates in British inner cities. This result was similarly reflected in other work with a differing methodology,[14] the findings of which agree that this intervention alone is insufficient to have an impact on low breast screening attendance in inner city areas.

Our intervention consisted primarily of a letter from the doctor to the patient recommending screening. We also placed a diary reminder in the patients' computer records. Although some women in the intervention group will have consulted during this short period, it seems that this element of the intervention had little or no impact on mammography attendance within three months after invitation. The computer reminder may have more impact in the long term, prompting discussion within the consultation and promoting opportunistic breast screening. Although women might have attended for screening after our arbitrary cut off period of three months, our brief intervention was unlikely to result in different attendance rates between the two groups beyond this time.

It is perhaps surprising that our intervention was ineffective as a prominent reason cited by women for not attending for mammography is that it was not recommended by their GP.[8,15] The main potential advantages of our intervention were that it did not require women to consult (so potentially reaching all women due to be screened) and bypassed doctors who may forget to recommend mammography during a busy consultation. Disadvantages of this approach were that the recommendation was not face to face and depended on factors such as patient literacy and first language. We cannot discount the possibility that women receiving the recommendation letter may have told friends in the control group about its contents, so contaminating the purity of our intervention. That we did not receive letters returned unopened suggests that letters were generally sent to the correct address. The lack of blinding on the part of the participating GPs would be likely to increase rather than decrease the chances of finding a significant effect of the recommendation letter.[16] Although our definition of the GP known best to women was arbitrary, again it would be likely to increase the effect of our intervention.

A systematic review of interventions to enhance screening for breast cancer recently reported that a recommendation by a doctor is one of the strongest predictors influencing a woman's decision to attend for screening.[8] Reminders for doctors and audit with feedback were the most effective, consistent with other reviews of strategies to change doctors' behaviour.[17] Reminders for patients and education were also effective, more so when in combination with reminders for doctors.

Apart from the methodological caveats cited above, there may be several other reasons for the discrepancy between our results and the conclusions of this systematic review. Firstly, our study took place in a London general practice with the attendant problems posed by an inner city population, such as lower levels of literacy and education, and language difficulties. Most of the studies cited in this systematic review were set in North American hospitals and studied mammography utilisation as well as clinical breast examination.[18,19] Most considered the effect of reminders for doctors and a minority, reminders for patients.[20] Secondly, systematic reviews may be subject to publication bias; possibly, negative studies addressing this topic may not have been published. Thirdly, effects of interventions may be overestimated through poor study, design, in particular by failure to conceal the allocation during randomisation.[16] Our study. benefited from stratification of prognostic factors affecting mammography attendance and from concealment of allocation during randomisation. Only one of the 20 studies cited in the review [8] used prognostic stratification and one used a concurrent control group rather than randomisation design.

Although our intervention failed to improve overall mammography uptake, our results showed that a greater proportion of women attended for mammography after intervention among those who received their invitation from the NHS breast screening service for the first time (29/53 (55%), intervention v 22/56 (39%), control). By contrast, for women who had failed to attend after their previous mammography invitation, the proportions of those attending in control and intervention groups were the same (24/73 (33%), intervention v 24/72 (33%), control). Although our study was not designed to have adequate statistical power to address these differences, these observations suggest, firstly, it may be worthwhile testing the effect of a doctor's recommendation letter targeted at women invited for the first time, and secondly, that a recommendation letter is unlikely to improve uptake in women who have failed to attend for their previous appointment.

We thank the Central and East London Breast Screening Service for their cooperation and help in dealing with our inquiries, Gene Feder for advice and help searching medical records; Sandra Cater (breast screening facilitator) for advice and help; partners, staff, and women participants at Lower Clapton Health Centre for their cooperation and willingness to support this project, and Professor Stephen Evans for use of the computer minimisation program.

References

1 Cancer Research Campaign. *Facts on cancer*. London: Scientific Year Book, 1993.

2 Secretary of State for Health. *Health of the Nation; a strategy for health in England*. London: HMSO, 1992.

3 Forrest A. *Breast cancer screening: report to the ministers of England, Wales, Scotland and Northern Ireland*. London: HMSO, 1986.

4 Chamberlain J, Moss SM, Kirkpatrick AE, *et al*. National Health Service breast screening programme results for 1991–2 . *BMJ* 1993;**307**:353–6.

5 National Health Service breast screening programme review 1996. (ISBN 1-87-1997-67-4.)

6 East London and City Health Authority. *Health in the East End*. Annual Public Health Report 1994/1995.

7 Healthy Eastenders Project. *Fair shares in health care. Healthy Eastenders project*. London: Department of General Practice and Primary Care, Queen Mary and Westfield College, 1996. (ISBN 1-897639-05-8.)

8 Mandellblatt J. Kanetsky PA. Effectiveness of interventions to enhance physician screening for breast cancer. *J Fam Pract* 1995;**40**:162–71.

9 Stephenson J. Non-responders can be encouraged to attend. *BMJ* 1995;**310**:1004–5.

10 Mugerwa F. *Refugees in Hackney: a study of health and welfare: summary of findings and recommendations*. London: Public Policy Research Unit, Queen Mary and Westfield College. 1997

11 NHS executive. *Health authority/general practitioner links. Review of benefits*. Leeds: Information Management Group, NHS Executive, 1996.

12 Schofield PE, Cockburn J, Hill DJ *et al*. Encouraging attendance at a screening mammography programme: determinants of response to different recruitment strategies. *J Med Screen* 1994;**1**:144–9.

13 Sharp DJ, Peters TJ, Bartholomew J, *et al*. Breast screening: a randomised control trial in UK general practice of three interventions designed to improve uptake. *J Epidemiol Community Health* 1996;**50**:72–6.

14 Majeed A, Given-Wilson R, Smith E. The impact of follow up letters on non-attenders for breast screening: a generalpractice based study. *J Med Screen* 1997;**4**:19–20

15 Fox SA, Murata PJ, Stein JA. The impact of physician compliance on screening mammography for older women. *Arch Intern Med* 1991;**151**:50–6.

16 Schultz KF, Grimes DA, Altman DG, *et al*. Blinding and exclusions after allocation in randomised controlled trials: a survey of published parallel group trials in obstetrics and gynacology. *BMJ* 1996;**312**:742–4.

17 Davis DA, Thomson MA, Oxman AD, *et al*. Changing physician performance: a systematic review of the effect of continuing medical education strategies. *JAMA* 1995;**274**:700–5.

18 McPhee SJ, Bird JA, Jenkins CN, *et al*. Promoting cancer screening. A randomised control trial of three interventions. *Arch Intern Med* 1989;**149**:1866–72.

19 Cheney C, Ramsdell JW. Effect of medical records' checklists on implementation of periodic health measures. *Am J Med* 1987;**83**:129–36.

20 Ornstein SM, Garr DR, Jenkins RG, *et al*. Computer generated physician and patient, reminders. Tools to improve population adherence to selected preventative services. *J Fam Pract* 1991;**32**:82–90.

This article was first published in the Lancet and is reproduced by permission of the Lancet

CORONARY ANGIOPLASTY VERSUS CORONARY ARTERY BYPASS SURGERY: THE RANDOMISED INTERVENTION TREATMENT OF ANGINA (RITA) TRIAL

Lancet 1993; **341**: 573–80

RITA Trial Participants

Executive (and Writing) Committee. Prof JR Hampton (chairman), Dr RA Henderson, Prof DG Julian, Mr J Parker, Prof SJ Pocock, Dr E Sowton, and Mr J Wallwork.
Data Monitoring Committee. Dr DA Chamberlain (chairman), Mr JF Dark, and Dr MD Joy.
Statistical Centre. Professor Pocock (director), Mr P Seed, and Mrs B Youard (London School of Hygiene and Tropical Medicine).
Steering Committee and trial participants listed at end of paper.
Correspondence to Prof John Hampton, Department of Medicine, D Floor, South Block, University Hospital, Nottingham NG7 2UH, UK.

The Randomised Intervention Treatment of Angina (RITA) trial is comparing the long-term effects of percutaneous transluminal coronary angioplasty (PTCA) and coronary artery bypass surgery (CABG) in patients with one, two, or three diseased coronary arteries in whom equivalent revascularisation was deemed achievable by either procedure. This first report is for a mean 2.5 years' follow-up on the 1011 patients randomised. 59% had grade 3 or 4 angina, 59% had experienced angina at rest, and 55% had two or more diseased coronary arteries. The intended procedure was done in 98% of patients. In 97% of CABG patients all intended vessels were grafted. Dilatation of all treatment vessels was attempted in 87% of PTCA patients with an angiographic success rate per vessel of 87% (90% excluding occluded vessels).

There have been 34 deaths (18 CABG, 16 PTCA) and the pre-defined combined primary event of death or definite myocardial infarction shows no evidence of a treatment difference (43 CABG, 50 PTCA; relative risk 0.88 [95% confidence interval 0.59–1.29]). 4% of PTCA patients required emergency CABG before discharge and a further 15% had CABG during follow-up. Within 2 years of randomisation 38% and 11% of the PTCA and CABG groups, respectively, required revascularisation procedure(s) or had a primary event (p < 0.001) and repeat coronary arteriography during follow-up was four times more common in PTCA than in CABG patients (31% *vs* 7%, p < 0.001). The prevalence of angina during follow-up was higher in the PTCA group (eg, 32% *vs* 11% at 6 months) but this difference became less marked after 2 years (31% *vs* 22%). Anti-anginal drugs were prescribed more frequently for PTCA patients.

At 1 month CABG patients were less physically active, with greater coronary related unemployment and lower mean exercise times than the PTCA patients. Thereafter employment status, breathlessness, and physical activity improved, with no significant differences between the two treatment groups. At 1 year mean exercise times had increased by 3 min for both groups.

These interim findings indicate that recovery after CABG, the more invasive procedure, takes longer than after PTCA. However, CABG leads to less risk of angina and fewer additional diagnostic and therapeutic interventions in the first 2 years than PTCA. So far, there is no significant difference in risk of death or myocardial infarction, and follow-up continues to at least five years.

INTRODUCTION

Percutaneous transluminal coronary angioplasty (PTCA) is used widely in the management of patients with coronary artery disease, and is an alternative to coronary artery bypass surgery (CABG) for selected patients with angina. The bypass operation is an effective treatment for angina, and randomised trials suggest that long-term survival is better than with medical treatment in some subgroups of patients.[1–3] By contrast information about the late results of PTCA is limited to registry studies [4–5] and the effect on prognosis is unknown.

In the late 1980s several randomised trials comparing the long-term effects of PTCA and CABG began.[6] In the UK the Randomised Intervention Treatment of Angina (RITA) trial was designed to compare the two methods in patients in whom equivalent myocardial revascularisation could be achieved by either treatment method.[7] This interim report describes the follow-up results at 2½ years.

PATIENTS AND METHODS

The design of the trial, including patient entry criteria, intervention procedures and outcome measures have been described in detail.[7] The protocol was approved by the ethics committees of the sixteen participating centres. RITA was designed to study the long-term effects of two different interventions for angina. A register of all patients undergoing coronary angiography under the care of participating cardiologists was maintained during the recruitment period to identify potentially randomisable patients. Patients with arteriographically proven coronary artery disease were considered if myocardial revascularisation was thought necessary on clinical grounds. Patients with stable or unstable angina were potentially eligible for the trial, but the trial procedures prevented patients with current symptoms requiring immediate intervention from being randomised. Eligible patients were not required to have angina if myocardial revascularisation was considered appropriate for reasons other than symptom relief. Patients with left-main-stern disease, previous coronary angioplasty or bypass surgery, haemodynamically significant valve disease, or a non-cardiac disease likely to limit long-term prognosis were excluded from the study.

The coronary arteriograms of potentially eligible patients were reviewed by a participating cardiologist and cardiothoracic surgeon, who jointly identified up to three major epicardial vessels requiring treatment. Patients were eligible if the investigators agreed that equivalent revascularisation was feasible by either method.[7] Each treatment vessel had at least one significant stenosis and was judged to supply 20% or more of the ventricular myocardium. Coronary stenoses were considered significant if there was at least 70% reduction in luminal diameter in one angiographic view or 50% reduction in two views. There was no requirement for all diseased vessels to be treated, but totally occluded vessels could be included as treatment vessels.

Eligible patients who gave written informed consent were randomised, by a telephone call to the Royal Free Hospital coronary care unit, to PTCA or CABG. There was prospective stratification by centre and by number of treatment vessels, using random permuted blocks within strata.

During the first 34 months of recruitment the coronary angiogram register recorded 27 975 patients with arteriographically proven coronary artery disease, of whom 3% were randomised to RITA. Overall myocardial revascularisation was considered necessary in 17 239 patients, of whom 69.9% were referred for CABG, 25.3% were referred for PTCA and 4.8% were randomised in the trial. The detailed findings of the register will be published separately.

Intervention procedure

Before joining the trial the sixteen participating hospitals, all regional cardiothoracic centres, were required to be performing coronary angioplasties with a high success and low complication rate. Operative methods were not standardised between centres, but angioplasty and surgery had to be done by experienced clinicians. Medication during or after either procedure was prescribed at the discretion of the supervising clinician. Patients assigned to multivessel angioplasty could have staged procedures but the plan was that all assigned intervention procedures be completed within 3 months of randomisation. PTCA was conventional balloon angioplasty, apart from 1 patient whose chronically occluded artery was treated by a low-speed rotational device.

Data collection

Every centre employed a research assistant to coordinate the study and collect data. The data were recorded on specially prepared forms and entered into a computerised database. Patients were examined and interviewed 1, 6 and 12 months after the intervention, and subsequent follow-up visits were scheduled at 2, 3, 4, and 5 years after randomisation.

The primary trial endpoint was predefined as the combined 5-year incidence of death and definite non-fatal myocardial infarction. All deaths and potential new myocardial infarcts were independently assessed by a central data review committee, blind to the patient's assigned treatment. Definite myocardial infarction was defined as the appearance of new abnormal Q waves within 7 days of an intervention (procedure-related myocardial infarction) or as a convincing clinical history at least 7 days after any intervention procedure, associated with new abnormal Q waves or activities of two cardiac enzymes (or of creatine kinase MB fraction alone) twice the upper limit of normal. Silent myocardial infarction was defined as the appearance of new abnormal Q waves on a follow-up electrocardiogram, without an accompanying clinical event.

All other major cardiovascular events and hospital admissions were documented. Following randomisation unstable angina was diagnosed when a patient was admitted with ischaemic cardiac pain at rest, without an increase in any cardiac enzyme or new abnormal Q waves. Patients were considered to have developed cardiac failure if they required new maintenance drug therapy for cardiac failure; for the purpose of the trial arrhythmias were considered significant when patients required a permanent pacemaker or new maintenance antiarrhythmic drug therapy. Stroke was diagnosed when a sudden focal disturbance of brain function of presumed vascular origin persisted for over 24 hours.

At follow-up visits angina was assessed by the Canadian Cardiovascular Society classification.[8] Physical activity was on a five-point scale ranging from sedentary (confined indoors) to vigorously active (regular exercise or heavy physical work). Breathlessness was assessed on a six-point scale from not breathless to breathless at rest. In most centres symptom-limited exercise treadmill tests were done using the modified Bruce protocol,[9] unless contraindicated by unstable angina or intercurrent illness. Left ventricular function was assessed by gated radionuclide left ventriculography in thirteen centres.

Statistics

The trial was intended to recruit 1000 patients, the main consideration being a reliable comparison of the 5-year incidence of death or non-fatal myocardial infarction.[7] Specifically, with a 20% incidence of this combined endpoint in one group, a trial of this size would have 80% power to detect a one-third reduction in the other group at the 5% significance level. 1011 patients were randomised during March, 1988, to November, 1991, and this report concerns their follow-up to June 30,

10

1992. All data have been analysed according to the original randomised group (intention-to-treat).

RESULTS

Baseline comparability

The characteristics at the time of randomisation for the 1011 patients entered are shown in table I. Overall there was good comparability between patients randomised to PTCA (n = 510) and CABG (n = 501).

A single treatment vessel was present in 45% of patients, while 12% had three treatment vessels. The median age was 57 years and 19% were women. Angina at least grade 3 (marked limitation of ordinary physical activity) was present in 59% of patients, and the median time since onset of angina was 9 months. During the 3 months before randomisation 40% had been admitted to hospital with angina, and 59% had experienced angina at rest. Also, a myocardial infarction had occurred previously in 43% of patients. 38% of patients were on three anti-anginal drugs (beta-blocker, calcium antagonist and long-acting nitrate) and 97% were on some anti-anginal medication at the time of randomisation.

Table I

Patient characteristics at the time of randomisation to CABG or PTCA

	CABG (n=501)	PTCA (n=510)	All patients (n=1011)
Treatment vessels			
One	222	234	456 (45%)
Two	218	213	431 (43%)
Three	61	63	124 (12%)
Age (yr)			
< 40	13	14	27 (3%)
40–49	88	91	179 (18%)
50–59	207	225	432 (43%)
60–69	169	156	325 (32%)
70–79	21	23	44 (4%)
Women	107	88	195 (19%)
Angina			
None	33	36	69 (7%)
Grade 1	33	44	77 (8%)
Grade 2	128	140	268 (27%)
Grade 3	155	159	314 (31%)
Grade 4	149	130	279 (28%)
At rest	275	282	557 (59%)
Causing hospital admission	187	189	376 (40%)
Median time since onset (lower and upper quartiles) (mo)	8 (4, 24)	9 (5, 24)	9 (4, 24)
Previous myocardial infarction	210	217	427 (43%)
Not working due to coronary disease	191	193	384 (38%)
Current medication			
Beta-blocker	369	383	752 (75%)
Calcium antagonist	363	365	728 (72%)
Long-acting nitrate	314	334	648 (64%)
Aspirin	353	370	723 (72%)
Antianginal drugs			
None	14	13	27 (3%)
One	116	95	211 (21%)
Two	174	216	390 (39%)
Three	194	185	379 (38%)

Randomised procedure

The intended randomised procedure was not done in 28 patients — in 11 (2%) randomised to CABG (patient refusal 6, symptomatic improvement 1, malignant disease diagnosed since randomisation 3, obesity 1, and in 17 (3%) randomised to PTCA (patient refusal 3, symptomatic improvement 4, malignant disease diagnosed since randomisation 1, lesion regression 3, disease severity 6). 5 patients received PTCA instead of the intended CABG and 7 patients were treated by CABG rather than randomised PTCA. On the intention-to-treat principle, these patients have been included in the original randomised groups for the follow-up results.

The assigned CABG and PTCA procedures were thus done in 490 (98%) and 493 (97%) patients, respectively. The median time from randomisation to procedure (and lower, upper quartiles) was 7 weeks (3, 11 weeks) for CAB G and 3 weeks (1, 6 weeks) for PTCA. It was intended that all assigned procedures be done within 3 months of randomisation, but for 79 CABG and 16 PTCA patients it took longer. The longer time to CABG is because of the need to accommodate trial patients in surgical waiting lists.

In 97% of patients who underwent CABG all vessels selected for treatment at randomisation were grafted. This rate depended on the number of treatment vessels and was 99%, 97%, and 87% for patients with one, two, and three treatment vessels, respectively. For 160 CABG patients (33%) the number of grafts was greater than the number of vessels selected for treatment, reflecting the need to graft all diseased vessels at a single operation. For instance 29% of patients had three or more grafts while only 12% had three treatment vessels at randomisation. An internal mammary artery graft was used in 74% of patients.

For patients who underwent an assigned PTCA, the number of vessels in which dilatation was attempted also sometimes differed from the number selected for treatment at randomisation. Dilatation of at least one vessel was attempted in all 493 patients, but dilatation of at least two was attempted in 81% of patients with two treatment vessels, and of at least three in 63% of those with three treatment vessels. Dilatation was attempted in fewer vessels than selected for treatment at randomisation in 62 patients (13%), but in more vessels in 32 (6%).

Angioplasty was attempted in 779 vessels with angiographic success (final diameter stenosis £50%) in 672 (87%). Dilatation was attempted in 64 occluded vessel, of which only 48% were successfully dilated. Successful dilatation was achieved in 90% of non-occluded vessels.

At least one vessel was successfully dilated in 90% of the 493 PTCA treated patients. Successful dilatation of all attempted vessels was achieved in 81% of patients (86% for patients with no occluded vessels). As expected, this success rate depended on the number of dilated vessels — 234/261 (90%), 132/158 (84%), and 36/47 (77%) for patients with one, two, or three non-occluded vessels attempted, respectively. Amongst the 493 PTCA patients, emergency CABG was required in 22 (4.5%) the definition of emergency was left to the individual operator. 7 other patients with unsuccessful but uncomplicated PTCA underwent elective CABG before discharge and a further 5 required a repeat PTCA before discharge. Amongst patients randomised to CABG pulmonary embolism occurred in 3 patients (0.6%) and wound-related complications delayed hospital discharge in 4.9%.

The median length of hospital stay (and lower, upper quartiles) for CABG and PTCA procedures were 12 days (10, 15 days) and 4 days (3, 8 days), respectively. The median hospital stay after the procedure (ie, excluding time spent in hospital before the procedure) was 9 days and 3 days, respectively, for CABG and PTCA. Of the 226 PTCA patients with more than one treated vessel, 15 (7%) had the procedure "staged" over more than one hospital admission.

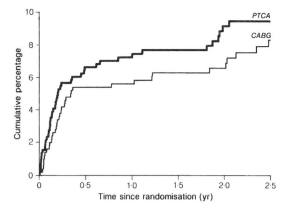

Fig 1 *Cumulative risk of death or myocardial infarction by treatment group.*

Patients numbers were:

Group						
	Time (yr)					
	0	0.5	1	1.5	2	2.5
CABG	501	501	441	388	322	250
PTCA	510	510	460	395	329	254

Extent of follow-up

All follow-ups and visits between randomisation and June 30, 1992, are included in this report. All patients have had 6 months follow-up and 50% have been followed up for over 2–5 years. No patient has been lost to follow-up for survival. However, 11 patients have withdrawn from further visits and are in follow-up by telephone only. A few patients fail to attend each planned visit. For instance, the visit at 6 months after procedure was achieved for 960 patients (95%); 13 were interviewed by telephone on questionnaire data, 15 gave information on clinical events, 10 were without data, and 13 had died.

Deaths and myocardial infarctions during follow-up

During a median follow-up time of 2.5 years 34 patients have died—18 (3.6%) in the CABG group and 16 (3.1%) in the PTCA group (table II). 10 died before discharge (6 after CABG and 4 after PTCA) and 6 of those deaths (4 CABG, 2 PTCA) were unequivocally procedure related. 2 died shortly after unsuccessful PTCA (1 stroke, 1 myocardial infarction), 1 died during elective CABG after unsuccessful PTCA, and 1 died during CABG of a myocardial infarction which began shortly before surgery. A further 8 cardiac deaths have occurred post-discharge

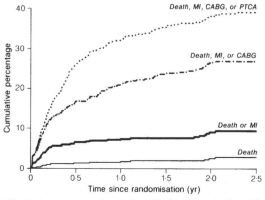

Fig 2 *Patients randomised to PTCA: cumulative risk of later PTCA, CABG, myocardial infarction, or death.*

Table II

Deaths, myocardial infarctions and new interventions during a median 2.5 years follow-up since randomisation

Event	CABG (n = 501)	PTCA (n = 510)
Death		
All causes	18	16
Pre-hospital discharge	6	4
Other cardiac death	4	4
Non-cardiac	8	8
*Non-fatal myocardial infarction**		
Definite	20	33
Silent	6	1
Patients with primary endpoint (death or myocardial infarction)	43	50
Subsequent interventions		
CABG	4	96
PTCA	16	93
Coronary arteriography,	39	159

*Each patient is included only once; 3 patients (2 CABG, 1 PTCA) each had two infarcts. Also 1 patient in CABG group had a non-fatal infarction and died subsequently.

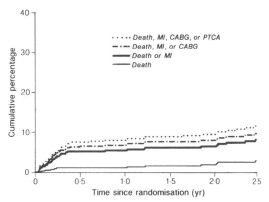

Fig 3 *Patients randomised to CABG: cumulative risk of later PTCA, CABG, myocardial infarction or death.*

(4 CABG, 4 PTCA). The 16 non-cardiac deaths (8 CABG, 8 PTCA) include 10 from malignant disease.

The numbers of patients having a non-fatal myocardial infarction since randomisation are shown in table II (26 and 34 definite or silent infarcts after CABG and PTCA, respectively). Of these, 12 and 18, respectively, occurred before hospital discharge. There were no deaths or myocardial infarctions during the time between randomisation and the assigned procedure.

The predefined combined primary end-point is death or definite or silent myocardial infarction, and so far 93 patients (43 CABG, 50 PTCA) have been so affected (fig 1). There is no evidence of a difference between CABG and PTCA groups (relative risk for CABG:PTCA is 0.88 with 95% CI 0.59–1.29; logrank p = 0.47), and follow-up continues to 5 years.

The risk of death or infarction appeared unrelated to the number of treatment vessels at randomisation, there being 40 primary endpoints in the 456 single vessel disease patients (16 CABG, 24 PTCA) and 53 primary endpoints in the 555 multi vessel patients (27 CABG, 26 PTCA). The relative risk single:multivessel is 0.91 (95% CI 0.60–1.40, p = 0.66). There is no evidence that any treatment difference depends on the number of diseased vessels (interaction test p = 0.35).

Subsequent interventions (table II)

Of the 510 patients randomised to PTCA, 96 (19%) have had a subsequent CABG. This includes 7 who had CABG instead of PTCA and 29 who required surgery before hospital discharge, as mentioned earlier. Fig 2 shows the cumulative life-table plot of time to CABG, myocardial infarction or death in the PTCA group, and indicates that within 2 years of randomisation an estimated 25% of PTCA patients have either required CABG or had a primary event.

93 (18%) of PTCA patients subsequently required at least one further repeat PTCA, 59 of these being with 6 months of randomisation. More than one new PTCA was done in 15 such patients and 1 patient had four such repeat RTCAs, 32 (33%) of the new CABGs mentioned above were after at least one additional PTCA had been attempted. The lifetable plot (fig 2) shows that within 2 years of randomisation an estimated 38% of PTCA patients experienced at least one of the

Table III

Secondary events during follow-up*

Event	Randomised group	Pre-discharge	Within 6 mo of discharge	After 6 mo
Unstable angina	CABG	0	5	5
	PTCA	14	28	15
Stroke	CABG	5	2	3
	PTCA	1	2	6
Cardiac failure	CABG	3	11	8
	PTCA	1	3	6
Arrhythmia	CABG	37	10	3
	PTCA	7	4	5

* Pre-discharge events are only for patients receiving their randomised procedure but data for latter two intervals are on an intention-to-treat basis. For each patient only first event of each kind is included.

following: further PTCA, CABG, myocardial infarction, or death. This risk of subsequent procedure or event was not significantly related to the number of treatment vessels at randomisation (36% in single vessel, 41% in multi-vessel patients, p = 0.27).

Amongst the 501 patients randomised to CABG, 4 have subsequently had a second CABG. 21 CABG patients have had subsequent PTCA, including the 5 who had PTCA instead of the randomised CABG. Within 2 years of randomisation, an estimated 11% of the CABG group had experienced further CABG, PTCA, myocardial infarction or death (fig 3) which is a much lower rate than the 38% in the PTCA group (p < 0.001).

157 PTCA patients (31%) and 37 CABG patients (7%) have had at least one repeat coronary arteriogram during the mean 2.5 years follow-up (p<0.001). This contrast is especially striking in the first 6 months when 96 PTCA and 5 CABG patients had arteriography.

Secondary events

Secondary events have been classified into three time bands: before discharge from randomised procedure, within 6 months of procedure, and beyond 6 months (table III). Unstable angina has been significantly more common in PTCA patients throughout follow-up but especially predischarge (14 PTCA, none CABG). Arrhythmia has been significantly more common in CABG patients, especially pre-discharge (37 CABG, 7 PTCA), as has cardiac failure, but there is no significant difference in strokes.

Angina and breathlessness

There was a striking improvement in reported angina in both treatment groups at all follow-up times (fig 4). However, at every time point there was a significant excess of patients with angina in the RTCA group. For instance at 6 months 11.0% of CABG patients have anginal symptoms compared with 31.6% of PTCA

Table IV

Anti-anginal medication over time

Time since randomised procedure	Rand-omised group	No of anti-anginal drugs				
		No	None	One	Two	Three
1 mo	CABG	489	334 *(68%)*	127	26	2 *(0.4%)*
	PTCA	497	72 *(14%)*	156	190	79 *(15.9%)*
6 mo	CABG	488	353 *(72%)*	107	26	2 *(0.4%)*
	PTCA	498	124 *(25%)*	187	134	53 *(10.6%)*
1 yr	CABG	407	277 *(68%)*	97	27	6 *(1.5%)*
	PTCA	436	136 *(31%)*	154	113	33 *(7.6%)*
2 yr	CABG	301	198 *(66%)*	76	22	5 *(1.7%)*
	PTCA	316	124 *(39%)*	106	67	19 *(6.0%)*

Table V

Physical activity over time

Time	CABG		PTCA	
	No	Physically active*	No	Physically active
Baseline	498	126 *(25%)*	509	135 *(27%)*
1 mo	481	184 *(38%)*	491	254 *(52%)*
6 mo	480	326 *(68%)*	490	299 *(61%)*
1 yr	402	268 *(67%)*	435	277 *(64%)*
2 yr	297	195 *(66%)*	312	196 *(63%)*

*At each visit patient's physical activity was scored on a five-point scale. Here the first two points (vigorously or moderately active) are combined into the one grading "physically active".

patients (RR = 0.35, 95% CI 0.26–0.47; p < 0.001). 2 years after randomisation the prevalence of angina in the CABG group had increased to 21.5% but this was still significantly less than the 31.3% for PTCA patients (p = 0.007). This difference in the prevalence of angina held for patients with a single treatment vessel (9% CABG, 29% PTCA at 6 months) and for those with two or more treatment vessels (12% CABG, 34% PTCA at 6 months).

A similar pattern emerges for severe angina (grade 3 or 4). Up to 1 year of follow-up severe angina was more than twice as common in the PTCA group. At two years both groups have a 6% prevalence of severe angina, but only 60% of patients have reached 2 years follow-up so far.

In both treatment groups, the prevalence of angina during follow-up was greater in patients with severe angina (grade 3 or 4) at randomisation. For instance, at 6 months in CABG patients, 16% of those with severe angina at baseline had angina still present compared with 6% of other CABG patients. 6 months after PTCA the prevalence of angina was 38% in those graded severe at baseline compared with 23% of the rest.

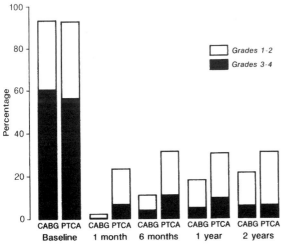

Fig 4 *Prevalence of angina (Canadian Cardiovascular Society classification) over time.*

Patients numbers were:

Group	Time (mo)				
	0	1	6	12	24
CABG	498	482	480	401	297
PTCA	509	491	491	433	310

Patients receiving PTCA had much greater use of anti-anginal drugs during follow-up compared to patients undergoing CABG (table IV). For instance, 6 months after their procedure 75% of PTCA patients were taking at least one anti-anginal drug and 11% were on triple drug therapy. 6 months after CABG 28% were receiving one or more anti-anginal drugs with just two such patients on triple drug therapy. By 2 years, this treatment difference in anti-anginal medication had narrowed but remained highly significant (eg, 61% of PTCA patients and 34% of CABG patients, respectively, on at least one anti-anginal drug).

There was a substantial reduction in breathlessness in both groups. At randomisation 35% of patients had been severely breathless (defined as breathless when walking at own pace, washing, dressing, or at rest); this fell to around 11% at all follow-up visits, with no evidence of a treatment difference.

Physical activity

There was a considerable increase m reported physical activity in both groups (table V). For instance only 26% of patients had moderate or vigorous activity at randomisation compared with 65% of patients after 1 year. As expected, one month after CABG there were fewer such physically active patients compared with one month after PTCA (38% *vs* 52%) but there is no evidence of a treatment difference thereafter.

Employment status

To avoid complications relating to normal retirement age and the employment intentions of women, we confine attention to men aged less than 63 at randomisation and their employment status up to 2 years later (table VI). At randomisation 47% of such men reported that they were not working because of coronary disease. In both groups this prevalence of coronary-related unemployment was increased 1 month after their procedure but then fell to below 30% during follow-up. At 1 month after CABG 79% of men were unemployed due to their coronary disease compared with 54% one month after PTCA. At later follow-up times there is a slight suggestion of a greater coronary-related unemployment rate in the PTCA group but this is not significant.

Table VI

Employment status over time (confined to men aged <63 at randomisation)

| Time | Not working due to coronary disease | |
	CABG	PTCA
Baseline	150/307 (49%)	147/325 (45%)
1 mo	235/299 (79%)	170/314 (54%)
6 mo	89/298 (30%)	99/317 (31%)
1 yr	54/253 (21%)	83/290 (29%)
2 yr	44/1188 (23%)	52/208 (25%)

There were changes in employment status in both directions. For instance, at 6 months 40% of the 290 patients not working due to coronary disease at baseline had returned to work. However, 12% of the 233 patients working at baseline were not working because of coronary disease 6 months after their procedure. At each occasion around 16% of the men were not working for other reasons.

Exercise testing

Exercise treadmill testing was done in 67% of patients in fourteen of the sixteen centres. Other test procedures were used in some centres, but here the results are confined to the modified Bruce protocol. At randomisation the mean exercise times in the CABG and PTCA groups were 10.3 min (SE 0.25; n = 332) and 10.9 min (SE 0.24; n = 345). Fig 5 shows, for four follow-up visits, the mean increases in exercise times compared with baseline, with adjustment for baseline

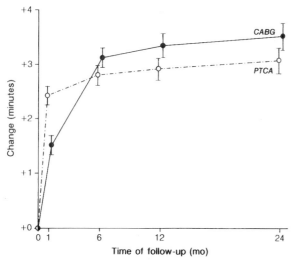

Fig 5 *Changes in modified Bruce exercise times (means and SE), with adjustment for baseline by analysis of covariance.*

Patients numbers and P-value for treatment difference were:

| Group | Time (mo) | | | |
	1	6	12	24
CABG	291	309	247	171
PTCA	318	322	276	191
p	0.0002	0.20	0.14	0.19

difference between groups by analysis of covariance. At all time points there is a substantial increase in mean exercise time for both treatment groups.

1 month after the procedure, the mean increase in exercise time is significantly greater in the PTCA group (2.35 min *vs* 1.62 min after CABG; p = 0.0002). At all subsequent visits up to 2 years there is a slightly greater mean increase in exercise time after CABG compared with after PTCA, but these differences are not significant.

Ejection fractions

Resting ejection fractions were studied in 47% of patients from thirteen centres. At both 1 month and 6 months after randomisation there was no evidence of a change in mean ejection fraction in either treatment group. For instance, at 6 months the mean changes were –0.1% and + 0.3% in the CABG and PTCA group (n = 239 and 233, respectively).

DISCUSSION

The RITA trial is one of several studies designed to compare the long-term effects of coronary angioplasty and coronary artery bypass surgery.[6] The principal objective of RITA is to compare the combined 5-year incidence of death and non-fatal myocardial infarction in the two treatment groups. This interim report, at a mean follow-up of 2.5 years. is presented because of wide interest in other outcome measures, including symptoms, exercise tolerance, and other cardiac events. Other smaller trials of CABG and PTCA have published preliminary reports (EAST, ERACI, GABI),[10–12] but the results of the Bypass Angioplasty Revascularisation Investigation (BARI) are awaited.[13]

Before randomisation in the RITA trial the participating cardiologist and surgeon were required to agree that equivalent revascularisation could be achieved by treating up to three target vessels. However, the trial is a pragmatic comparison of treatment intentions, and during the trial angioplasty was attempted in all target vessels in 87% of patients (angiographic success rate of 87%). By contrast, all target arteries were grafted in 97% of surgically treated patients. This reflects an intrinsic difference between the two myocardial revascularisation procedures: the risk of coronary angioplasty is increased in patients with multivessel disease 14 and in the study many cardiologists apparently accepted partial revascularisation rather than subject such patients to multiple angioplasty procedures.

The rates of myocardial infarction and death during hospital admission for the randomised intervention procedures were low in both treatment groups, and are consistent with previously published reports.[2,3,14,15] The in-hospital mortality rate amongst the CABG patients was especially low at 1.2%, possibly reflecting the type of patients selected for inclusion. The rate of emergency coronary artery bypass surgery amongst PTCA patients was 4.5%, and this figure is slightly higher than in some recent reports.[15] However, direct comparison with observational studies is difficult because without the constraints imposed by a clinical trial there is always the potential for underreporting of complications. The RITA trial data indicate that emergency surgery remains an important risk of coronary angioplasty.

After a mean follow-up of 2.5 years there is no evidence of a treatment difference in the combined incidence of death or myocardial infarction. However, the trial design was based on a follow-up period of at least 5 years, and the confidence intervals for the estimated rates of death and myocardial infarction are currently wide. Further long-term follow-up will be required before the risk of death or myocardial infarction can be reliably compared between the two treatment strategies.

During the study there were major differences in the rates of repeat coronary arteriography and re-intervention between the two treatment groups. Thus 31% of PTCA patients but only 7% of CABG patients have so far required repeat coronary arteriography. 19% of PTCA patients required CABG and angioplasty was repeated in a further 12%. By contrast, the re-intervention rate amongst surgically treated patients was only 5%. These findings are reflected in a major difference in event-free survival between the two groups: an estimated 62% of the PTCA group and 89% of the CABG group remained free from all major cardiac events and interventions 2 years after randomisation. The ERACI trial randomised 127 patients with multivessel disease to PTCA or CABG and has reported similar results after one year.[11] The difference in event-free survival in our trial may be due to differences in the extent of revascularisation achieved at the randomised intervention procedure, and restenosis in many PTCA patients. The high re-intervention rate potentially exposes PTCA patients to additional risk, but this was not reflected in an increased risk of death or non-fatal myocardial infarction in the PTCA group as a whole.

The incidence of unstable angina was higher amongst PTCA patients than amongst CABG patients during follow-up, but the mechanism for this difference is unclear. Following balloon dilatation some coronary lesions may be dissected and about one third develop significant restenosis, [16,17] and perhaps these changes predispose PTCA patients to greater risk of unstable angina.

Both revascularisation procedures were associated with a marked improvement in angina during the first two years of follow-up. Nevertheless, at every follow-up assessment around 30% of PTCA patients remained symptomatic with angina. A substantial proportion of PTCA patients also remained on anti-anginal medication, but some of these drugs may have been prescribed as part of post-angioplasty treatment protocols at individual participating centres, rather than for specific anginal symptoms. Further investigation is required to evaluate the extent to which the high prevalence of angina after angioplasty is due to incomplete revascularisation or due to restenosis. By contrast, one month after surgical

revascularisation only 2% of patients complained of angina. During later follow-up angina gradually recurred amongst surgically treated patients, and at two years the difference in angina status and requirement for anti-anginal medication between the two treatment groups is less marked. The extent to which angina recurrence amongst CABG patients is due to graft occlusion [18,19] or progression of native coronary artery disease is uncertain.

These data suggest that CABG is a more effective treatment for angina than PTCA in the medium term. However, this modest treatment advantage is not associated with a major difference in functional capacity: as would be expected, one month after revascularisation surgically treated patients had shorter exercise times, more breathlessness, lower levels of physical activity and a lower rate of return to work than PTCA patients. Thereafter there was no treatment difference in breathlessness score, level of physical activity or employment status. The small differences in exercise treadmill time at one and two years were not significant.

As yet there is no evidence that patients with single or multivessel disease differ substantially in terms of the risk of death or myocardial infarction, the prevalence of angina or the need for further intervention. The RITA trial is the only study comparing CABG and PTCA to include patients with single vessel disease,[6] and a more detailed subgroup analysis will be presented at a later date.

During the initial randomisation procedure the surgically treated patients remained in hospital for twice as long as the PTCA patients. Similar findings have been reported from the German Angioplasty Bypass-Surgery Investigation (GABI).[12] We intend to undertake a more extensive comparison of treatment costs and subsequent resource use in the RITA trial, incorporating data on all hospital admissions, interventions and prescribed medication.

During the recruitment phase of the RITA trial 4–8% of patients referred for myocardial revascularisation by the participating cardiologists were randomised, and similar randomisation rates have been observed in other coronary intervention trials.[3,20] However, in the RITA trial many angiographically eligible patients were not randomised for non-clinical reasons (eg, consent refused). The trial patients are therefore likely to be representative of the relatively large subgroup of patients who are suitable for either CABG or PTCA, particularly patients in whom equivalent revascularisation is considered feasible by either treatment method.

Not all patients currently treated by coronary angioplasty are also candidates for bypass surgery. The Angioplasty Compared to Medicine (ACME) trial is a randomised comparison of coronary angioplasty and continued medical care, and recently reported outcome in 212 patients with single vessel disease. At 6 months PTCA was associated with greater symptomatic improvement than medical therapy, but the difference in exercise tolerance between the two treatment strategies was modest.[20] In the UK a major trial comparing treatment strategies of coronary angioplasty and conservative (medical) care (RITA-2) is currently recruiting patients, and should further define the role of PTCA in the management of patients with coronary artery disease.

The RITA trial has demonstrated substantial differences in clinical outcome between two groups of patients with coronary artery disease who are randomised to initial treatment policies of PTCA or CABG. Both methods of myocardial revascularisation are associated with similar risk of death or non-fatal myocardial infarction during 2.5 years follow-up, but data from further follow-up (and from other trials) will elucidate a more precise and longer term treatment comparison. CABG involves a longer hospitalisation and convalescence, but thereafter surgically treated patients enjoy better relief of angina and require fewer anti-anginal drugs. PTCA offers a simpler initial procedure, but subsequently patients so treated are more likely to complain of angina, take anti-anginal medication, and undergo repeat coronary arteriography and a further myocardial revascularisation procedure.

RITA trial participants. E Sowton (chairman),* AK Yates,* PVL Curry, PB Deverall, G Jackson (Guy's Hospital, London, 140 patients randomised); CW Pumphrey,* DJ Parker,* T Treasure,* J Pepper, J Smith, DE Ward (St George's Hospital, London, 118); N Brooks,* H Moussalli,* D Bennett, C Bray, C Campbell, AK Deiraniya, M Jones, R Lawson, A Rahman, C Ward (Wythenshaw Hospital, Manchester, 112), R Balcon,* P Magee,* C Layton, AD Timmis, JEC Wright (London Chest Hospital, 103); RH Swanton,* W Pugsley,* (Middlesex Hospital, London, 76); PJB Hubner,* RK Firmin,* AH Gershlick, T Spyt (Groby Road Hospital, Leicester, 71); DB O'Keffe,* H O'Kane,* J Cleland, DJ Gladstone, P Morton, JG Murtagh, ME Scott (Belfast City Hospital, 58); SM Cobbe,* DJ Wheatley,* FG Dunn, I. Hutton, AR Lorimer, AP Rae, WS Hillis (Royal Infirmary, Glasgow, 56); DS Dymond,* SJ Edmondson,* SO Banim, DW Davies, AW Nathan, G Reece, RAJ Spurrell (St Bartholomew's Hospital, London, 55); DC Cumberland,* GH Smith,* GDG Oakley (Northern General Hospital, Sheffield, 51); DE Jewitt,* JRW Keates, * CA Bucknall, AT Forsyth (King's College Hospital, London, 50;. RJ Wainwright,* FP Shabbo,* JB O'Riorden (Brook Hospital, London, 47); P Bloomfield,* EWJ Cameron,* D de Bono (Royal Infirmary of Edinburgh, 29); MT Rothman,* AJ Wood,* AH MacDonald, PG Mills, T Lewis (Royal London Hospital, 20); RA Foale,* R Stanbridge* (St Mary's Hospital, London, 18); KAA Fox,* IM Breckenridge* (University Hospital of Wales, Cardiff, 7).
*Indicates Steering Committee.

The most important acknowledgment is to the 1011 patients who agreed to accept randomisation. The RITA Steering Committee also recognises the dedicated work of the research assistants who collected the trial data and the Royal Free Hospital coronary care unit who provided the randomisation service. The RITA trial is supported by grants from the British Heart Foundation, British Cardiac Society, and Department of Health. Additional financial support has been provided by Advanced Cardiovascular Systems, Inc (USA), Medtronic Ltd (UK), and Schneider (UK).

References

[1] The VA Coronary Artery Bypass Surgery Cooperative Study Group. Eighteen-year follow-up in the Veterans Affairs cooperative study of coronary artery bypass surgery for stable angina. *Circulation* 1992; **86**: 121–30.

[2] Varnauskas E, and the European Coronary Surgery Study Group. Twelve year follow-up of survival in the randomized European Coronary Surgery Study. *N Engl J Med* 1988; **319**: 332–37.

[3] Alderman EL, Bourassa MG, Cohen LS, *et al.* Ten-year follow-up of survival and myocardial infarction in the randomized coronary artery surgery study. *Circulation* 1990; **82**: 1629–46.

[4] Gruentzig AR, King SB, Schlumpf M, Siegenthaler W. Long-term follow-up after percutaneous transluminal coronary angioplasty: the early Zurich experience. *N Engl J Med* 1987; **316**: 1127–32.

[5] Detre K, Holubkov R, Kelsey S, *et al.* One-year follow-up results in the 1985–1986 National Heart, Lung and Blood Institute's percutaneous transluminal coronary angioplasty registry. *Circulation* 1989; **80**: 421–28.

[6] Editorial. BARI, CABRI, EAST, GABI, and RITA: coronary angioplasty on trial. *Lancet* 1990; **335**: 1315–16.

[7] Henderson RA, for the Randomised Intervention Treatment of Angina trial. The Randomised Intervention Treatment of Angina (RITA) protocol; a long term study of coronary angioplasty and coronary bypass surgery in patients with angina. *Br Heart J* 1989; **62**: 411–14.

[8] Cambeau L. Grading of angina pectoris. *Circulation* 1976; **54**: 522–23.

[9] Sheffield LT. Graded exercise test (GXT) for ischaemic heart disease: a submaximal test to a target heart rate. In: exercise testing and training of apparently healthy individuals: a handbook for physicians. New York: American Heart Association Committee on Exercise, 1972: 35–38.

[10] King SB, Lembo NJ, Hall EC, and the EAST Investigators.The Emory angioplasty *vs* surgery trial (EAST): analysis of baseline patient characteristics. *Circulation* 1992; **82** (suppl I): 508–1 (abstr).

[11] Rodriguez A, Boullon F, Paviotti C, *et al.* Argentine randomized trial coronary angioplasty *vs* bypass surgery in multiple vessel disease (ERACI). In hospital results and one year follow-up. *J Am Coll Cardiol* 1992; **19**: 24A (abstr).

[12] Hamm CW, Ischinger T, Reimers J, Dietz U, Rupprecht HJ for the GABI study group. Angioplasty *vs* bypass-surgery in patients with multivessel disease: in-hospital outcome in the GABI trial. *Circulation* 1992; **82** (suppl I): 373–I (abstr).

[13] Anon. Protocol for the Bypass Angioplasty Revascularisation Investigation. *Circulation* 1991; **84** (suppl V): V1-V27.

[14] Detre K, Holubkov R, Kelsey S, *et al.* Percutanous transluminal coronary angioplasty in 1985–1986 and 1977–1981. *N Engl J Med* 1988; **318**: 265–70.

[15] Hubner P. Cardiac interventional procedures in the United Kingdom during 1989. *Br Heart J* 1991; **66**: 469–71.

[16] Serruys PW, Luijten HE, Beatt KJ, *et al.* Incidence of restenosis after successful coronary angioplasty: a time-related phenomenon. A quantitative angiographic study in 342 consecutive patients at 1, 2, 3, and 4 months. *Circulation* 1988; 77: 361–71.

[17] Nobuyoshi M, Kimura T, Nosaka H, *et al.* Restenosis after successful coronary angioplasty: serial angiographic follow-up of 229 patients. *J Am Coll Cardiol* 1988; **12**: 616–23.

[18] Fitzgibbon GM, Leach AJ, Kafka HP, Keon WJ. Coronary bypass graft fate: long-term angiographic study. *J Am Coll Cardiol* 1991; **17**: 1075–80.

[19] Lyde BW, Loop FD, Cosgrove DM, Radiff NB, Easley K, Taylor PC. Long-term (5 to 12 years) serial studies of internal mammary artery and saphenous vein coronary bypass grafts. *J Thorac Cardiovasc Surg* 1985; **89**: 248–58.

[20] Parisi AF, Folland ED, Hartigan P, on behalf of the Veterans Affairs ACME investigators. A comparison of angioplasty with medical therapy in the treatment of single-vessel coronary artery disease. *N Engl J Med* 1992; **326**: 10–16.

This article was first published in the Lancet and is reproduced with permission of the Lancet

CORONARY ANGIOPLASTY VERSUS MEDICAL THERAPY FOR ANGINA: THE SECOND RANDOMISED INTERVENTION TREATMENT OF ANGINA (RITA-2) TRIAL

Lancet 1997; **350**: 461–68

RITA-2 trial participants listed at end of article

Correspondence to: Prof Stuart Pocock, London School of Hygiene & Tropical Medicine, London WC1E 7HT, UK

SUMMARY

Background The role of percutaneous transluminal coronary angioplasty (PTCA) in the management of patients with angina remains controversial, particularly in patients whose symptoms are adequately controlled by medical treatment.

Methods RITA-2 is a randomised trial comparing the long-term effects of PTCA and conservative (medical) care in patients with coronary artery disease considered suitable for either treatment option. 1018 patients were recruited from 20 cardiology centres in UK and Ireland. The 504 randomised to PTCA were intended to have dilatation within 3 months. The 514 assigned to medical treatment received antianginal drugs; those whose symptoms were not controlled by optimum medical therapy could cross-over to myocardial revascularisation. The primary endpoint was the combined frequency of death from all causes and definite non-fatal myocardial infarction.

Findings This report covers a median 2.7 years' follow-up. At randomisation 53% of patients had grade 2 or worse angina, and 40% had two or more diseased coronary arteries. 93% of patients randomised to PTCA had this procedure carried out, within a median of 5 weeks. Death or definite myocardial infarction occurred in 32 patients (6.3%) treated with PTCA and in 17 patients (3.3%) with medical care (absolute difference 3.0% [95% CI 0.4–5.7%], p=0.02). This difference was mainly due to one death and seven non-fatal myocardial infarctions related to the randomised procedures. There were 18 deaths (11 PTCA, seven medical) of which ten were not due to heart disease. Of the patients in the PTCA group, 40 (7.9%) required coronary artery bypass grafting (CABG), including nine instead of PTCA and seven emergencies following unsuccessful PTCA. 56 other PTCA Patients (11.1%) required further non-randomised PTCA. In the medical group 118 patients (23.0%) underwent a revascularisation procedure during follow-up, mostly because of worsening symptoms. Angina improved in both groups, but more so in the PTCA group. There was a 16.5% absolute excess of grade 2 or worse angina in the medical group 3 months after randomisation (p<0.001), which attenuated to 7.6% after 2 years. Total exercise time (Bruce protocol) also improved in both groups, again with a treatment difference in favour of PTCA: mean advantage of 35 s at 3 months (p<0–001). These benefits of PTCA were greater in patients with more severe angina at baseline, judged by high initial grade of angina and short initial exercise-time.

Interpretation In patients with coronary artery disease considered suitable for either PTCA or medical care, early intervention with PTCA was associated with greater symptomatic improvement, especially in patients with more severe angina. When managing individuals with angina, clinicians must balance these benefits against the small excess hazard associated with PTCA due to procedure-related complications.

INTRODUCTION

For patients with angina w o require revascularisation, randomised trials comparing the long-term effects of coronary angioplasty and coronary artery bypass surgery [1-3] have provided important information for clinical management. Randomised trials are also needed to determine whether patients in whom myocardial revascularisation is not essential should be treated by early angloplasty, or can have revascularisation deferred. The Veterans Administration Angioplasty Compared to Medicine trial[4] is relevant but had limited power to detect clinically important differences.

The second Randomised Intervention Treatment of Angina (RITA-2) trial was designed to compare the effects of initial strategies of coronary angioplasty and conservative (medical) care over at least 5 years' follow-up in patients deemed suitable for either treatment. We present the interim results of RITA-2 after a median 2.7 years' follow-up.

PATIENTS AND METHODS

Patients

Patients were recruited at 20 centres in the UK and Ireland. The ethics committee of each centre approved the protocol. Patients with coronary artery disease proven arteriographically were considered if the supervising cardiologist thought that both continued medical therapy and coronary angloplasty were acceptable alternatives. All eligible patients had a significant stenosis in at least one major epicardial vessel that appeared technically amenable to balloon dilatation.

11

Patients had to be over 18 years of age, but there was no upper age limit and patients of either sex were considered. Patients were not required to have current symptoms but patients with severe symptoms, were potentially eligible if they would consider an initial strategy of conservative therapy. Patients with multivessel disease, occluded coronary arteries, or impaired left ventricular function were eligible. Patients with recent unstable angina could also be included; this was defined as an episode of ischaemic chest pain associated with electrocardiographic changes with admission within the preceding 90 days, but entry was restricted to those whose most recent episode was at least 7 days before randomisation and who had not developed new pathological Q waves or increases in serum cardiac enzymes to twice normal.

Patients in whom early myocardial revascularisation (coronary angioplasty or coronary bypass surgery) was considered necessary for symptom relief or for prognostic benefit and patients with previous myocardial revascularisation, left main stem disease, or haemodynamically significant valve disease were not eligible. Patients with life-threatening non-cardiac disease likely to limit survival or have a major influence on compliance were not eligible.

During the recruitment phase, patients undergoing coronary arteriography under the care of the participating cardiologists were entered into a log. The main purpose of the log was to identify eligible patients, but since the log was not completely maintained in all centres we can only give estimated numbers screened and eligible. Across all centres, around 70 000 patients underwent coronary arteriography for any reason during the trial recruitment phase (figure 1). Of these, around 2750 were considered eligible for RITA-2, of whom 1018 (37%) were randomised. Clinician's subjective choice was inevitably a major contributor to deciding whether patients were eligible and whether to randomise or not. This may be the principal reason why recruitment was low. Of course, myocardial revascularisation is mandated on prognostic or symptomatic grounds for many patients who have undergone coronary arteriography. In addition, patients' refusal was the documented reason for about half the eligible patients who were not randomised. For all patients undergoing arteriography, the consequent planned treatment was declared to be medical (35%), percutaneous transluminal coronary angioplasty (PTCA) (19%), coronary artery bypass grafting (CABG) (35%), other (6%), or unknown (4%).

Before randomisation the coronary arteriograms of eligible patients were reviewed by an interventional cardiologist who identified at least one significant coronary lesion in a major epicardial vessel which would be dilated if the patient were assigned to treatment by angioplasty. A significant coronary lesion was defined as a 50% or greater diameter stenosis in at least two radiographic projections or 70% diameter stenosis in one projection. Major coronary vessels were defined as the

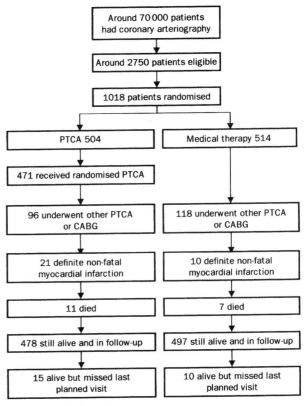

Figure 1: Trial profile

left anterior descending artery or large diagonal branches, and a circumflex artery or large obtuse marginal branches, and a balanced or dominant right coronary artery.

Patients who satisfied the eligibility criteria and provided informed consent to participate in the trial were randomised by telephone call to the Royal Free Hospital's coronary care unit. The randomisation used permuted blocks within strata defined by centre, by extent of disease (single vessel or multivessel), and whether the patient had had recent unstable angina.

Treatment

The protocol required that patients assigned to coronary angioplasty underwent dilatation of the prospectively identified stenosis or stenoses within 3 months of randomisation. Methods for PTCA were not standardised between centres but all angioplasty procedures had to be carried out by experienced operators, usually consultant interventional cardiologists or occasionally fully-trained senior cardiac registrars. There was no requirement for all coronary stenoses to be dilated, but multivessel dilatation could be staged over more than one procedure. In all cases the intended strategy was based on conventional balloon dilatation, but stents and other coronary interventional techniques (eg, coronary atherectomy) were permissible if the initial angioplasty result was unsatisfactory. Angioplasty of a coronary stenosis was considered successful if there was a reduction in stenosis severity of at least 20%, with less than 50% residual stenosis and good distal flow on the final arteriogram. Following intervention, medication was determined by individual clinical circumstances, but clinicians were encouraged to discontinue antianginal drugs for patients without angina. During follow-up, coronary arteriography and additional intervention procedures were carried out when indicated, with the objective of detecting and treating patients with restenosis. The trial did not reimburse centres for costs related to intervention procedures.

Patients assigned to initial medical therapy were prescribed antianginal medication for symptom relief. During follow-up, coronary arteriography was repeated only for compelling clinical reasons, and the indications for a change from the assigned non-interventional strategy were recorded on a cross-over form. The protocol required that myocardial revascularisation procedures were reserved for patients whose symptoms were not adequately controlled by optimal medical therapy, which usually included a b-adrenoceptor blocker, with a calcium antagonist and/or long-acting nitrate in maximally tolerated doses.

During the study all patients were treated with aspirin unless contraindicated. Patients were recruited before the results of randomised trials of the clinical effects of hydroxy-methylglutaryl co-enzyme A (HMG Co-A) reductase inhibitors were published,[5] and lipid-lowering drugs were prescribed at the discretion of the supervising clinician.

Data collection

Patients were assessed at baseline, and at 3 months, at 6 months, and yearly after randomisation. Demographic information, risk factors, and coronary arteriographic data were recorded at baseline. Left ventricular function was assessed from a right anterior oblique contrast left ventricular angiogram with a wallmotion score.[6] Contraction was scored on a six-point scale (normal=1, mild/moderate hypokinesia=2, severe hypokinesia=3, akinesia=4, dyskinesia=5, aneurysmal=6) for each of five left ventricular segments (anterobasal, anteroapical, apical, inferoapical, and inferobasal). The sum of the scores (ranging from 5–30) provided an index of overall left ventricular function.

The primary endpoint was defined as the combined frequency of death (from all causes) and definite non-fatal myocardial infarction. An independent event-validation committee reviewed all deaths and reported myocardial infarcts, blind to the patient's assigned treatment. The cause of death was classified as cardiac or non-cardiac. Definite myocardial infarction was diagnosed if new pathological Q waves (>30 ms in duration) appeared on an electrocardiogram within 7 days of any myocardial revascularisation procedure (procedure-related infarction) or during subsequent follow-up. Definite myocardial infarction was also diagnosed if a convincing clinical history was associated with electrocardiographic changes compatible with non-Q-wave infarction and the serum activities of at least two cardiac enzymes were above twice normal. Possible myocardial infarction was diagnosed within 7 days of

any myocardial revascularisation procedure or in association with a convincing clinical history if changes consistent with a diagnosis of non-Q-wave myocardial infarction appeared on a follow-up electrocardiogram or if the serum activities of at least two cardiac enzymes were above twice normal.

All major cardiovascular events and hospital admissions were documented. Unstable angina was defined as admission for ischaemic cardiac pain associated with electrocardiographic signs of myocardial ischaemia, but without elevation of serum cardiac enzymes or the appearance of new Q waves. Stroke was defined as a sudden focal disturbance of brain function of presumed vascular origin persisting longer than 24 hours. For transient stroke the clinical syndrome persisted less than 24 hours. Patients were considered to have developed cardiac failure if they required new maintenance drug therapy for heart failure. An arrhythmia occurring after randomisation was considered significant if the patient required new maintenance antiarrhythmic drug therapy or permanent pacemaker implantation.

Angina was assessed with the Canadian Cardiovascular Society classification,[7] and by documentation of antianginal drug use. Breathlessness and physical activity were assessed by ordinal scales.[2] Symptom-limited treadmill tests (Bruce protocol[8]) were carried out at 3 and 6 months and at 1 and 3 years after randomisation. Interim analyses were reviewed by the data-monitoring committee about every 6 months, each time with a recommendation that the trial continue as planned.

Statistics

The accrual target of 1400 patients was calculated on the basis of previous reports[9–12] which suggested that the combined 5-year rate of death and definite non-fatal myocardial infarction in the trial would be around 15%. A trial of this size would have 80% Power to detect a one-third reduction in the event rate in one treatment arm compared with the other at (two-sided) 5% significance. The recruitment rate was slower than anticipated, largely because the treatment policies were distinct, which makes the clinician's willingness and patient's consent to randomisation no easy matter. 1018 patients were randomised from July, 1992, to May, 1996, when accrual was terminated to avoid extension of recruitment beyond 4 years. Our trial has substantial power to provide precise comparison of the two treatment strategies for symptoms and exercise tolerance. All data were analysed according to the original treatment assignment (intention-to-treat).

RESULTS

1018 patients were randomised to coronary angioplasty (504) or continued medical treatment (514). This report concerns follow-up to Nov 30, 1996, which was complete for 98% of patients. Minimum and median follow-ups were 6 months and 2.7 years respectively.

11

Table 1

Patients' characteristics at randomisation

	PTCA (n=504)	Medical (n=514)	All patients (n=1018)
Diseased vessels			
1	311	300	611 (60%)
2	163	175	338 (33%)
3	30	39	69 (7%)
Recent unstable angina	47	52	99 (10%)
Angina grade			
None	103	97	200 (20%)
1	116	157	273 (27%)
2	180	154	334 (33%)
3	62	61	123 (12%)
4	43	43	86 (8%)
Antianginal drugs			
None	24	47	71 (7%)
1	217	195	412 (41%)
2	188	193	381 (37%)
3	74	79	153 (15%)
Current medication			
β-blocker	344	335	679 (67%)
Calcium antagonist	238	273	511 (50%)
Long-acting nitrate	233	210	443 (44%)
Aspirin	439	447	886 (87%)
Lipid-lowering drug	70	60	130 (13%)
ACE inhibitor	46	56	102 (10%)
Age (years)			
<50	101	106	207 (20%)
50–59	180	197	377 (37%)
60–69	190	181	371 (37%)
≥70	31	29	60 (6%)
Women	93	90	183 (18%)
Previous myocardial infarction	235	236	471 (47%)
On diabetic treatment	48	42	90 (9%)
Left ventricular score			
5	276	269	545 (54%)
6–9	194	201	395 (39%)
≥10	27	36	63 (6%)

ACE=angiotensin-converting enzyme.

Table 2

Deaths, myocardial infarctions, and new interventions during median 2.7 years' follow-up

	PTCA	Medical
Deaths		
All causes	11	7
Cardiac	5	3
Non-cardiac	6	4
Definite non-fatal myocardial infarctions*		
Total	21	10
Related to randomised PTCA	7	–
Related to other intervention	3	2
Other	11	8
Possible non-fatal myocardial infarctions*		
Total	3	5
Related to randomised PTCA	1	—
Related to other intervention	1	1
Other	1	4
Patients with primary endpoint (death or definite myocardial infarction)	32	17
Subsequent interventions		
Non-randomised PTCA	62	101
CABG	40	30
Coronary arteriography	133	92

*Each patient is included only once.

Baseline comparability

Overall, there was close similarity between patients randomised to PTCA and medical treatment (table 1). The median age was 58 years and 18% were women. Angina grade 3 or worse (marked limitation of ordinary physical activity) was present in 21% of patients. A fifth of patients reported no anginal symptoms at the time of randomisation but since all patients had undergone coronary arteriography most would have had symptoms earlier. During the 3 months before randomisation 16% had been admitted with angina. A previous myocardial infarction had occurred in 47% of patients, 22% of these being within the previous 3 months.

Randomised PTCA

The intended randomised PTCA was performed in 471 (93%) of patients in the PTCA group. Reasons for not undergoing PTCA in the other 33 were: lesion regression (12), symptomatic improvement (four), disease progression (ten, of whom nine underwent CABG), patient refused (seven).

The median time from randomisation to PTCA was 5 weeks; 5% of PTCAs were done within a week and 91% within 12 weeks of randomisation. In total, angioplasty was attempted in 642 vessel segments of which 93% were successfully dilated. A single-vessel segment was treated in 335 patients with 92% success. 107 and 29 patients, respectively, had two and three or more vessel segments treated, with all segments successfully dilated in 86% and 90% of such patients, respectively. Dilatation was attempted in 65 occluded vessels with 69% success.

Patients' recruitment began before the widespread use of coronary stents, which were used during 12 (4%) of the 311 randomised PTCAs during 1992–94 compared with 32 (20%) of the 160 randomised PTCAs during 1995–96.

PTCA was complicated by emergency CABG in seven patients (1.5%), including two in whom stents were inserted. Another patient underwent elective CABG before discharge from hospital. The median length of hospital stay for the group randomised to angioplasty was 3 days, with 15% staying only 1 day and 8% over a week.

Death and myocardial infarction

During follow-up, 18 patients have died: 11 (2.2%) in the PTCA group and seven (1.4%) in the medical group (table 2, p=0.32).

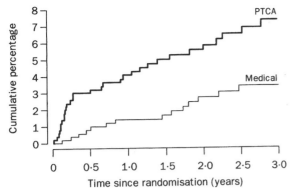

Figure 2 *Cumulative risk of death or definite myocardial infarction*

Number of patients

PTCA	504	488	437	390	324	254	181
Medical	514	509	468	411	345	276	209

The five cardiac deaths in the PTCA group included a randomised-procedure-related death from severe haemorrhagic complications of standard-dose heparin, a death due to complications of CABG following non-randomised PTCA, two sudden deaths 12 weeks and 2 years after PTCA, and a death from myocardial infarction 46 weeks after randomisation in a patient not undergoing PTCA because of lesion regression. The three cardiac deaths in the medical group were sudden in two and followed myocardial infarction in one patient.

There were 21 and ten definite non-fatal myocardial infarctions in the PTCA and medical groups, respectively, this difference being largely explained by the seven randomised-procedure-related infarcts in the PTCA group (for two of whom stents were inserted). Three of the other definite infarcts in the PTCA group were related to later non-randomised PTCA or CABG. During follow-up, death or definite myocardial infarction occurred in 32 PTCA patients (6.3%) and 17 medical patients (3.3%) (figure 2, table 2). The relative risk was 1.92 with 95% CI 1.08 to 3.41 (p=0.02). The absolute treatment difference in risk of death and myocardial infarction was 3.0% (95% CI 0.4–5.7%).

Subsequent interventions

Since randomisation, 40 patients randomised to PTCA (7.9%) and 30 patients randomised to medical treatment (5.8%) had a CABG (table 2). This includes the seven

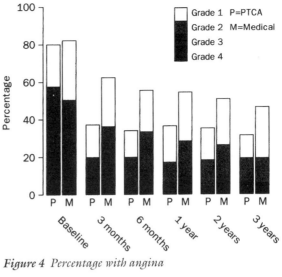

Figure 4 *Percentage with angina*

Number of patients

PTCA	504	503	501	448	333	188
Medical	514	514	513	471	348	206

emergency CABGs following the randomised PTCA and the nine CABGs performed instead of the intended randomised PTCA mentioned earlier. Three patients (two PTCA, one medical) underwent a second CABG. Figure 3 shows the accumulating risk of death, myocardial infarction, or CABG for patients randomised to PTCA and medical treatment. The combined risk after 2 years' follow-up was 12.3% and 7.1% in the PTCA and medical groups, respectively. Additional non-randomised PTCA has been required in 62 patients randomised to PTCA of whom six also had CABG. The estimated life-table risk of requiring repeat PTCA or CABG within a year of the initial randomised PTCA was 14.9%.

In the medical group, 101 patients subsequently underwent PTCA of whom 13 also needed CABG. The accumulating risks of PTCA together with death, myocardial infarction, and CABG are also shown in figure 3. The risk of requiring PTCA or CABG within a year of randomisation was 15.4%. Most of the medical group "cross-overs" to PTCA or CABG were because the patient's angina was not adequately controlled by medical therapy. Of the 117 medical group patients who have undergone revascularisation, 75% had grade 3 or 4 angina and 83% were taking two or more antianginal

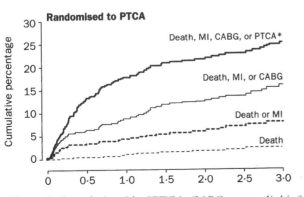

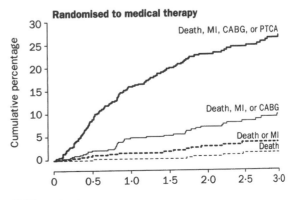

Figure 3 *Cumulative risk of PTCA, CABG, myocardial infarction (MI), or death*

*in addition to randomised PTCA.

Table 3

Secondary events during follow-up*

Event	Total	Time since randomisation		
		Within 3 months	3 months to 1 year	Over 1 year
Unstable angina				
PTCA	50	18	20	21
Medical	47	14	20	21
Cardiac failure				
PTCA	8	3	5	1
Medical	15	5	5	6
Arrhythmia				
PTCA	15	5	6	4
Medical	7	1	7	3
Stroke				
PTCA	1	1	0	0
Medical	6	2	3	4
Transient stroke				
PTCA	1	0	0	1
Medical	5	0	0	5

*Entry in each cell refers to number of patients experiencing event in that period.

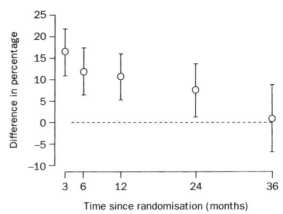

***Figure 5** Difference in percentage with grade 2 or worse angina*

Medical minus PTCA, 95% CI.

drugs at the time of change in treatment strategy. As for the randomised procedures, the use of coronary stents during non-randomised PTCA increased by calendar year: 9/95 (9%) in 1993–94, 16/59 (27%) in 1995, and 15/32 (47%) in 1996.

Secondary events

The occurrence of other clinical events is shown overall and in three time bands: first 3 months, rest of the year, and beyond a year since randomisation (table 3). The pattern of unstable angina was similar in both randomised groups (9.5%). Cardiac failure was slightly more common in the medical group (p=0.15) while arrhythmias were more frequent in the PTCA group (p=0.08). The incidence of stroke and transient stroke was low, each with a non-significantly greater rate in the medical group.

Angina and breathlessness

Throughout follow-up there was a substantial improvement in reported angina in both groups, but this improvement was significantly greater in the PTCA group (figure 4). This treatment difference was greater early on (figure 5), with a 16.5% excess of grade 2+ angina in the medical group 3 months after randomisation (p<0.001). After 2 years' follow-up, the medical group had only a 7.6% excess of grade 2+ angina (p=0.02), which represents a significant attenuation in the treatment difference over these 21 months (p=0.05).

This trend can be partly explained by the fact that patients with worsening symptoms underwent cardiac interventions subsequently in both treatment groups. For instance, in the medical group, of the 68 patients reporting grade 2+ angina at 3 months who improved

to less than grade 2 at 2 years, 26 (38%) underwent PTCA and/or CABG in the intervening 21 months. Similarly, in the PTCA group, of the 42 patients experiencing the same improvement, 12 (29%) had had a coronary intervention meantime.

Centres differed in the baseline rate of angina grade 2 or more (heterogeneity test, p<0.001), which reflects differences in attitude as to what severity of angina was appropriate for inclusion in RITA-2. However, there was no evidence of between-centre heterogeneity in the treatment difference in angina frequency at 3 months (p=0.12), although such a test inevitably lacks statistical power.

Patients in the medical group had greater use of antianginal drugs during follow-up compared with patients in the PTCA group (table 4). Even so the use of triple-drug therapy never exceeded 20% in the medical group, and over two-thirds of PTCA patients were still taking at least one antianginal drug after 2 years' follow-up. There was no difference between the

Table 4

Antianginal medication

Time since randomisation	Number	Number of antianginal drugs			
		None	1	2	3
3 months					
PTCA	501	99 (20%)	218	132	52 (10%)
Medical	508	36 (7%)	184	195	93 (18%)
6 months					
PTCA	499	115 (23%)	223	122	39 (8%)
Medical	508	37 (7%)	170	206	95 (19%)
1 year					
PTCA	144	112 (25%)	199	100	33 (7%)
Medical	466	45 (10%)	155	193	73 (16%)
2 years					
PTCA	328	101 (31%)	136	66	25 (8%)
Medical	343	43 (13%)	111	137	52 (15%)
3 years					
PTCA	188	68 (36%)	73	36	11 (6%)
Medical	203	28 (14%)	67	78	30 (15%)

Table 5

Angina grade and exercise time at 6 months

Baseline feature	Number*	Angina grade 2+ at 6 months (%)		Mean (SE) exercise time at 6 months	
		PTCA	Medical	PTCA	Medical
Angina grade at baseline					
0 or 1	473	13.8	17.4	9.16 (0.18)	9.25 (0.19)
2	334	20.6	42.4	8.79 (0.21)	7.86 (0.23)
3 or 4	209	36.5	57.8	8.44 (0.29)	7.45 (0.29)
Exercise time at baseline (min)					
<6	263	23.2	45.5	6.85 (0.24)	5.87 (0.20)
6–9	359	19.6	35.4	8.88 (0.17)	8.15 (0.15)
9	332	19.5	19.9	10.49 (0.17)	10.92 (0.18)
Sex					
Male	835	20.5	31.4	9.34 (0.13)	8.90 (0.15)
Female	183	22.8	39.8	6.72 (0.25)	6.52 (0.26)
Age years)					
<60	584	20.9	31.0	9.54 (0.16)	9.19 (0.17)
≥60	431	20.7	35.7	8.04 (0.18)	7.48 (0.20)

*For simplicity, this combines both treatment groups. Angina grade at 6 months and exercise time at 6 months were not reported for 9 and 118 patients, respectively.

two treatment groups in the use of aspirin or lipid-lowering drugs during follow-up.

During follow-up, breathlessness was reduced in the PTCA group (42% at 3 months *vs* 57% in the medical group, P<0–001). Similarly, severe breathlessness (defined as breathless when walking at own pace, washing, dressing, or at rest) was less common in the PTCA group compared with the medical group at 3 months (13% *vs* 17%, p=0.04) but these differences became less marked over time.

There was no significant difference in reported physical activity. Also the rates of unemployment due to coronary disease did not differ between the PTCA and medical groups, staying at around 25% for men aged under 65 at randomisation throughout 2 years' follow-up.

Exercise testing

The Bruce test was performed in about 90% of patients at each follow-up. At baseline, the mean exercise time was 7 min 41 s in both groups (SD 2 min 47 s). Figure 6 shows the mean changes in exercise time in relation to baseline. After 3 months the PTCA group had a larger improvement in exercise time compared with the medical group, mean difference 35 s (95% CI 20–51 s), but this attenuated (non-significantly) to 25 s (7–42 s) by 1 year. At 3 months, the numbers of patients who improved their exercise time by over 2 min compared with baseline were 124 (30%) and 74 (17%) in the PTCA and medical groups, respectively.

Subgroup analyses

The most striking findings are the strong influences of baseline grade of angina and baseline exercise time on the treatment differences (table 5). For patients with baseline angina grade 2 or more there was a marked benefit of PTCA at 6 months with a 20% lower frequency of angina and a 1-min longer mean exercise time than in the medical group patients. By contrast, for patients with no angina or grade 1 angina at baseline, there was negligible difference between PTCA and medical policies (Interaction tests for angina and exercise outcomes, respectively, p=0.03 and p=0.01). Similarly the beneficial effects of PTCA on angina and exercise times at 6 months were confined to patients with a baseline exercise time of 9 min or less (interaction tests for angina and exercise outcomes, respectively, p=0.007 and p<0.001).

We simultaneously analysed the influences of angina grade and exercise time at baseline on these treatment differences at 6 months. The benefits of PTCA over medical treatment were largely concentrated in patients with both severe angina and poor exercise time at baseline. For the 366 patients with both angina grade 2 or more and exercise time of 9 min or less at baseline, the frequency of angina grade 2 or more at 6 months was 27.6% greater in the medical group than in the PTCA group. By contrast, for the 183 patients with both angina grade 0 or 1 and exercise time over 9 min at baseline, the medical group had 1.6% fewer patients with angina grade 2 or more at 6 months. For patients in an intermediate situation (either angina grade 2 or more at baseline or exercise time of 9 min or under at baseline), the medical group had 8.0% more patients with angina grade 2 or more at 6 months. A similar pattern of differential treatment effects emerged when we analysed mean exercise time at 6 months by baseline exercise time and baseline grade of angina. These results were confirmed by multiple logistic regression analysis of angina outcome and quantitative multiple-regression analyses of exercise time outcome.

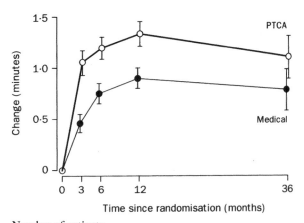

Number of patients

PTCA	469	418	425	369	154
Medical	485	446	436	399	177

Figure 6 *Changes in Bruce exercise times*
Mean and SE.

There were no significant interactions between treatment and six other baseline features: age, sex, number of diseased vessels, recent unstable angina, previous myocardial infarction, and left ventricular abnormality. Mean exercise times were substantially lower in women and older patients in both treatment groups. There were insufficient data for reliable evaluation of the primary endpoint by such subgroups.

DISCUSSION

RITA-2 was designed to compare initial policies of PTCA and medical care in patients with coronary artery disease in whom both treatments were deemed acceptable. Our patients ranged from those with no angina and single-vessel disease to those with severe symptoms and multivessel disease. Most had mild symptoms, one-vessel or two-vessel disease and preserved left-ventricular-function scores, and would be predicted to be at low cardiovascular risk.[6,13,14] The patients were therefore not representative of all patients undergoing percutaneous coronary intervention, but represented a substantial group for whom medical therapy or angioplasty appear appropriate and for whom optimal treatment has been uncertain.

After 2.7 years, the PTCA group had a significantly greater risk of death or non-fatal infarction, the main endpoint. Even so, the absolute risk was low in both groups (3.3% in the medical arm versus 6.3% in the PTCA arm), and most of this difference occurred within 3 months of randomisation.

The randomised PTCA procedures were carried out with high success and low complication rates, with one procedure-related death (0.2%). RITA-2 lacks statistical power to detect small but potentially important differences in long-term mortality. Indeed, having recruited fewer patients than intended, we had reduced power for the main endpoint, which was nevertheless statistically significant.

RITA-2 patients were not systematically screened for myocardial infarction, and small procedure-related

infarcts, which may be associated with increased cardiovascular risk,[15] were not included in the main endpoint. The true infarct rate in RITA-2 may therefore have been underestimated.

The excess risk of definite non-fatal infarction in the PTCA group was mainly due to procedure-related events but might also be partly explained by closer supervision of the PTCA patients. We doubt that this inevitable difference in follow-up could result in substantial bias. The risk of unheralded myocardial infarction in the medical group was low, although all patients had a significant coronary stenosis in a major epicardial artery. These data are consistent with evidence that myocardial infarction is often not due to pre-existing flow-limiting stenoses.[16,17] To date, the RITA-2 results provide no evidence to support the widely held belief that successful PTCA of a severe coronary stenosis reduces the risk of myocardial infarction. We await the long-term survival effects of the excess of non-fatal infarcts among PTCA Patients, but a detrimental effect on prognosis is plausible.

The prognostic advantage of revascularisation by PTCA or CABG in ACIP[18] may reflect the fact that the patients were at higher cardiovascular risk, as judged by age and disease severity, than our patients. Moreover, 41% of patients assigned to revascularisation underwent coronary bypass surgery, which has prognostic advantages in particular groups.[13,14]

We demonstrated that PTCA improves symptoms (angina and breathlessness), reduces the requirement for antianginal medication, and improves exercise tolerance compared with medical therapy. These differences attenuated over 2–3 years' follow-up, partly because the patients with severe symptoms in the medical group eventually underwent myocardial revascularisation. Symptomatic improvement in the medical group may also be partly due to modification of antianginal therapy, disease regression, development of coronary collaterals, and regression to the mean. In the PTCA group the initial decrease in the occurrence of angina was maintained over 3 years, but during this period additional revascularisation procedures were carried out in over a fifth of these patients.

Subgroup analyses indicated that the beneficial effects of PTCA on angina and exercise tolerance are greatest in patients with severe symptoms or limited exercise tolerance at baseline; these findings have important implications for management. Patients without severe angina initially did not gain substantial symptomatic benefit from PTCA, and one might argue that in these patients revascularisation may reasonably be deferred unless more severe symptoms supervene. Moreover, exercise tolerance did not improve appreciably in patients with good exercise tolerance at baseline, and since these patients are at low cardiovascular risk[19,20] they are unlikely to gain major prognostic advantage from coronary angioplasty. For patients with more severe symptoms or impaired exercise tolerance, PTCA seems more warranted, but the beneficial effects must be balanced against the small procedure-related hazard. These observations suggest that the current clinical enthusiasm for early PTCA in low-risk cohorts in some countries needs to be reappraised.

Other small trials have also compared the effects of PTCA and medical treatment.[4,21-23] None has sufficient power to compare the two strategies for risk of death or myocardial infarction, but their results could be combined with RITA-2 in a meta-analysis.

Since RITA-2 began in 1992 there have been important advances in the medical and interventional treatment of patients with coronary artery disease. HMG CoA reductase inhibitors reduce cardiovascular risk in patients with coronary artery disease,[5,24] and the use of these drugs increased during RITA-2.

Nevertheless, more aggressive use of lipid-lowering therapy in both groups might have resulted in better prognosis with fewer additional revascularisation procedures. Glycoprotein IIb/IIIa receptor blockers [25,26] and coronary stents [27-30] improve the acute and long-term results of coronary interventions. The use of stents increased during RITA-2 reflecting routine clinical practice in the UK and other countries. In some centres, stents are used in 50–70% of percutaneous coronary interventions, but the long-term implications of such a policy are unknown.

By addressing the balance between symptomatic benefit and procedure-related risk, RITA-2 has helped to define optimal treatment strategies for an important subgroup of patients with angina.

Contributors

Executive and writing committee: DA Chamberlain, KAA Fox, RA Henderson, DG Julian, DJ Parker, SJ Pocock.
Data monitoring committee: TW Meade, SM Cobbe, SJW Evans, JR Hampton.
Endpoint validation committee: M D Joy, S Holmberg, D B Shaw.
Statistical coordinating centre: T Clayton, C Marley, SJ Pocock, B Youard.

RITA-2 trialists

C Ilsley, T Farrel, V Paul, R Knight (Harefield Hospital, Middlesex, 168 patients randomised); N Brooks, D Bennett, C Bray, R Levy, C Ward, T Coppinger (Wythenshawe Hospital, Manchester, 130); C Pumphrey, S Brecker, D Ward, A-M Murtagh (St George's Hospital, London, 102); C Bucknall, D Brennand-Roper, J Chambers, R Cooke, G Jackson, P Holt, N Sulke, K Tan, S Karani (Guy's Hospital, London, 95); DB O'Keefe, JG Murtagh, SG Richardson, ME Scott, S Graffin (Belfast City Hospital, 74); R Balcon, C Layton, P Mills, M Rothman, A Timmis, C Atkins (London Chest Hospital, 64); AF Mackintosh, H Larkin, RV Lewis, JB Stoker, LB Tan, GJ Williams, Y Brown (Killingbeck Hospital, Leeds, 59); J Pitts-Crick, E Barnes, P Borcham, R Chamberlain-Webber, M Papouchado, M Halestrap, J Tagney (Bristol Royal Infirmary, 52); RH Swanton, JM Walker, E Firman (Middlesex Hospital, London, 46); D Reid, PC Adams, R Bexton, K Evemy, S Furniss, D Williams, A McDermott (Freeman Hospital, Newcastle upon Tyne, 42); D Jewitt, P Richardson, M Thomas, RJ Wainwright, A Jacob, (King's College Hospital, London, 38); B Maurer, A Buckley, E Dinn, F Begley (St Vincent's Hospital, Dublin, 31); R Watson, SP Singh, L Cadd (City Hospital, Birmingham, 29); R Perry, G Epstein, R Carey (Broadgreen Hospital, Liverpool, 24); P Crean, N Ghaisas, D Hughes (St James's Hospital, Dublin, 21); D Dymond, S Banim, A W Nathan, R A J Spurrell, H Jones, J Elstob (St Bartholomew's Hospital, London, 18); B Gribbin, C Forfar, O Ormerod, T Longney (John Radcliffe Hospital, Oxford, 17); H Gray, K Dawkins, J Seymour, I Simpson, M McGuirk (Southampton General Hospital, 5), MF Shiu (Walsgrave Hospital, Coventry, 2); D Sugrue, B Egan, B Holigan (Mater Misericordiae Hospital, Dublin, 1).

Acknowledgments

We thank the 1018 patients who participated in the trial. We also acknowledge the dedicated work of Bronwen Youard (trial co-ordinator 1992–96), and the Royal Free Hospital's coronary care unit, which provided the randomisation service. The trial was supported by grants from the British Heart Foundation and the Medical Research Council. Additional financial support was provided by Advanced Cardiovascular Systems Inc (USA), Intervention Ltd (UK), Cordis Ltd, Schneider (UK), and Nycomed Ltd.

References

1 The Bypass Angioplasty Revascularization Investigation (BARI) investigators. Comparison of coronary bypass surgery with angioplasty in patients with multivessel disease. *N Engl J Med* 1996; **335**: 217–25.

2 RITA trial participants. Coronary angioplasty versus coronary artery bypass surgery: the Randomised Intervention Treatment of Angina (RITA) trial. *Lancet* 1993; **341**: 573–80.

3 Pocock SJ, Henderson RA, Rickards AF, *et al*. Meta-analysis of randomised trials comparing coronary angioplasty with bypass surgery. *Lancet* 1995; **346**: 1184–89.

4 Folland ED, Hartigan PM, Parisi AF. Percutaneous transluminal coronary angioplasty versus medical therapy for stable angina pectoris: outcomes for patients with double-vessel versus single-vessel coronary artery disease in a Veterans Affairs Cooperative Randomized Trial. *J Am Coll Cardiol* 1997; **29**: 1505–11.

5 Scandinavian simvastatin survival study group. Randomised trial of cholesterol lowering in 4444 patients with coronary heart disease: the Scandinavian simvastatin survival study (4S). *Lancet* 1994; **344**: 1383–89.

6 Ringqvist I, Fisher LD, Mock M, *et al*. Prognostic value of angiographic indices of coronary artery disease from the coronary artery surgery study. *J Clin Invest* 1983; **71**: 1854–66.

7 Campeau L. Grading of angina pectoris. *Circulation* 1976; **54**: 522–23.

8 Bruce RA, Blackman JR, Jones JW, Strait G. Exercise testing in adult normal subjects and cardiac patients. *Pediatrics* 1963; **32**: 742.

9 Califf RM, Tomabechi Y, Lee KL, *et al*. Outcome in one-vessel coronary artery disease. *Circulation* 1983; **67**: 283–90.

10 Hlatky MA, Califf RM, Kong Y, Harrell FE, Rosati RA. Natural history of patients with single vessel disease suitable for percutaneous transluminal coronary angioplasty. *Am J Cardiol* 1983; **52**: 225–29.

11

[11] Ellis SG, Fisher L, Dushman-Ellis S, *et al.* Comparison of coronary angioplasty with medical treatment for single- and double-vessel disease with left anterior descending coronary involvement: long-term outcome based on an Emory-CASS registry study. *Am Heart J* 1989; **118**: 208–20.

[12] Alderman EL, Bourassa MG, Cohen LS, *et al.* Ten-year follow-up of survival and myocardial infarction in the randomised coronary artery surgery study. *Circulation* 1990; **82**: 1629–46.

[13] Yusuf S, Zucker D, Peduzzi P, *et al.* Effect of coronary artery bypass graft surgery on survival: overview of 10-year results from randomised trials by the Coronary Artery Bypass Graft Surgery Trialists Collaboration. *Lancet* 1994; **344**: 563–70.

[14] Jones RH, Kesler K, Phillips HR, *et al.* Long-term survival benefits of coronary artery bypass grafting and percutaneous transluminal angioplasty in patients with coronary artery disease. *J Thor Cardiovas Surg* 1996; **111**: 1013–25.

[15] Abdelmegid AE, Ellis SG, Sapp SK, Whitlow PL, Topol EJ. Defining the appropriate threshold of creatine kinase elevation after percutaneous coronary interventions. *Am Heart J* 1996; **131**: 1097–105.

[16] Giroud D, Li JM, Urban P, *et al.* Relation of the site of acute myocardial infarction to the most severe coronary arterial stenosis at prior angiography. *Am J Cardiol* 1992; **69**: 729–32.

[17] Nobuyoshi M, Tanaka M, Nosaka H, *et al.* Progression of coronary atherosclerosis: is coronary spasm related to progression? *J Am Coll Cardiol* 1991; **18**: 904–10.

[18] Davies RF, Goldberg AD, Forman S, *et al.* Asymptomatic cardiac ischaemia pilot (ACIP) study two-year follow-up: outcomes of patients randomized to initial strategies of medical therapy versus revascularization. *Circulation* 1997; **95**: 2037–43.

[19] Weiner DA, Ryan TJ, McCabe CH, *et al.* Prognostic importance of a clinical profile and exercise test in medically treated patients with coronary artery disease. *J Am Coll Cardiol* 1984; **3**: 772–79.

[20] Mark DB, Hlatky MA, Harrell FE, Lee KL, Califf RM, Pryor DB. Exercise treadmill score for predicting prognosis in coronary artery disease. *Ann Intern Med* 1987; **106**: 793–800.

[21] Hueb W, Bellotti G, Almeida de Oliveira S, *et al.* The medicine, angioplasty or surgery study (MASS): a prospective, randomised trial of medical therapy, balloon angioplasty or bypass surgery for single proximal left anterior descending artery stenoses. *J Am Coll Cardiol* 1995; **25**: 1600–05.

[22] Sievers B, Hamm CW, Herzner A, Kuck KH. Medical therapy versus PTCA: a prospective, randomized trial in patients with asymptomatic coronary single vessel disease. *Circulation* 1993; **88**: I–296 (abstr).

[23] Pansi AF, Folland ED, Hartigan P, on behalf of the Veterans Affairs ACME Investigators. A comparison of angioplasty with medical therapy in the treatment of single-vessel coronary artery disease. *N Engl J Med* 1992; **326**: 10–16.

[24] Sacks FM, Pfeffer MA, Moyé LA, *et al.* The effect of pravastatin on coronary events after myocardial infarction in patients with average cholesterol levels. *N Engl J Med* 1996, **335**: 1001–09.

[25] IMPACT-II Investigators. Randomised placebo-controlled trial of effect of eptifibatide on complications of percutaneous coronary intervention: IMPACT-II. *Lancet* 1997; **349**: 1422–28.

[26] EPILOG Investigators. Platelet glycoprotein IIb/IIIa receptor blockade and low dose heparin during percutaneous coronary revascularization. *N Engl J Med* 1997; **336**: 1689–96.

[27] Serruys PW, de Jaegere P, Kiemeneij F, *et al.* A comparison of balloon-expandable-stent implantation with balloon angioplasty in patients with coronary artery disease. *N Engl J Med* 1994; **331**: 489–95.

[28] Fischman DL, Leon MB, Baim DS, *et al.* A randomized comparison of coronary-stent placement and balloon angioplasty in the treatment of coronary artery disease. *N Engl J Med* 1994; **331**: 496–501.

[29] Simes PA, Golf S, Myreng Y, *et al.* Stenting in chronic coronary occlusion (SICCO): a randomized controlled trial of adding stent implantation after successful angioplasty. *J Am Coll Cardiol* 1996, **28**: 1444–51.

[30] Versaci F, Gaspardone A, Tomai F, Crea F, Chiariello L, Gioffrè PA. A comparison of coronary-artery stenting with angioplasty for isolated stenosis of the proximal left anterior descending coronary artery. *N Engl J Med* 1997; **336**: 817–22.

11

This article was first published in Family Practice and is reproduced by permission of Oxford University Press

EMPOWERING RESEARCH:
STATISTICAL POWER IN GENERAL PRACTICE RESEARCH

Nick Fox and Nigel Mathers

Family Practice 1997; **14**: 324–329.

Received 16 December 1996; Accepted 3 April 1997.

Institute of General Practice and Primary Care, School of Health and Related Research, University of Sheffield.

Correspondence to N Fox at Community Sciences Centre, Northern General Hospital, Herries Road, Sheffield S5 7AU, UK.

Background. Statistical power is a measure of the extent to which a study is capable of discerning differences or associations which exist within the population under investigation, and is of critical importance whenever a hypothesis is tested by statistics. Conventionally, studies should reach a power level of 0.8, such that four times out of five a false null hypothesis will be rejected by a study. Statistical power may most easily be increased by increasing sample size.
Objective. We aimed to assess the level of statistical power of general practice research.
Methods. A total of 1422 statistical tests in 85 quantitative original papers in the *British Journal of General Practice* were analysed for statistical power.
Results. The median power of tests analysed was 0.71, representing a slightly greater than two-thirds likelihood of rejecting false null hypotheses. Of 85 studies, 37 (44%) attained power of 0.8 or more. Ten studies had power of more than 0.99 suggesting 'over-powering'. Twenty-one of the papers surveyed (25%) had a likelihood of gaining significant results poorer than that obtained by tossing a coin when a null hypothesis is false.
Conclusion. While achieving higher power than studies in similar surveys of other disciplines, the power of general practice research fails short of the 0.8 convention. Adequate power is essential so that effects which exist are not missed. Recommendations are made concerning power calculations prior to the start of research and reporting of results in journal articles.
Keywords. General practice research, research publication, sampling, statistical power.

INTRODUCTION

In quantitative research, decisions about sample size are crucial. Purely at the level of resource costs, the size of sample has an impact: achieving larger sample sizes generally entails increased costs in terms of staffing for data collection and analysis, and other research expenses. In addition, certain research topics will impose their own constraints about the size of sample which can realistically be achieved. For example, a study based upon a single GP patient population may face diminishing numbers of respondents who may be recruited when a condition is relatively uncommon or a particular treatment regimen is undertaken. Even where an initial sample size is quite large, subsequent stratifications by factors such as gender and age may soon reduce the sample to small numbers.

The objective of tests of statistical inference is to generalize study findings to the population under investigation. Statistical tests of differences between groups or associations between variables seek to disprove a null hypothesis (H_0) which states that there is no difference or no association within the population. If a null hypothesis can be rejected, it means that some difference or some association may be inferred from the study to the wider population. However, the potential for a statistical test to disprove a null hypothesis depends upon the power of the study, and as such, statistical power is crucial to quantitative research. The need for a study to possess adequate power can be illustrated by considering the four situations which can arise when the data from a study are analysed using statistical tests of inference. These are illustrated in Figure 1.

Each cell in the figure represents a possible relationship between the findings of the study and the 'real-life' situation in the population under investigation (but which of course cannot be known other than through statistical inference). Cells 1 and 4 represent desirable outcomes, while cells 2 and 3 represent potential outcomes of a study which are undesirable and need to be minimized.

POPULATION

Null Hypothesis is:	False	True
S **False**	Correct Result	Type I Error (alpha)
T **U** **D** **Y** **True**	Type II Error (beta)	Correct Result

Figure 1 The null hypothesis (H_0) statistical significance and statistical power

Cell 1

The null hypothesis has been disproved by the results of the study (that is, there is support for a hypothesis which suggests some differences between groups or association between variables). This is also the situation in the population. Thus, we can be satisfied that the study is reflecting the world outside the limits of the study and it is to be accepted as a 'correct' result.

Cell 4

The results from the study support the null hypothesis. This is the situation which pertains in the population, so we can be satisfied that our study reflects the circumstances in the population. Once again, this is a 'correct' result.

Cell 2

In this cell, as in cell 1, the study results falsify the null hypothesis, indicating some kind of difference or association between variables. However, in the world beyond the study, the null hypothesis is actually true and there is no effect. This is known as a Type I error: the error of wrongly rejecting a true null hypothesis. The likelihood of committing a Type I error is known as the alpha (a) value or the statistical significance of the test. Many readers will be more familiar with alpha as the quoted *P* level of significance of a test. The *P* value marks the probability of committing a Type I error; thus a *P* value of 0.05 indicates a 5% (or 1 in 20) chance of committing a Type I error. Cell 2 thus reflects an incorrect finding from a study, and the alpha value represents the likelihood of this occurring.

Cell 3

This cell similarly reflects an undesirable outcome of a study. Here, as in Cell 4, a study supports the null hypothesis, implying that there is no difference or association in the population under investigation. But in reality, the null hypothesis is false and there is some kind of difference or association which the study is missing. This mistake is known as a Type II error and is the error of wrongly accepting a false null hypothesis. The likelihood of committing a Type II error is the beta value of a statistical test, the complement $(1-\beta)$ is the statistical power of the test. Thus, the statistical power of a test is the likelihood of avoiding a Type II error

when the null hypothesis is false. Conventionally, a value of 0.80 or 80% is the target value for statistical power, representing a likelihood that four times out of five a false null hypothesis will be correctly rejected. Outcomes of studies which fall into cell 3 are incorrect; β, or its complement power are the measures of the likelihood of such an outcome of a study.

All research should seek to avoid both Type I and Type II errors, which lead to incorrect inferences about the world beyond the study. In practice, there is a trade-off. Reducing the likelihood of committing a Type I error by increasing the level of significance at which one is willing to accept a positive finding reduces the statistical power of the test, increasing the possibility of a Type II error, and vice versa. However, both statistical significance and statistical power are affected by sample size. While researchers are usually aware that the chances of gaining a significant result will depend on the size of a study's sample, explicit power calculations are often not undertaken prior to the start of a study, and the evidence from various fields of study is that many studies do not meet the 0.8 conventional target for power.[1-4] Such under-powered studies have much reduced likelihoods of being able to discern the effects which they set out to seek: a study with a power of 0.66 will only detect an effect two times out of three, while studies with power of 0.5 or less will detect effects at levels less frequent than those achieved by tossing a coin. A non-significant finding of a study may thus simply reflect the inadequate power of the study to detect differences or associations at levels which are conventionally accepted as statistically significant.

Statistical power calculations can be undertaken after a study has been completed, and this paper reports such analyses on general practice research. More importantly, such calculations need to be undertaken prior to a study to avoid both the wasteful consequences of under-powering, and of overpowering in which sample sizes are excessively large, leading to very high power at the expense of higher than necessary study costs.

Power is a function of three variables: the level of significance (α) the effect size (the measure of 'how wrong' a null. hypothesis is),[4] and the sample size.

While calculation of power entails recourse to tables of values for these variables, the calculation is relatively straightforward in most cases.

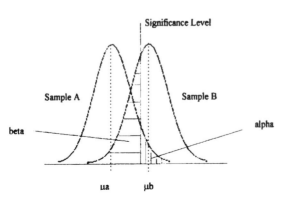

Figure 2 *The risk of Type I and Type II errors for* α = 0.05

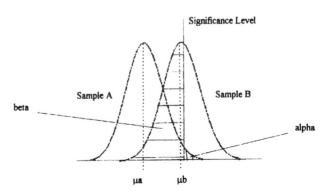

Figure 3 *The risk of Type I and Type II errors for* α = 0.01

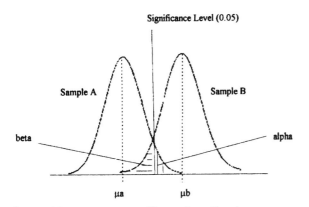

Figure 4 Impact on power of increasing effect size

Firstly, power depends on the level of statistical significance chosen by the researchers. The more stringent the level of significance chosen, the lower the power. The trade-off between significance and power is illustrated by Figures 2 and 3 which represent the distributions of two differing samples A and B, for instance the heights of female and male adults. If the mean of population A is *ma* and that of population B is μb, then the null hypothesis that there is no difference between population means, H_0: $\mu a = \mu b$, while the hypothesis that the mean of B is greater than that of A, H_1: $\mu b > \mu a$.

In Figure 2, the one-tailed a value of 0.05 has been selected and is represented by the vertical cut-off line. By drawing this line we are saying that all scores to the right of this line come from sample B. In this example, we are likely to be right much of the time. However, the scores to the right of this cut-off line include the shaded portion containing 5% of sample A scores. At this level of significance, 5% of sample A is likely to be mistakenly allocated to sample B. This is the chance of a Type I error, of concluding that the sample comes from B when it does not. In addition, the shaded area to the left of the cut-off represents scores from sample B which do not achieve the desired significance level, and thus are mistakenly allocated to sample A. This portion represents the β value, that is, the likelihood of missing a real difference between the two distributions, of committing a Type II error.

In Figure 3, the α value has been set at a value of 0.01, and as can be seen, the shaded area to the right of the line is smaller, while that to the left is substantially larger. Thus as α is reduced β increases, and the concomitant power (1–β) is lower. Researchers need to decide the relative consequences of committing a Type I error (for example, missing a real improvement in management of a condition supplied by a new but costly treatment) and committing a Type II error (for instance, missing subtle side effects of a proposed new drug), and set the α value accordingly. If the α value is more stringent sample size will need to be increased to compensate. If the directionality of a hypothesis can be stated then it is legitimate to use one-tailed as opposed to two-tailed tests (where possible) and this will increase power.

The second factor is the effect size (ES) which is under investigation in the study. Except in research which is effectively repeating earlier studies, the size of an effect will not be known, as it reflects the very population variation which a piece of research sets out to study. However it is essential that estimates of ES are made, because unless an effect size is large then many studies with small sample sizes are likely to be under-powered. Once again this can be illustrated graphically. Figure 2 demonstrates a relatively small effect between two distributions for which a *t*-test might be used to explore the extent of difference. In Figure 4, the a value remains at 0.05, but now the ES (reflected in the difference between the means of the two distributions) is larger. As can be seen, the shaded area representing β is much reduced, and the power increased.

Accurate estimation of effect sizes is essential for calculating power before a study begins, particularly where multiple hypotheses are being tested. It is sometimes possible to increase effect size, but usually this is the intractable element in the equation. So researchers need to consider how large sample sizes will need to be to adequately test all the hypotheses in a study, and this assessment will affect considerations of research design. The effect of increasing the size of a sample is illustrated in Figure 5. While the effect size (μa–μb) remains the same as in Figure 2, the variance (represented by the area under the curves) is reduced and, for an a of 0.05, β is reduced.

An ES can be estimated in four ways:[4] first, from a review of the literature or meta-analysis, which can suggest the size of ES which may be expected; second, by means of a pilot study which can gather data from which the size of effect may be estimated; third, one can make a decision about the smallest size of effect which it is worth identifying — for example, if we wish to assess the relative effectiveness two rival drugs, if we are willing to accept the two drugs as equivalent if there is no more than a 10% difference in their efficacy, then this effect size may be set, acknowledging that smaller effects will not be discernible. Finally, as a last resort, one can use a 'guesstimate' as to whether an ES is 'small', 'medium', or 'large'. Definitions and values for 'small', 'medium' and 'large' effects for a range of statistical tests, based on figures in Ref. 5, are set out in Table 1, along with formulae for calculating these

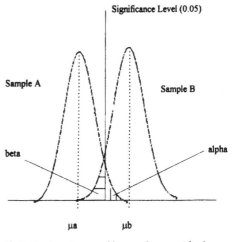

Figure 5 Impact on power of increasing sample size

effects for each test. A 'medium' effect is defined as one which is 'visible to the naked eye' — in other words, one which could be discerned from everyday experience without recourse to formal measurement. For example, the difference between male and female adult heights in the UK would be counted as a medium ES. Using the formula in Table 1 for calculating an ES for a t-test, if mean heights for women and men are 160 and 175 cm respectively, and the pooled standard deviation is 7.5 cm, the ES = 175 –160/7.5 = 0.5.

Most effects encountered in biomedical and social research should be assumed to be small, unless there is a good reason to claim a medium effect, while a 'large' effect size would probably need to be defined as one which is so large that it hardly seems necessary to undertake research into something so well established. Cohen offers the example of the difference between the heights of 13- and 18-year-old girls as a 'large' effect.[5]

Power calculations may also be used as part of the critical appraisal of research papers. Unfortunately it is rare to see b values quoted for tests in research reports; indeed, the results reported are often inadequate to calculate effect sizes. In the last part of this paper, we offer recommendations to journal editors and contributors on how results should be presented to enable readers to assess the power of a study. Formulae for calculating effect sizes vary from test to test (see Table 1), but most are relatively easy to calculate, and more information can be obtained from various texts on the subject.[5,6] Appraisal of study power can be particularly difficult where negative results are simply reported as 'not significant' without supplying any details of test statistics, raw results or degrees of freedom. Statistically non-significant results can be highly significant clinically. However, if a study fails to reject a null hypothesis, it is important to know whether this is because the null hypothesis is correct or whether the test is simply under-powered and thus unlikely to produce statistically significant results.

SURVEY OF STATISTICAL POWER IN GENERAL PRACTICE RESEARCH

To explore the power of general practice research, we analysed all the statistical tests reported in the *British Journal of General Practice* (BJGP) over a period of 18

months. Power was calculated for each test based on the reported sample size. This enabled calculation of the power of each quantitative study published during this period, to assess the adequacy of sample sizes to supply sufficient power.

Methods

All original research papers published in the BJGP during the period January 1994 to June 1995 inclusive were analysed in terms of the power of statistical tests reported. Table 2 indicates the breakdown of papers by type. Qualitative papers were excluded, as were meta-analyses and articles which, although reporting quantitative data, did not report any formal statistical analysis even though in some instances such tests could have been undertaken. A further six papers were excluded because they did not use standard statistical tests for which power tables were available. This left 85 papers, involving 1422 tests for which power could be calculated using power tables.[5,6] Power was calculated for each test following conventions of similar research into statistical power.[1–4] Where adequate data were available (for example details of group means and standard deviations, or results of x^2 tests) precise effect sizes could be calculated. Where this was not possible (in particular for results simply reported as 'non-significant') the following assumptions were made, all of which considerably over-estimate the power of the test. First, for significant results, the effect size was assumed to be 'medium', which as noted earlier means an effect 'visible to the naked eye'. Non-significant results were assumed to have a 'small' ES. Second, a values were set at the lowest possible conventional level of 0.05, and where a directional test was used, a one-tailed a was used (equivalent to two-tailed a of 0.1).

From the calculations of power for individual tests, a mean power for each paper was derived. This strategy has been adopted in other studies into statistical power:[1–4] what is reported is study power, rather than test-by-test power, providing an estimate of the quality of studies in terms of overall adequacy of their statistical power.

Results

Eighty-five papers comprising 1422 tests were analysed. The median number of tests per paper was 12, with a

Table 1

Effect size definitions[a] and formulae

Test	'Small'	'Medium'	'Large'	Formula
t-test	0.2	0.5	0.8	$d = \mu a – \mu b / \sigma$
F test	0.1	0.25	0.4	σ of means/pooled σ
Correlation (Pearson)	0.1	0.3	0.5	r
x^2	0.1	0.3	0.5	$(x^2/N)^{-1}$
Multiple regression	0.02	0.15	0.35	$(R^2/1–R^2)^{-1}$

[a] Effect sizes for non-parametric tests may be assumed to be as for their parametric equivalents.

μ_a = mean of sample a; σ = standard deviation; r = correlation coefficient; x^2 = chi square test statistic; R^2 = multiple R squared.

Table 2

Types of research paper published in period January 1994–June 1995

Type of paper	N
Qualitative	7
Meta-analysis or discursive	4
Quantitative without hypothesis testing	35
Quantitative: non-standard tests	6
Quantitative	85
Total	137

Table 3

Power of studies (n = 85)

Power band	N	%
<0.25	2	2
0.26–0.49	19	22
0.50–0.79	27	32
0.80–0.96	21	25
≥0.97	16	19

minimum of one test and a maximum of 90. The median power of the 85 studies was 0.71, representing a slightly greater than two-thirds probability of rejecting null hypotheses. The proportions of tests in different power bands is summarized in Table 3. Of the 85 studies, 37 (44%) had power of ≥ 0.8, while 48 (56%) fell below this conventional target. The lowest power rating was 0.24, while 10 studies (12%) reached power values of 0.99 or more. Unlike some earlier studies of statistical power, no attempt has been made to subdivide studies into those with large, medium and small effect sizes, partly because in a number of cases, the effect sizes were probably over-estimated as 'medium', and because within a single paper, many different variables with differing effect sizes might be under investigation.

Discussion

The results of this survey of general practice research published in the BJGP indicates somewhat higher power ratings than those reported for other disciplines, including nursing,[4] psychology,[2] education,[1] management[3] and in some medical journals. However, over half of the studies fell below the conventional figure of 0.8, and 25% had a power of 0.5 or less, suggesting a chance of gaining significant results poorer than that obtained by tossing a coin.

Scrutiny of the distribution of powers indicated bimodality. Sixteen of the 37 papers meeting or exceeding the 0.8 target had a power of > 97 %. Such high powers were achieved by the use of very large samples. Given that it is necessary to double the sample size to increase power from 0.8 to 0.97, it is reasonable to argue that as such the studies were overpowered, and used sample sizes which were excessively expensive in terms of researcher time for data collection and analysis. In some cases these studies used pre-existing data sets and so this criticism is less pertinent; elsewhere, researchers may have devoted far greater efforts in terms of time and obtaining goodwill from subjects than may strictly have been necessary to achieve adequate power. The importance of pre-study calculations of necessary sample size to achieve statistical power of 0.8 or thereabouts is relevant both for those studies demonstrated to be under-powered and those for whom power is excessive.

Conclusions and recommendations

More than half of the published quantitative papers in general practice research surveyed in this study possessed inadequate statistical power. This means that during the statistical analysis there was a substantial risk of missing significant results. Twenty-five per cent of papers surveyed had a chance of gaining significant results (when there was a false null hypothesis) poorer than that obtained from tossing a coin. With regard to the use of statistical power analysis in general practice research, we would recommend that all primary care and general practice researchers should undertake power calculations, referring to relevant texts or to a statistician, to decide on the necessary sample size before starting research. Furthermore, we would tactfully suggest to editors of general practice journals that they should request authors to report the value of each test statistic with the a and b values as well as sample size, to enable readers to assess the power of a study. All such values for non-significant results should also be reported.

12

References

1 Brewer J. On the power of statistical tests in the American Educational Research Journal. *Am Educ Res J* 1972; **9**: 391–401.
2 Chase J, Chase B. A statistical power analysis of applied psychological research. *J Appl Psychol* 1976; **61**: 234–237.
3 Mazen AM, Graf LE, Kellog CE, Hemmasi M. Statistical power in contemporary management research. *Acad Man J* 1987; **30**: 369–380
4 Polit DF, Sherman RE. Statistical power in nursing research. *Nurs Res* 1990; **39**: 365–369
5 Cohen J. *Statistical Power Analysis for the Behavioural Sciences*. New York, NY: Academic Press, 1977.
6 Machin D, Campbell MJ. *Statistical Tables for the Design of Clinical Trials*. Oxford: Blackwell Scientific, 1987.
7 Reed JF, Slaichert W. Statistical proof in inconclusive 'negative' trials. *Arch Intern Med* 1981; **141**: 1307–1310.

TABLE 3.1

SAMPLE SIZES FOR COMPARISON OF PROPORTIONS.
IN: SAMPLE SIZES FOR CLINICAL STUDIES.
OXFORD: BLACKWELL SCIENCE, 1997

Machin D, Campbell MJ, Fayers P and Pinol APY

13

Table 3.1 Sample sizes for comparison of proportions *(continued)*.

π^2	α 2-sided	1-sided	0.50	0.65	0.70	0.75	0.80	0.85	0.90	0.95	0.99
						$\pi_1 = 0.05$					
0.10	0.01	0.005	369	487	533	586	647	723	824	986	1329
	0.02	0.010	301	408	451	499	556	626	721	872	1197
	0.05	0.025	214	305	342	385	435	497	582	719	1015
	0.10	0.050	151	229	261	298	343	398	474	598	871
	0.20	0.100	92	154	181	212	250	298	363	473	719
0.15	0.01	0.005	120	158	173	190	209	233	266	318	427
	0.02	0.010	98	132	146	162	180	202	232	281	385
	0.05	0.025	70	99	111	125	141	161	188	231	326
	0.10	0.050	49	74	85	97	111	129	153	193	280
	0.20	0.100	30	50	59	69	81	96	117	152	231
0.20	0.01	0.005	65	85	93	102	113	125	143	170	228
	0.02	0.010	53	71	79	87	97	109	125	151	206
	0.05	0.025	38	54	60	67	76	86	101	124	174
	0.10	0.050	27	40	46	52	60	69	82	103	149
	0.20	0.100	16	27	32	37	43	52	63	81	123
0.25	0.01	0.005	43	56	61	67	73	82	93	111	148
	0.02	0.010	35	47	52	57	63	71	81	98	133
	0.05	0.025	25	35	39	44	49	56	65	80	113
	0.10	0.050	18	26	30	34	39	45	53	67	96
	0.20	0.100	11	18	21	24	28	34	41	53	79
0.30	0.01	0.005	31	40	44	48	53	59	67	79	106
	0.02	0.010	26	34	37	41	46	51	58	70	95
	0.05	0.025	18	25	28	32	36	40	47	58	80
	0.10	0.050	13	19	22	25	28	32	38	48	69
	0.20	0.100	8	13	15	18	20	24	29	38	56
0.35	0.01	0.005	24	31	34	37	41	45	51	60	80
	0.02	0.010	20	26	29	31	35	39	44	53	72
	0.05	0.025	14	20	22	24	27	31	36	44	61
	0.10	0.050	10	15	17	19	21	25	29	36	52
	0.20	0.100	6	10	12	13	16	18	22	29	43
0.40	0.01	0.005	19	25	27	29	32	36	40	48	63
	0.02	0.010	16	21	23	25	28	31	35	42	57
	0.05	0.025	11	16	17	19	22	24	28	34	48
	0.10	0.050	8	12	13	15	17	20	23	29	41
	0.20	0.100	5	8	9	11	12	15	18	22	33
0.45	0.01	0.005	16	20	22	24	26	29	33	39	51
	0.02	0.010	13	17	19	21	23	25	29	34	46
	0.05	0.025	10	13	14	16	18	20	23	28	38
	0.10	0.050	7	10	11	12	14	16	19	23	33
	0.20	0.100	4	7	8	9	10	12	14	18	27
0.50	0.01	0.005	14	17	19	20	22	24	27	32	42
	0.02	0.010	11	14	16	17	19	21	24	28	38
	0.05	0.025	8	11	12	13	15	17	19	23	32
	0.10	0.050	6	8	9	10	12	13	15	19	27
	0.20	0.100	4	6	6	7	8	10	12	15	22
0.55	0.01	0.005	12	15	16	17	19	20	23	27	35
	0.02	0.010	10	12	13	15	16	18	20	24	31
	0.05	0.025	7	9	10	11	12	14	16	19	26
	0.10	0.050	5	7	8	9	10	11	13	16	22
	0.20	0.100	3	5	5	6	7	8	10	12	18
π^2	α 2-sided	1-sided	0.50	0.65	0.70	0.75	0.80	0.85	0.90	0.95	0.99

The cells of the table give the number of patients required *in each treatment arm*.

Table 3.1 Sample sizes for comparison of proportions *(continued)*.

π^2	α 2-sided	α 1-sided	Power 1−β 0.50	0.65	0.70	0.75	0.80	0.85	0.90	0.95	0.99
					$\pi_1 = 0.05$						
0.60	0.01	0.005	10	13	14	15	16	17	19	23	29
	0.02	0.010	8	11	11	12	14	15	17	20	26
	0.05	0.025	6	8	9	10	11	12	14	16	22
	0.10	0.050	4	6	7	7	8	9	11	13	19
	0.20	0.100	3	4	5	5	6	7	8	10	15
0.65	0.01	0.005	9	11	12	13	14	15	17	19	25
	0.02	0.010	7	9	10	11	12	13	14	17	22
	0.05	0.025	5	7	8	8	9	10	12	14	18
	0.10	0.050	4	5	6	6	7	8	9	11	16
	0.20	0.100	3	4	4	5	5	6	7	9	13
0.70	0.01	0.005	8	10	10	11	12	13	14	16	21
	0.02	0.010	7	8	9	9	10	11	12	14	19
	0.05	0.025	5	6	7	7	8	9	10	12	16
	0.10	0.050	4	5	5	6	6	7	8	10	13
	0.20	0.100	2	3	4	4	5	5	6	7	11
0.75	0.01	0.005	7	8	9	10	10	11	12	14	18
	0.02	0.010	6	7	8	8	9	10	11	12	16
	0.05	0.025	4	5	6	6	7	8	8	10	13
	0.10	0.050	3	4	4	5	5	6	7	8	11
	0.20	0.100	2	3	3	4	4	4	5	6	9
0.80	0.01	0.005	6	7	8	8	9	10	11	12	15
	0.02	0.010	5	6	7	7	8	8	9	11	13
	0.05	0.025	4	5	5	6	6	7	7	8	11
	0.10	0.050	3	4	4	4	5	5	6	7	9
	0.20	0.100	2	3	3	3	3	4	4	5	7
0.85	0.01	0.005	6	7	7	7	8	8	9	10	13
	0.02	0.010	5	6	6	6	7	7	8	9	11
	0.05	0.025	3	4	4	5	5	6	6	7	9
	0.10	0.050	3	3	3	4	4	4	5	6	8
	0.20	0.100	2	2	2	3	3	3	4	4	6
0.90	0.01	0.005	5	6	6	6	7	7	8	9	10
	0.02	0.010	4	5	5	5	6	6	7	8	9
	0.05	0.025	3	4	4	4	4	5	5	6	7
	0.10	0.050	2	3	3	3	4	4	4	5	6
	0.20	0.100	2	2	2	2	3	3	3	4	5
0.95	0.01	0.005	5	5	5	6	6	6	7	7	8
	0.02	0.010	4	4	5	5	5	5	6	6	7
	0.05	0.025	3	3	3	4	4	4	4	5	6
	0.10	0.050	2	3	3	3	3	3	3	4	5
	0.20	0.100	2	2	2	2	2	2	3	3	4
					$\pi_1 = 0.10$						
0.15	0.01	0.005	581	767	841	924	1021	1140	1300	1556	2098
	0.02	0.010	474	643	711	787	877	988	1137	1377	1889
	0.05	0.025	337	481	540	607	686	785	918	1135	1603
	0.10	0.050	237	361	412	470	540	628	748	945	1376
	0.20	0.100	144	243	285	335	394	469	574	747	1135
0.20	0.01	0.005	170	224	245	269	297	331	377	451	608
	0.02	0.010	139	187	207	229	255	287	330	399	547
	0.05	0.025	98	140	157	177	199	228	266	329	464
	0.10	0.050	69	105	120	137	157	182	217	274	398
	0.20	0.100	42	71	83	97	115	136	166	216	328
π^2	α 2-sided	α 1-sided	Power 1−β 0.50	0.65	0.70	0.75	0.80	0.85	0.90	0.95	0.99

The cells of the table give the number of patients required *in each treatment arm*.

Table 3.1 Sample sizes for comparison of proportions *(continued)*.

π^2	α 2-sided	1-sided	0.50	0.65	0.70	0.75	Power 1−β 0.80	0.85	0.90	0.95	0.99
					$\pi_1 = 0.10$						
0.25	0.01	0.005	86	112	123	135	149	166	189	226	303
	0.02	0.010	70	94	104	115	128	144	165	200	273
	0.05	0.025	50	71	79	89	100	114	133	164	231
	0.10	0.050	35	53	60	69	79	91	109	137	198
	0.20	0.100	22	36	42	49	57	68	83	108	163
0.30	0.01	0.005	54	70	77	84	92	103	117	140	187
	0.02	0.010	44	59	65	72	79	89	102	123	168
	0.05	0.025	31	44	49	55	62	71	82	101	142
	0.10	0.050	22	33	38	43	49	57	67	84	122
	0.20	0.100	14	22	26	30	36	42	51	67	100
0.35	0.01	0.005	38	49	53	58	64	71	81	96	129
	0.02	0.010	31	41	45	50	55	62	71	85	116
	0.05	0.025	22	31	34	38	43	49	57	70	98
	0.10	0.050	16	23	26	30	34	39	46	58	84
	0.20	0.100	10	16	18	21	25	29	35	46	69
0.40	0.01	0.005	28	36	40	43	48	53	60	71	95
	0.02	0.010	23	31	34	37	41	46	52	63	85
	0.05	0.025	17	23	26	29	32	36	42	52	72
	0.10	0.050	12	17	20	22	25	29	34	43	62
	0.20	0.100	7	12	14	16	18	22	26	34	50
0.45	0.01	0.005	22	28	31	34	37	41	46	55	73
	0.02	0.010	18	24	26	29	32	36	40	48	65
	0.05	0.025	13	18	20	22	25	28	33	40	55
	0.10	0.050	9	14	15	17	20	22	26	33	47
	0.20	0.100	6	9	11	12	14	17	20	26	39
0.50	0.01	0.005	18	23	25	27	30	33	37	44	58
	0.02	0.010	15	19	21	23	25	28	32	39	52
	0.05	0.025	11	14	16	18	20	22	26	32	44
	0.10	0.050	8	11	12	14	16	18	21	26	37
	0.20	0.100	5	7	9	10	11	13	16	21	30
0.55	0.01	0.005	15	19	20	22	24	27	30	35	47
	0.02	0.010	12	16	17	19	21	23	26	31	42
	0.05	0.025	9	12	13	15	16	18	21	26	35
	0.10	0.050	6	9	10	11	13	15	17	21	30
	0.20	0.100	4	6	7	8	9	11	13	17	24
0.60	0.01	0.005	13	16	17	19	20	22	25	29	38
	0.02	0.010	10	13	14	16	17	19	22	26	34
	0.05	0.025	7	10	11	12	14	15	17	21	29
	0.10	0.050	5	8	8	9	11	12	14	17	24
	0.20	0.100	3	5	6	7	8	9	11	14	20
0.65	0.01	0.005	11	13	15	16	17	19	21	24	32
	0.02	0.010	9	11	12	13	15	16	18	21	28
	0.05	0.025	6	9	9	10	11	13	15	18	24
	0.10	0.050	5	6	7	8	9	10	12	14	20
	0.20	0.100	3	4	5	6	7	8	9	11	16
0.70	0.01	0.005	9	12	12	13	15	16	18	21	26
	0.02	0.010	8	10	11	11	12	14	15	18	24
	0.05	0.025	6	7	8	9	10	11	12	15	20
	0.10	0.050	4	6	6	7	8	9	10	12	17
	0.20	0.100	3	4	4	5	6	6	8	9	13
π^2	α 2-sided	1-sided	0.50	0.65	0.70	0.75	Power 1−β 0.80	0.85	0.90	0.95	0.99

13

The cells of the table give the number of patients required *in each treatment arm*.

Table 3.1 Sample sizes for comparison of proportions *(continued)*.

π^2	α 2-sided	1-sided	Power $1-\beta$ 0.50	0.65	0.70	0.75	0.80	0.85	0.90	0.95	0.99
						$\pi_1 = 0.10$					
0.75	0.01	0.005	8	10	11	12	12	14	15	17	22
	0.02	0.010	7	8	9	10	11	12	13	15	20
	0.05	0.025	5	6	7	8	8	9	10	12	16
	0.10	0.050	4	5	5	6	7	7	8	10	14
	0.20	0.100	2	3	4	4	5	5	6	8	11
0.80	0.01	0.005	7	9	9	10	11	12	13	15	19
	0.02	0.010	6	7	8	8	9	10	11	13	16
	0.05	0.025	4	6	6	7	7	8	9	10	14
	0.10	0.050	3	4	5	5	6	6	7	8	11
	0.20	0.100	2	3	3	4	4	5	5	7	9
0.85	0.01	0.005	6	8	8	9	9	10	11	12	15
	0.02	0.010	5	6	7	7	8	9	9	11	14
	0.05	0.025	4	5	5	6	6	7	7	9	11
	0.10	0.050	3	4	4	4	5	5	6	7	9
	0.20	0.100	2	3	3	3	3	4	5	5	8
0.90	0.01	0.005	6	7	7	7	8	8	9	10	13
	0.02	0.010	5	6	6	6	7	7	8	9	11
	0.05	0.025	4	4	5	5	5	6	6	7	9
	0.10	0.050	3	3	3	4	4	5	5	6	8
	0.20	0.100	2	2	2	3	3	3	4	5	6
0.95	0.01	0.005	5	6	6	6	7	7	8	9	10
	0.02	0.010	4	5	5	5	6	6	7	8	9
	0.05	0.025	3	4	4	4	4	5	5	6	7
	0.10	0.050	2	3	3	3	4	4	4	5	6
	0.20	0.100	2	2	2	2	3	3	3	4	5
						$\pi_1 = 0.15$					
0.20	0.01	0.005	767	1013	1110	1220	1348	1506	1717	2055	2770
	0.02	0.010	626	849	938	1040	1158	1305	1502	1819	2495
	0.05	0.025	444	635	713	801	906	1036	1212	1498	2118
	0.10	0.050	313	476	543	621	714	829	988	1248	1817
	0.20	0.100	190	321	377	442	520	620	758	987	1500
0.25	0.01	0.005	213	281	307	337	373	416	474	567	764
	0.02	0.010	174	235	260	288	320	361	415	502	688
	0.05	0.025	123	176	197	222	250	286	335	413	583
	0.10	0.050	87	132	151	172	197	229	273	344	501
	0.20	0.100	53	89	104	122	144	171	209	272	413
0.30	0.01	0.005	103	136	149	163	180	201	229	273	367
	0.02	0.010	84	114	126	139	155	174	200	242	331
	0.05	0.025	60	85	96	107	121	138	161	199	280
	0.10	0.050	42	64	73	83	95	111	131	166	240
	0.20	0.100	26	43	51	59	69	83	101	131	198
0.35	0.01	0.005	63	82	90	98	109	121	137	164	220
	0.02	0.010	51	69	76	84	93	105	120	145	198
	0.05	0.025	37	52	58	65	73	83	97	119	168
	0.10	0.050	26	39	44	50	57	66	79	99	144
	0.20	0.100	16	26	31	36	42	50	60	78	118
0.40	0.01	0.005	43	56	61	67	74	82	93	111	148
	0.02	0.010	35	47	52	57	63	71	81	98	133
	0.05	0.025	25	35	39	44	49	56	65	80	113
	0.10	0.050	18	26	30	34	39	45	53	67	96
	0.20	0.100	11	18	21	24	28	34	41	53	79
π^2	α 2-sided	1-sided	Power $1-\beta$ 0.50	0.65	0.70	0.75	0.80	0.85	0.90	0.95	0.99

The cells of the table give the number of patients required *in each treatment arm*.

Table 3.1 Sample sizes for comparison of proportions (continued).

π^2	α 2-sided	1-sided	Power 1-β 0.50	0.65	0.70	0.75	0.80	0.85	0.90	0.95	0.99
					$\pi^1 = 0.15$						
0.45	0.01	0.005	31	41	45	49	54	59	67	80	107
	0.02	0.010	26	34	38	41	46	51	59	71	96
	0.05	0.025	18	26	29	32	36	41	47	58	81
	0.10	0.050	13	19	22	25	28	33	39	48	69
	0.20	0.100	8	13	15	18	21	24	29	38	57
0.50	0.01	0.005	24	31	34	37	41	45	51	61	81
	0.02	0.010	20	26	29	32	35	39	45	54	73
	0.05	0.025	14	20	22	24	27	31	36	44	61
	0.10	0.050	10	15	17	19	22	25	29	37	52
	0.20	0.100	6	10	12	14	16	19	22	29	43
0.55	0.01	0.005	19	25	27	29	32	36	40	48	63
	0.02	0.010	16	21	23	25	28	31	35	42	57
	0.05	0.025	11	16	17	19	22	24	28	34	48
	0.10	0.050	8	12	13	15	17	20	23	29	41
	0.20	0.100	5	8	9	11	12	15	17	22	33
0.60	0.01	0.005	16	20	22	24	26	29	32	38	50
	0.02	0.010	13	17	19	20	22	25	28	34	45
	0.05	0.025	9	13	14	16	17	20	23	28	38
	0.10	0.050	7	10	11	12	14	16	18	23	32
	0.20	0.100	4	7	8	9	10	12	14	18	26
0.65	0.01	0.005	13	17	18	20	21	24	26	31	41
	0.02	0.010	11	14	15	17	18	20	23	27	36
	0.05	0.025	8	11	12	13	14	16	19	22	31
	0.10	0.050	6	8	9	10	11	13	15	18	26
	0.20	0.100	4	5	6	7	8	10	11	14	21
0.70	0.01	0.005	11	14	15	16	18	20	22	26	33
	0.02	0.010	9	12	13	14	15	17	19	23	30
	0.05	0.025	7	9	10	11	12	13	15	18	25
	0.10	0.050	5	7	7	8	9	11	12	15	21
	0.20	0.100	3	5	5	6	7	8	9	12	17
0.75	0.01	0.005	10	12	13	14	15	16	18	21	28
	0.02	0.010	8	10	11	12	13	14	16	19	25
	0.05	0.025	6	8	8	9	10	11	13	15	21
	0.10	0.050	4	6	6	7	8	9	10	13	17
	0.20	0.100	3	4	4	5	6	7	8	10	14
0.80	0.01	0.005	8	10	11	12	13	14	15	18	23
	0.02	0.010	7	9	9	10	11	12	13	16	20
	0.05	0.025	5	6	7	8	8	9	11	13	17
	0.10	0.050	4	5	5	6	7	7	9	10	14
	0.20	0.100	2	3	4	4	5	6	7	8	11
0.85	0.01	0.005	7	9	9	10	11	12	13	15	19
	0.02	0.010	6	7	8	9	9	10	11	13	17
	0.05	0.025	4	6	6	7	7	8	9	11	14
	0.10	0.050	3	4	5	5	6	6	7	9	12
	0.20	0.100	2	3	3	4	4	5	5	7	9
0.90	0.01	0.005	6	8	8	9	9	10	11	12	15
	0.02	0.010	5	6	7	7	8	9	9	11	14
	0.05	0.025	4	5	5	6	6	7	7	9	11
	0.10	0.050	3	4	4	4	5	5	6	7	9
	0.20	0.100	2	3	3	3	3	4	5	5	8
π^2	α 2-sided	1-sided	Power 1-β 0.50	0.65	0.70	0.75	0.80	0.85	0.90	0.95	0.99

The cells of the table give the number of patients required *in each treatment arm*.

Table 3.1 Sample sizes for comparison of proportions *(continued)*.

π^2	α 2-sided	α 1-sided	Power 1–β 0.50	0.65	0.70	0.75	0.80	0.85	0.90	0.95	0.99
					π^1= 0.15						
0.95	0.01	0.005	6	7	7	7	8	8	9	10	13
	0.02	0.010	5	6	6	6	7	7	8	9	11
	0.05	0.025	3	4	4	5	5	6	6	7	9
	0.10	0.050	3	3	3	4	4	4	5	6	8
	0.20	0.100	2	2	2	3	3	3	4	4	6
0.25	0.01	0.005	926	1223	1340	1473	1628	1819	2074	2482	3347
	0.02	0.010	755	1026	1133	1256	1399	1576	1814	2197	3015
	0.05	0.025	536	767	861	968	1094	1251	1464	1810	2558
	0.10	0.050	378	575	656	750	862	1002	1193	1507	2196
	0.20	0.100	230	388	455	534	628	749	915	1193	1812
0.30	0.01	0.005	249	329	360	396	437	488	556	665	896
	0.02	0.010	203	276	305	337	376	423	486	589	807
	0.05	0.025	145	206	231	260	294	336	392	485	684
	0.10	0.050	102	155	176	201	231	269	320	404	587
	0.20	0.100	62	104	122	143	169	201	245	319	484
0.35	0.01	0.005	118	155	170	187	206	230	262	313	421
	0.02	0.010	96	130	144	159	177	199	229	277	379
	0.05	0.025	69	98	109	123	138	158	185	228	321
	0.10	0.050	48	73	83	95	109	127	150	190	275
	0.20	0.100	30	49	58	68	79	95	115	150	227
0.40	0.01	0.005	70	92	101	110	122	136	154	184	247
	0.02	0.010	57	77	85	94	105	117	135	163	222
	0.05	0.025	41	58	65	72	82	93	109	134	188
	0.10	0.050	29	43	49	56	64	75	89	111	161
	0.20	0.100	18	29	34	40	47	56	68	88	133
0.45	0.01	0.005	47	61	67	74	81	90	102	122	163
	0.02	0.010	38	52	57	63	70	78	90	108	147
	0.05	0.025	27	39	43	48	54	62	72	89	124
	0.10	0.050	19	29	33	37	43	50	59	74	107
	0.20	0.100	12	20	23	27	31	37	45	58	88
0.50	0.01	0.005	34	44	48	53	58	65	73	87	116
	0.02	0.010	28	37	41	45	50	56	64	77	104
	0.05	0.025	20	28	31	35	39	44	52	63	88
	0.10	0.050	14	21	24	27	31	35	42	52	76
	0.20	0.100	9	14	17	19	22	26	32	41	62
0.55	0.01	0.005	26	33	36	40	44	49	55	65	87
	0.02	0.010	21	28	31	34	38	42	48	58	78
	0.05	0.025	15	21	23	26	29	33	39	47	66
	0.10	0.050	11	16	18	20	23	27	31	39	56
	0.20	0.100	7	11	12	14	17	20	24	31	46
0.60	0.01	0.005	20	26	28	31	34	38	43	50	67
	0.02	0.010	17	22	24	26	29	33	37	44	60
	0.05	0.025	12	17	18	20	23	26	30	36	51
	0.10	0.050	9	12	14	16	18	21	24	30	43
	0.20	0.100	5	9	10	11	13	15	19	24	35
0.65	0.01	0.005	17	21	23	25	27	30	34	40	53
	0.02	0.010	14	18	19	21	23	26	30	35	47
	0.05	0.025	10	13	15	16	18	21	24	29	40
	0.10	0.050	7	10	11	13	14	16	19	24	34
	0.20	0.100	4	7	8	9	10	12	15	19	28
π^2	α 2-sided	α 1-sided	Power 1–β 0.50	0.65	0.70	0.75	0.80	0.85	0.90	0.95	0.99

The cells of the table give the number of patients required *in each treatment arm*.

Table 3.1 Sample sizes for comparison of proportions *(continued)*.

π^2	α 2-sided	1-sided	Power $1-\beta$								
			0.50	0.65	0.70	0.75	0.80	0.85	0.90	0.95	0.99
					$\pi^1 = 0.20$						
0.70	0.01	0.005	14	17	19	20	22	24	27	32	42
	0.02	0.010	11	15	16	17	19	21	24	28	38
	0.05	0.025	8	11	12	13	15	17	19	23	32
	0.10	0.050	6	8	9	10	12	13	16	19	27
	0.20	0.100	4	6	6	7	8	10	12	15	22
0.75	0.01	0.005	11	14	15	17	18	20	22	26	34
	0.02	0.010	9	12	13	14	16	17	20	23	31
	0.05	0.025	7	9	10	11	12	14	16	19	26
	0.10	0.050	5	7	8	9	10	11	13	16	22
	0.20	0.100	3	5	5	6	7	8	10	12	18
0.80	0.01	0.005	10	12	13	14	15	17	19	22	28
	0.02	0.010	8	10	11	12	13	14	16	19	25
	0.05	0.025	6	8	8	9	10	11	13	15	21
	0.10	0.050	4	6	6	7	8	9	10	13	18
	0.20	0.100	3	4	5	5	6	7	8	10	14
0.85	0.01	0.005	8	10	11	12	13	14	15	18	23
	0.02	0.010	7	9	9	10	11	12	13	16	20
	0.05	0.025	5	6	7	8	8	9	11	13	17
	0.10	0.050	4	5	5	6	7	7	9	10	14
	0.20	0.100	2	3	4	4	5	6	7	8	11
0.90	0.01	0.005	7	9	9	10	11	12	13	15	19
	0.02	0.010	6	7	8	8	9	10	11	13	16
	0.05	0.025	4	6	6	7	7	8	9	10	14
	0.10	0.050	3	4	5	5	6	6	7	8	11
	0.20	0.100	2	3	3	4	4	5	5	7	9
0.95	0.01	0.005	6	7	8	8	9	10	11	12	15
	0.02	0.010	5	6	7	7	8	8	9	11	13
	0.05	0.025	4	5	5	6	6	7	7	8	11
	0.10	0.050	3	4	4	4	5	5	6	7	9
	0.20	0.100	2	3	3	3	3	4	4	5	7
					$\pi_1 = 0.25$						
0.30	0.01	0.005	1059	1398	1533	1684	1862	2080	2371	2838	3828
	0.02	0.010	864	1173	1296	1436	1600	1802	2074	2513	3448
	0.05	0.025	613	877	984	1107	1251	1431	1674	2070	2926
	0.10	0.050	432	658	750	858	986	1146	1365	1724	2511
	0.20	0.100	262	443	520	610	719	856	1047	1364	2073
0.35	0.01	0.005	279	368	403	443	490	547	623	745	1004
	0.02	0.010	228	309	341	378	421	474	545	660	904
	0.05	0.025	162	231	259	291	329	376	440	543	767
	0.10	0.050	114	173	198	226	259	301	358	452	658
	0.20	0.100	69	117	137	161	189	225	275	358	543
0.40	0.01	0.005	130	171	187	205	227	253	288	344	463
	0.02	0.010	106	143	158	175	195	219	252	305	417
	0.05	0.025	75	107	120	135	152	174	203	251	354
	0.10	0.050	53	80	92	105	120	139	166	209	303
	0.20	0.100	33	54	64	74	88	104	127	165	250
0.45	0.01	0.005	76	100	109	120	132	147	167	200	268
	0.02	0.010	62	84	92	102	113	127	146	177	241
	0.05	0.025	44	63	70	79	89	101	118	145	204
	0.10	0.050	31	47	53	61	70	81	96	121	175
	0.20	0.100	19	32	37	43	51	60	74	95	144

π^2	α 2-sided	1-sided	Power $1-\beta$								
			0.50	0.65	0.70	0.75	0.80	0.85	0.90	0.95	0.99

The cells of the table give the number of patients required *in each treatment arm*.

13

Table 3.1 Sample sizes for comparison of proportions *(continued)*.

π^2	2-sided	1-sided	0.50	0.65	0.70	0.75	0.80	0.85	0.90	0.95	0.99
					$\pi_1 = 0.25$						
0.50	0.01	0.005	50	66	72	79	87	96	110	131	175
	0.02	0.010	41	55	61	67	74	84	96	115	157
	0.05	0.025	29	41	46	52	58	66	77	95	133
	0.10	0.050	21	31	35	40	46	53	63	79	114
	0.20	0.100	13	21	24	29	33	40	48	62	94
0.55	0.01	0.005	36	47	51	56	61	68	77	92	123
	0.02	0.010	29	39	43	47	53	59	68	81	110
	0.05	0.025	21	29	33	37	41	47	54	67	93
	0.10	0.050	15	22	25	28	32	37	44	55	80
	0.20	0.100	9	15	17	20	24	28	34	44	66
0.60	0.01	0.005	27	35	38	42	46	51	57	68	91
	0.02	0.010	22	29	32	35	39	44	50	60	81
	0.05	0.025	16	22	24	27	31	35	40	49	69
	0.10	0.050	11	17	19	21	24	28	33	41	59
	0.20	0.100	7	11	13	15	18	21	25	32	48
0.65	0.01	0.005	21	27	29	32	35	39	44	52	69
	0.02	0.010	17	23	25	27	30	34	38	46	62
	0.05	0.025	12	17	19	21	24	27	31	38	52
	0.10	0.050	9	13	14	16	19	21	25	31	45
	0.20	0.100	6	9	10	12	14	16	19	25	37
0.70	0.01	0.005	17	21	23	25	28	31	35	41	54
	0.02	0.010	14	18	20	22	24	27	30	36	48
	0.05	0.025	10	14	15	17	19	21	24	29	41
	0.10	0.050	7	10	11	13	15	17	20	24	35
	0.20	0.100	5	7	8	9	11	12	15	19	28
0.75	0.01	0.005	14	17	19	20	22	25	28	33	43
	0.02	0.010	11	15	16	17	19	21	24	29	38
	0.05	0.025	8	11	12	13	15	17	19	23	32
	0.10	0.050	6	8	9	10	12	13	16	19	27
	0.20	0.100	4	6	7	7	9	10	12	15	22
0.80	0.01	0.005	11	14	15	17	18	20	22	26	34
	0.02	0.010	9	12	13	14	16	17	20	23	31
	0.05	0.025	7	9	10	11	12	14	16	19	26
	0.10	0.050	5	7	8	9	10	11	13	16	22
	0.20	0.100	3	5	5	6	7	8	10	12	18
0.85	0.01	0.005	10	12	13	14	15	16	18	21	28
	0.02	0.010	8	10	11	12	13	14	16	19	25
	0.05	0.025	6	8	8	9	10	11	13	15	21
	0.10	0.050	4	6	6	7	8	9	10	13	17
	0.20	0.100	3	4	4	5	6	7	8	10	14
0.90	0.01	0.005	8	10	11	12	12	14	15	17	22
	0.02	0.010	7	8	9	10	11	12	13	15	20
	0.05	0.025	5	6	7	8	8	9	10	12	16
	0.10	0.050	4	5	5	6	7	7	8	10	14
	0.20	0.100	2	3	4	4	5	5	6	8	11
0.95	0.01	0.005	7	8	9	10	10	11	12	14	18
	0.02	0.010	6	7	8	8	9	10	11	12	16
	0.05	0.025	4	5	6	6	7	8	8	10	13
	0.10	0.050	3	4	4	5	5	6	7	8	11
	0.20	0.100	2	3	3	4	4	4	5	6	9

π^2	2-sided	1-sided	0.50	0.65	0.70	0.75	0.80	0.85	0.90	0.95	0.99

The cells of the table give the number of patients required *in each treatment arm*.

Table 3.1 Sample sizes for comparison of proportions *(continued)*.

π^2	α 2-sided	1-sided	Power 1–β 0.50	0.65	0.70	0.75	0.80	0.85	0.90	0.95	0.99
						$\pi_1 = 0.30$					
0.35	0.01	0.005	1165	1539	1686	1853	2049	2289	2609	3123	4212
	0.02	0.010	950	1290	1426	1580	1760	1983	2283	2765	3794
	0.5	0.025	675	965	1083	1218	1377	1575	1842	2278	3220
	0.10	0.050	475	723	826	944	1084	1261	1502	1897	2764
	0.20	0.100	289	488	572	671	791	942	1152	1501	2281
0.40	0.01	0.005	302	399	437	480	530	592	675	808	1088
	0.02	0.010	247	335	370	409	456	513	590	715	980
	0.05	0.025	175	250	281	315	356	407	477	589	831
	0.10	0.050	124	188	214	244	281	326	388	490	713
	0.20	0.100	75	127	148	174	205	244	298	388	589
0.45	0.01	0.005	139	183	200	219	242	270	308	368	495
	0.02	0.010	113	153	169	187	208	234	269	326	446
	0.05	0.025	81	115	128	144	163	186	217	268	378
	0.10	0.050	57	86	98	112	128	149	177	223	324
	0.20	0.100	35	58	68	80	94	111	136	177	267
0.50	0.01	0.005	80	105	115	126	139	155	177	211	283
	0.02	0.010	65	88	97	108	120	134	154	186	255
	0.05	0.025	47	66	74	83	93	107	124	153	216
	0.10	0.050	33	50	56	64	74	85	101	128	185
	0.20	0.100	20	34	39	46	54	64	78	101	152
0.55	0.01	0.005	52	68	75	82	90	101	114	136	183
	0.02	0.010	43	57	63	70	78	87	100	121	164
	0.05	0.025	31	43	48	54	61	69	81	99	139
	0.10	0.050	22	32	37	42	48	55	66	82	119
	0.20	0.100	13	22	26	30	35	41	50	65	98
0.60	0.01	0.005	37	48	53	57	63	70	80	95	127
	0.02	0.010	30	40	44	49	54	61	70	84	114
	0.05	0.025	22	30	34	38	42	48	56	69	97
	0.10	0.050	15	23	26	29	33	39	46	57	83
	0.20	0.100	10	15	18	21	24	29	35	45	68
0.65	0.01	0.005	28	36	39	42	47	52	59	69	93
	0.02	0.010	23	30	33	36	40	45	51	61	83
	0.05	0.025	16	22	25	28	31	35	41	50	70
	0.10	0.050	12	17	19	22	25	28	33	42	60
	0.20	0.100	7	11	13	15	18	21	26	33	49
0.70	0.01	0.005	21	27	30	32	36	39	44	53	70
	0.02	0.010	17.	23	25	28	30	34	39	46	63
	0.05	0.025	13	17	19	21	24	27	31	38	53
	0.10	0.050	9	13	15	17	19	22	25	32	45
	0.20	0.100	6	9	10	12	14	16	19	25	37
0.75	0.01	0.005	17	21	23	25	28	31	35	41	54
	0.02	0.010	14	18	20	22	24	27	30	36	48
	0.05	0.025	10	14	15	17	19	21	24	29	41
	0.10	0.050	7	10	11	13	15	17	20	24	35
	0.20	0.100	5	7	8	9	11	12	15	19	28
0.80	0.01	0.005	14	17	19	20	22	24	27	32	42
	0.02	0.010	11	15	16	17	19	21	24	28	38
	0.05	0.025	8	11	12	13	15	17	19	23	32
	0.10	0.050	6	8	9	10	12	13	16	19	27
	0.20	0.100	4	6	6	7	8	10	12	15	22
π^2	α 2-sided	1-sided	Power 1–β 0.50	0.65	0.70	0.75	0.80	0.85	0.90	0.95	0.99

13

The cells of the table give the number of patients required *in each treatment arm*.

Table 3.1 Sample sizes for comparison of proportions *(continued)*.

	α						Power 1–β				
π^2	2-sided	1-sided	0.50	0.65	0.70	0.75	0.80	0.85	0.90	0.95	0.99
					$\pi_1 = 0.30$						
0.85	0.01	0.005	11	14	15	16	18	20	22	26	33
	0.02	0.010	9	12	13	14	15	17	19	23	30
	0.05	0.025	7	9	10	11	12	13	15	18	25
	0.10	0.050	5	7	7	8	9	11	12	15	21
	0.20	0.100	3	5	5	6	7	8	9	12	17
0.90	0.01	0.005	9	12	12	13	15	16	18	21	26
	0.02	0.010	8	10	11	11	12	14	15	18	24
	0.05	0.025	6	7	8	9	10	11	12	15	20
	0.10	0.050	4	6	6	7	8	9	10	12	17
	0.20	0.100	3	4	4	5	6	6	8	9	13
0.95	0.01	0.005	8	10	10	11	12	13	14	16	21
	0.02	0.010	7	8	9	9	10	11	12	14	19
	0.05	0.025	5	6	7	7	8	9	10	12	16
	0.10	0.050	4	5	5	6	6	7	8	10	13
	0.20	0.100	2	3	4	4	5	5	6	7	11
					$\pi_1 = 0.35$						
0.40	0.01	0.005	1245	1644	1802	1980	2189	2445	2788	3337	4501
	0.02	0.010	1015	1379	1524	1688	1881	2119	2439	2954	4054
	0.05	0.025	721	1031	1157	1301	1471	1682	1969	2434	3440
	0.10	0.050	508	773	882	1008	1159	1347	1604	2027	2953
	0.20	0.100	308	521	612	717	845	1007	1231	1604	2437
0.45	0.01	0.005	319	421	461	507	560	625	712	852	1148
	0.02	0.010	260	353	390	432	481	542	623	754	1034
	0.05	0.025	185	264	296	333	376	430	503	621	877
	0.10	0.050	130	198	226	258	296	344	410	517	753
	0.20	0.100	79	134	157	183	216	257	314	409	621
0.50	0.01	0.005	145	190	208	229	253	282	321	384	517
	0.02	0.010	118	160	176	195	217	244	281	340	465
	0.05	0.025	84	120	134	150	170	194	227	280	395
	0.10	0.050	59	90	102	117	134	155	185	233	338
	0.20	0.100	36	61	71	83	98	116	142	184	279
0.55	0.01	0.005	83	108	119	130	144	160	182	217	292
	0.02	0.010	67	91	100	111	123	139	159	192	263
	0.05	0.025	48	68	76	85	96	110	128	158	223
	0.10	0.050	34	51	58	66	76	88	105	132	191
	0.20	0.100	21	35	40	47	55	66	80	104	157
0.60	0.01	0.005	53	70	76	84	92	103	117	139	187
	0.02	0.010	44	59	65	71	79	89	102	123	168
	0.05	0.025	31	44	49	55	62	71	82	101	142
	0.10	0.050	22	33	37	43	49	56	67	84	122
	0.20	0.100	14	22	26	30	36	42	51	66	100
0.65	0.01	0.005	37	49	53	58	64	71	81	96	128
	0.02	0.010	31	41	45	49	55	62	70	85	115
	0.05	0.025	22	31	34	38	43	49	57	70	98
	0.10	0.050	16	23	26	30	34	39	46	58	83
	0.20	0.100	10	16	18	21	25	29	35	46	69
0.70	0.01	0.005	28	36	39	42	47	52	59	69	93
	0.02	0.010	23	30	33	36	40	45	51	61	83
	0.05	0.025	16	22	25	28	31	35	41	50	70
	0.10	0.050	12	17	19	22	25	28	33	42	60
	0.20	0.100	7	11	13	15	18	21	26	33	49
	α						Power 1–β				
π^2	2-sided	1-sided	0.50	0.65	0.70	0.75	0.80	0.85	0.90	0.95	0.99

The cells of the table give the number of patients required *in each treatment arm*.

Table 3.1 Sample sizes for comparison of proportions *(continued)*.

π^2	2-sided	1-sided	0.50	0.65	0.70	0.75	0.80	0.85	0.90	0.95	0.99
	α					Power $1-\beta$					
						$\pi_1 = 0.35$					
0.75	0.01	0.005	21	27	29	32	35	39	44	52	69
	0.02	0.010	17	23	25	27	30	34	38	46	62
	0.05	0.025	12	17	19	21	24	27	31	38	52
	0.10	0.050	9	13	14	16	19	21	25	31	45
	0.20	0.100	6	9	10	12	14	16	19	25	37
0.80	0.01	0.005	17	21	23	25	27	30	34	40	53
	0.02	0.010	14	18	19	21	23	26	30	35	47
	0.05	0.025	10	13	15	16	18	21	24	9	40
	0.10	0.050	7	10	11	13	14	16	19	24	34
	0.20	0.100	4	7	8	9	10	12	15	19	28
0.85	0.01	0.005	13	17	18	20	21	24	26	31	41
	0.02	0.010	11	14	15	17	18	20	23	27	36
	0.05	0.025	8	11	12	13	14	16	19	22	31
	0.10	0.050	6	8	9	10	11	13	15	18	26
	0.20	0.100	4	5	6	7	8	10	11	14	21
0.90	0.01	0.005	11	13	15	16	17	19	21	24	32
	0.02	0.010	9	11	12	13	15	16	18	21	28
	0.05	0.025	6	9	9	10	11	13	15	18	24
	0.10	0.050	5	6	7	8	9	10	12	14	20
	0.20	0.100	3	4	5	6	7	8	9	11	16
0.95	0.01	0.005	9	11	12	13	14	15	17	19	25
	0.02	0.010	7	9	10	11	12	13	14	17	22
	0.05	0.025	5	7	8	8	9	10	12	14	18
	0.10	0.050	4	5	6	6	7	8	9	11	16
	0.20	0.100	3	4	4	5	5	6	7	9	13
						$\pi_1 = 0.40$					
0.45	0.01	0.005	1298	1714	1879	2065	2282	2550	2907	3480	4693
	0.02	0.010	1059	1438	1589	1760	1961	2210	2543	3080	4227
	0.05	0.025	752	1075	1206	1356	1534	1754	2053	2538	3587
	0.10	0.050	529	806	920	1051	1208	1405	1673	2114	3079
	0.20	0.100	322	543	638	748	881	1050	1283	1672	2541
0.50	0.01	0.005	329	434	475	522	577	645	735	879	1184
	0.02	0.010	268	364	402	445	496	559	643	778	1067
	0.05	0.025	191	272	305	343	388	443	519	641	905
	0.10	0.050	134	204	233	266	305	355	423	533	777
	0.20	0.100	82	138	161	189	223	265	324	422	641
0.55	0.01	0.005	148	194	213	234	258	288	328	392	527
	0.02	0.010	120	163	180	199	222	249	287	347	475
	0.05	0.025	86	122	137	153	173	198	231	286	403
	0.10	0.050	60	91	104	119	136	158	188	238	345
	0.20	0.100	37	62	72	85	100	118	144	188	285
0.60	0.01	0.005	83	110	120	131	145	162	184	220	295
	0.02	0.010	68	92	101	112	125	140	161	194	266
	0.05	0.025	49	69	77	86	97	111	130	160	225
	0.10	0.050	34	52	59	67	77	89	106	133	193
	0.20	0.100	21	35	41	48	56	66	82	105	159
0.65	0.01	0.005	53	70	76	84	92	103	117	139	187
	0.02	0.010	44	59	65	71	79	89	102	123	168
	0.05	0.025	31	44	49	55	62	71	81	101	142
	0.10	0.050	22	33	37	43	49	56	67	84	122
	0.20	0.100	14	22	26	30	36	42	51	66	100
π^2	2-sided	1-sided	0.50	0.65	0.70	0.75	0.80	0.85	0.90	0.95	0.99
	α					Power $1-\beta$					

13

The cells of the table give the number of patients required *in each treatment arm*.

Table 3.1 Sample sizes for comparison of proportions *(continued)*.

π^2	α 2-sided	α 1-sided	Power 1−β 0.50	0.65	0.70	0.75	0.80	0.85	0.90	0.95	0.99
					$\pi_1 = 0.40$						
0.70	0.01	0.005	37	48	53	57	63	70	80	95	127
	0.02	0.010	30	40	44	49	54	61	70	84	114
	0.05	0.025	22	30	34	38	42	48	56	69	97
	0.10	0.050	15	23	26	29	33	39	46	57	83
	0.20	0.100	10	15	18	21	24	29	35	45	68
0.75	0.01	0.005	27	35	38	42	46	51	57	68	91
	0.02	0.010	22	29	32	35	39	44	50	60	81
	0.05	0.025	16	22	24	27	31	35	40	49	69
	0.10	0.050	11	17	19	21	24	28	33	41	59
	0.20	0.100	7	11	13	15	18	21	25	32	48
0.80	0.01	0.005	20	26	28	31	34	38	43	50	67
	0.02	0.010	17	22	24	26	29	33	37	44	60
	0.05	0.025	12	17	18	20	23	26	30	36	51
	0.10	0.050	9	12	14	16	18	21	24	30	43
	0.20	0.100	5	9	10	11	13	15	19	24	35
0.85	0.01	0.005	16	20	22	24	26	29	32	38	50
	0.02	0.010	13	17	19	20	22	25	28	34	45
	0.05	0.025	9	13	14	16	17	20	23	28	38
	0.10	0.050	7	10	11	12	14	16	18	23	32
	0.20	0.100	4	7	8	9	10	12	14	18	26
0.90	0.01	0.005	13	16	17	19	20	22	25	29	38
	0.02	0.010	10	13	14	16	17	19	22	26	34
	0.05	0.025	7	10	11	12	14	15	17	21	29
	0.10	0.050	5	8	8	9	11	12	14	17	24
	0.20	0.100	3	5	6	7	8	9	11	14	20
0.95	0.01	0.005	10	13	14	15	16	17	19	23	29
	0.02	0.010	8	11	11	12	14	15	17	20	26
	0.05	0.025	6	8	9	10	11	12	14	16	22
	0.10	0.050	4	6	7	7	8	9	11	13	19
	0.20	0.100	3	4	5	5	6	7	8	10	15
					$\pi_1 = 0.45$						
0.50	0.01	0.005	1324	1749	1917	2107	2329	2602	2966	3551	4789
	0.02	0.010	1080	1467	1621	1796	2001	2255	2595	3143	4314
	0.05	0.025	767	1097	1231	1384	1565	1790	2095	2590	3661
	0.10	0.050	540	822	939	1073	1233	1433	1707	2157	3142
	0.20	0.100	328	554	651	763	899	1071	1309	1707	2593
0.55	0.01	0.005	332	438	480	528	583	651	742	888	1196
	0.02	0.010	271	368	406	450	501	564	649	786	1077
	0.05	0.025	193	275	308	347	392	448	524	647	914
	0.10	0.050	136	206	235	269	309	359	427	539	784
	0.20	0.100	83	139	163	191	225	268	327	426	647
0.60	0.01	0.005	148	194	213	234	258	288	328	392	527
	0.02	0.010	120	163	180	199	222	249	287	347	475
	0.05	0.025	86	122	137	153	173	198	231	286	403
	0.10	0.050	60	91	104	119	136	158	188	238	345
	0.20	0.100	37	62	72	85	100	118	144	188	285
0.65	0.01	0.005	83	108	119	130	144	160	182	217	292
	0.02	0.010	67	91	100	111	123	139	159	192	263
	0.05	0.025	48	68	76	85	96	110	128	158	223
	0.10	0.050	34	51	58	66	76	88	105	132	191
	0.20	0.100	21	35	40	47	55	66	80	104	157
π^2	α 2-sided	α 1-sided	Power 1−β 0.50	0.65	0.70	0.75	0.80	0.85	0.90	0.95	0.99

The cells of the table give the number of patients required *in each treatment arm*.

Table 3.1 Sample sizes for comparison of proportions (*continued*).

π^2	α 2-sided	1-sided	Power $1-\beta$ 0.50	0.65	0.70	0.75	0.80	0.85	0.90	0.95	0.99
					$\pi_1 = 0.45$						
0.70	0.01	0.005	52	68	75	82	90	101	114	136	183
	0.02	0.010	43	57	63	70	78	87	100	121	164
	0.05	0.025	31	43	48	54	61	69	81	99	139
	0.10	0.050	22	32	37	42	48	55	66	82	119
	0.20	0.100	13	22	26	30	35	41	50	65	98
0.75	0.01	0.005	36	47	51	56	61	68	77	92	123
	0.02	0.010	29	39	43	47	53	59	68	81	110
	0.05	0.025	21	29	33	37	41	47	54	67	93
	0.10	0.050	15	22	25	28	32	37	44	55	80
	0.20	0.100	9	15	17	20	24	28	34	44	66
0.80	0.01	0.005	26	33	36	40	44	49	55	65	87
	0.02	0.010	21	28	31	34	38	42	48	58	78
	0.05	0.025	15	21	23	26	29	33	39	47	66
	0.10	0.050	11	16	18	20	23	27	31	39	56
	0.20	0.100	7	11	12	14	17	20	24	31	46
0.85	0.01	0.005	19	25	27	29	32	36	40	48	63
	0.02	0.010	16	21	23	25	28	31	35	42	57
	0.05	0.025	11	16	17	19	22	24	28	34	48
	0.10	0.050	8	12	13	15	17	20	23	29	41
	0.20	0.100	5	8	9	11	12	15	17	22	33
0.90	0.01	0.005	15	19	20	22	24	27	30	35	47
	0.02	0.010	12	16	17	19	21	23	26	31	42
	0.05	0.025	9	12	13	15	16	18	21	26	35
	0.10	0.050	6	9	10	11	13	15	17	21	30
	0.20	0.100	4	6	7	8	9	11	13	17	24
0.95	0.01	0.005	12	15	16	17	19	20	23	27	35
	0.02	0.010	10	12	13	15	16	18	20	24	31
	0.05	0.025	7	9	10	11	12	14	16	19	26
	0.10	0.050	5	7	8	9	10	11	13	16	22
	0.20	0.100	3	5	5	6	7	8	10	12	18
					$\pi_1 = 0.50$						
0.55	0.01	0.005	1324	1749	1917	2107	2329	2602	2966	3551	4789
	0.02	0.010	1080	1467	1621	1796	2001	2255	2595	3143	4314
	0.05	0.025	767	1097	1231	1384	1565	1790	2095	2590	3661
	0.10	0.050	540	822	939	1073	1233	1433	1707	2157	3142
	0.20	0.100	328	554	651	763	899	1071	1309	1707	2593
0.60	0.01	0.005	329	434	475	522	577	645	735	879	1184
	0.02	0.010	268	364	402	445	496	559	643	778	1067
	0.05	0.025	191	272	305	343	388	443	519	641	905
	0.10	0.050	134	204	233	266	305	355	423	533	777
	0.20	0.100	82	138	161	189	223	265	324	422	641
0.65	0.01	0.005	145	190	208	229	253	282	321	384	517
	0.02	0.010	118	160	176	195	217	244	281	340	465
	0.05	0.025	84	120	134	150	170	194	227	280	395
	0.10	0.050	59	90	102	117	134	155	185	233	338
	0.20	0.100	36	61	71	83	98	116	142	184	279
0.70	0.01	0.005	80	105	115	126	139	155	177	211	283
	0.02	0.010	65	88	+7	108	120	134	154	186	255
	0.05	0.025	47	66	74	83	93	107	124	153	216
	0.10	0.050	33	50	56	64	74	85	101	128	185
	0.20	0.100	20	34	39	46	54	64	78	101	152

π^2	α 2-sided	1-sided	Power $1-\beta$ 0.50	0.65	0.70	0.75	0.80	0.85	0.90	0.95	0.99

The cells of the table give the number of patients required *in each treatment arm*.

Table 3.1 Sample sizes for comparison of proportions *(continued)*.

π^2	α 2-sided	α 1-sided	0.50	0.65	0.70	0.75	Power 1−β 0.80	0.85	0.90	0.95	0.99
					$\pi_1 = 0.50$						
0.75	0.01	0.005	50	66	72	79	87	96	110	131	175
	0.02	0.010	41	55	61	67	74	84	96	115	157
	0.05	0.025	29	41	46	52	58	66	77	95	133
	0.10	0.050	21	31	35	40	46	53	63	79	114
	0.20	0.100	13	21	24	29	33	40	48	62	94
0.80	0.01	0.005	34	44	48	53	58	65	73	87	116
	0.02	0.010	28	37	41	45	50	56	64	77	104
	0.05	0.025	20	28	31	35	39	44	52	63	88
	0.10	0.050	14	21	24	27	31	35	42	52	76
	0.20	0.100	9	14	17	19	22	26	32	41	62
0.85	0.01	0.005	24	31	34	37	41	45	51	61	81
	0.02	0.010	20	26	29	32	35	39	45	54	73
	0.05	0.025	14	20	22	24	27	31	36	44	61
	0.10	0.050	10	15	17	19	22	25	29	37	52
	0.20	0.100	6	10	12	14	16	19	22	29	43
0.90	0.01	0.005	18	23	25	27	30	33	37	44	58
	0.02	0.010	15	19	21	23	25	28	32	39	52
	0.05	0.025	11	14	16	18	20	22	26	32	44
	0.10	0.050	8	11	12	14	16	18	21	26	37
	0.20	0.100	5	7	9	10	11	13	16	21	30
0.95	0.01	0.005	14	17	19	20	22	24	27	32	42
	0.02	0.010	11	14	16	17	19	21	24	28	38
	0.05	0.025	8	11	12	13	15	17	19	23	32
	0.10	0.050	6	8	9	10	12	13	15	19	27
	0.20	0.100	4	6	6	7	8	10	12	15	22
					$\pi_1 = 0.55$						
0.60	0.01	0.005	1298	1714	1879	2065	2282	2550	2907	3480	4693
	0.02	0.010	1059	1438	1589	1760	1961	2210	2543	3080	4227
	0.05	0.025	752	1075	1206	1356	1534	1754	2053	2538	3587
	0.10	0.050	529	806	920	1051	1208	1405	1673	2114	3079
	0.20	0.100	322	543	638	748	881	1050	1283	1672	2541
0.65	0.01	0.005	319	421	461	507	560	625	712	852	1148
	0.02	0.010	260	353	390	432	481	542	623	754	1034
	0.05	0.025	185	264	296	333	376	430	503	621	877
	0.10	0.050	130	198	226	258	296	344	410	517	753
	0.20	0.100	79	134	157	183	216	257	314	409	621
0.70	0.01	0.005	139	183	200	219	242	270	308	368	495
	0.02	0.010	113	153	169	187	208	234	269	326	446
	0.05	0.025	81	115	128	144	163	186	217	268	378
	0.10	0.050	57	86	98	112	128	149	177	223	324
	0.20	0.100	35	58	68	80	94	111	136	177	267
0.75	0.01	0.005	76	100	109	120	132	147	167	200	268
	0.02	0.010	62	84	92	102	113	127	146	177	241
	0.05	0.025	44	63	70	79	89	101	118	145	204
	0.10	0.050	31	47	53	61	70	81	96	121	175
	0.20	0.100	19	32	37	43	51	60	74	95	144
0.80	0.01	0.005	47	61	67	74	81	90	102	122	163
	0.02	0.010	38	52	57	63	70	78	90	108	147
	0.05	0.025	27	39	43	48	54	62	72	89	124
	0.10	0.050	19	29	33	37	43	50	59	74	107
	0.20	0.100	12	20	23	27	31	37	45	58	88
π^2	α 2-sided	α 1-sided	0.50	0.65	0.70	0.75	Power 1−β 0.80	0.85	0.90	0.95	0.99

The cells of the table give the number of patients required *in each treatment arm*.

Table 3.1 Sample sizes for comparison of proportions *(continued)*.

π²	α 2-sided	1-sided	0.50	0.65	0.70	0.75	Power 1–β 0.80	0.85	0.90	0.95	0.99
						π₁= 0.55					
0.85	0.01	0.005	31	41	45	49	54	59	67	80	107
	0.02	0.010	26	34	38	41	46	51	59	71	96
	0.05	0.025	18	26	29	32	36	41	47	58	81
	0.10	0.050	13	19	22	25	28	33	39	48	69
	0.20	0.100	8	13	15	18	21	24	29	38	57
0.90	0.01	0.005	22	28	31	34	37	41	46	55	73
	0.02	0.010	18	24	26	29	32	36	40	48	65
	0.05	0.025	13	18	20	22	25	28	33	40	55
	0.10	0.050	9	14	15	17	20	22	26	33	47
	0.20	0.100	6	9	11	12	14	17	20	26	39
0.95	0.01	0.005	16	20	22	24	26	29	33	39	51
	0.02	0.010	13	17	19	21	23	25	29	34	46
	0.05	0.025	10	13	14	16	18	20	23	28	38
	0.10	0.050	7	10	11	12	14	16	19	23	33
	0.20	0.100	4	7	8	9	10	12	14	18	27
						π₁ = 0.60					
0.65	0.01	0.005	1245	1644	1802	1980	2189	2445	2788	3337	4501
	0.02	0.010	1015	1379	1524	1688	1881	2119	2439	2954	4054
	0.05	0.025	721	1031	1157	1301	1471	1682	1969	2434	3440
	0.10	0.050	508	773	882	1008	1159	1347	1604	2027	2953
	0.20	0.100	308	521	612	717	845	1007	1231	1604	2437
0.70	0.01	0.005	302	399	437	480	530	592	675	808	1088
	0.02	0.010	247	335	370	409	456	513	590	715	980
	0.05	0.025	175	250	281	315	356	407	477	589	831
	0.10	0.050	124	188	214	244	281	326	388	490	713
	0.20	0.100	75	127	148	174	205	244	298	388	589
0.75	0.01	0.005	130	171	187	205	227	253	288	344	463
	0.02	0.010	106	143	158	175	195	219	252	305	417
	0.05	0.025	75	107	120	135	152	174	203	251	354
	0.10	0.050	53	80	92	105	120	139	166	209	303
	0.20	0.100	33	54	64	74	88	104	127	165	250
0.80	0.01	0.005	70	92	101	110	122	136	154	184	247
	0.02	0.010	57	77	85	94	105	117	135	163	222
	0.05	0.025	41	58	65	72	82	93	109	134	188
	0.10	0.050	29	43	49	56	64	75	89	111	161
	0.20	0.100	18	29	34	40	47	56	68	88	133
0.85	0.01	0.005	43	56	61	67	74	82	93	111	148
	0.02	0.010	35	47	52	57	63	71	81	98	133
	0.05	0.025	25	35	39	44	49	56	65	80	113
	0.10	0.050	18	26	30	34	39	45	53	67	96
	0.20	0.100	11	18	21	24	28	34	41	53	79
0.90	0.01	0.005	28	36	40	43	48	53	60	71	95
	0.02	0.010	23	31	34	37	41	46	52	63	85
	0.05	0.025	17	23	26	29	32	36	42	52	72
	0.10	0.050	12	17	20	22	25	29	34	43	62
	0.20	0.100	7	12	14	16	18	22	26	34	50
0.95	0.01	0.005	19	25	27	29	32	36	40	48	63
	0.02	0.010	16	21	23	25	28	31	35	42	57
	0.05	0.025	11	16	17	19	22	24	28	34	48
	0.10	0.050	8	12	13	15	17	20	23	29	41
	0.20	0.100	5	8	9	11	12	15	18	22	33
π²	α 2-sided	1-sided	0.50	0.65	0.70	0.75	Power 1–β 0.80	0.85	0.90	0.95	0.99

The cells of the table give the number of patients required *in each treatment arm*.

13

Table 3.1 Sample sizes for comparison of proportions *(continued)*.

π²	α 2-sided	1-sided	0.50	0.65	0.70	0.75	0.80	0.85	0.90	0.95	0.99
						Power 1–β					

$\pi_1 = 0.65$

π²	2-sided	1-sided	0.50	0.65	0.70	0.75	0.80	0.85	0.90	0.95	0.99
0.70	0.01	0.005	1165	1539	1686	1853	2049	2289	2609	3123	4212
	0.02	0.010	950	1290	1426	1580	1760	1983	2283	2765	3794
	0.05	0.025	675	965	1083	1218	1377	1575	1842	2278	3220
	0.10	0.050	475	723	826	944	1084	1261	1502	1897	2764
	0.20	0.100	289	488	572	671	791	942	1152	1501	2281
0.75	0.01	0.005	279	368	403	443	490	547	623	745	1004
	0.02	0.010	228	309	341	378	421	474	545	660	904
	0.05	0.025	162	231	259	291	329	376	440	543	767
	0.10	0.050	114	173	198	226	259	301	358	452	658
	0.20	0.100	69	117	137	161	189	225	275	358	543
0.80	0.01	0.005	118	155	170	187	206	230	262	313	421
	0.02	0.010	96	130	144	159	177	199	229	277	379
	0.05	0.025	69	98	109	123	138	158	185	228	321
	0.10	0.050	48	73	83	95	109	127	150	190	275
	0.20	0.100	30	49	58	68	79	95	115	150	227
0.85	0.01	0.005	63	82	90	98	109	121	137	164	220
	0.02	0.010	51	69	76	84	93	105	120	145	198
	0.05	0.025	37	52	58	65	73	83	97	119	168
	0.10	0.050	26	39	44	50	57	66	79	99	144
	0.20	0.100	16	26	31	36	42	50	60	78	118
0.90	0.01	0.005	38	49	53	58	64	71	81	96	129
	0.02	0.010	31	41	45	50	55	62	71	85	116
	0.05	0.025	22	31	34	38	43	49	57	70	98
	0.10	0.050	16	23	26	30	34	39	46	58	84
	0.20	0.100	10	16	18	21	25	29	35	46	69
0.95	0.01	0.005	24	31	34	37	41	45	51	60	80
	0.02	0.010	20	26	29	31	35	39	44	53	72
	0.05	0.025	14	20	22	24	27	31	36	44	61
	0.10	0.050	10	15	17	19	21	25	29	36	52
	0.20	0.100	6	10	12	13	16	18	22	29	43

$\pi_1 = 0.70$

π²	2-sided	1-sided	0.50	0.65	0.70	0.75	0.80	0.85	0.90	0.95	0.99
0.75	0.01	0.005	1059	1398	1533	1684	1862	2080	2371	2838	3828
	0.02	0.010	864	1173	1296	1436	1600	1802	2074	2513	3448
	0.05	0.025	613	877	984	1107	1251	1431	1674	2070	2926
	0.10	0.050	432	658	750	858	986	1146	1365	1724	2511
	0.20	0.100	262	443	520	610	719	856	1047	1364	2073
0.80	0.01	0.005	249	329	360	396	437	488	556	665	896
	0.02	0.010	203	276	305	337	376	423	486	589	807
	0.05	0.025	145	206	231	260	294	336	392	485	684
	0.10	0.050	102	155	176	201	231	269	320	404	587
	0.20	0.100	62	104	122	143	169	201	245	319	484
0.85	0.01	0.005	103	136	149	163	180	201	229	279	367
	0.02	0.010	84	114	126	139	155	174	200	242	331
	0.05	0.025	60	85	96	107	121	138	161	199	280
	0.10	0.050	42	64	73	83	95	111	131	166	240
	0.20	0.100	26	43	51	59	69	83	101	131	198
0.90	0.01	0.005	54	70	77	84	92	103	117	140	187
	0.02	0.010	44	59	65	72	79	89	102	123	168
	0.05	0.025	31	44	49	55	62	71	82	101	142
	0.10	0.050	22	33	38	43	49	57	67	84	122
	0.20	0.100	14	22	26	30	36	42	51	67	100

π²	α 2-sided	1-sided	0.50	0.65	0.70	0.75	0.80	0.85	0.90	0.95	0.99
						Power 1–β					

The cells of the table give the number of patients required *in each treatment arm*.

Table 3.1 Sample sizes for comparison of proportions *(continued)*.

π^2	2-sided	1-sided	0.50	0.65	0.70	0.75	0.80	0.85	0.90	0.95	0.99
	α						Power $1-\beta$				
					$\pi_1 = 0.70$						
0.95	0.01	0.005	31	40	44	48	53	59	67	79	106
	0.02	0.010	26	34	37	41	46	51	58	70	95
	0.05	0.025	18	25	28	32	36	40	47	58	80
	0.10	0.050	13	19	22	25	28	32	38	48	69
	0.20	0.100	8	13	15	18	20	24	29	38	56
					$\pi_1 = 0.75$						
0.80	0.01	0.005	926	1223	1340	1473	1628	1819	2074	2482	3347
	0.02	0.010	755	1026	1133	1256	1399	1576	1814	2197	3015
	0.05	0.025	536	767	861	968	1094	1251	1464	1810	2558
	0.10	0.050	378	575	656	750	862	1002	1193	1507	2196
	0.20	0.100	230	388	455	534	628	749	915	1193	1812
0.85	0.01	0.005	213	281	307	337	373	416	474	567	764
	0.02	0.010	174	235	260	288	320	361	415	502	688
	0.05	0.025	123	176	197	222	250	286	335	413	583
	0.10	0.050	87	132	151	172	197	229	273	344	501
	0.20	0.100	53	89	104	122	144	171	209	272	413
0.90	0.01	0.005	86	112	123	135	149	166	189	226	303
	0.02	0.010	70	94	104	115	128	144	165	200	273
	0.05	0.025	50	71	79	89	100	114	133	164	231
	0.10	0.050	35	53	60	69	79	91	109	137	198
	0.20	0.100	22	36	42	49	57	68	83	108	163
0.95	0.01	0.005	43	56	61	67	73	82	93	111	148
	0.02	0.010	35	47	52	57	63	71	81	98	133
	0.05	0.025	25	35	39	44	49	56	65	80	113
	0.10	0.050	18	26	30	34	39	45	53	67	96
	0.20	0.100	11	18	21	24	28	34	41	53	79
					$\pi_1 = 0.80$						
0.85	0.01	0.005	767	1013	1110	1220	1348	1506	1717	2055	2770
	0.02	0.010	626	849	938	1040	1158	1305	1502	1819	2495
	0.05	0.025	444	635	713	801	906	1036	1212	1498	2118
	0.10	0.050	313	476	543	621	714	829	988	1248	1817
	0.20	0.100	190	321	377	442	520	620	758	987	1500
0.90	0.01	0.005	170	224	245	269	297	331	377	451	608
	0.02	0.010	139	187	207	229	255	287	330	399	547
	0.05	0.025	98	140	157	177	199	228	266	329	464
	0.10	0.050	69	105	120	137	157	182	217	274	398
	0.20	0.100	42	71	83	97	115	136	166	216	328
0.95	0.01	0.005	65	85	93	102	113	125	143	170	228
	0.02	0.010	53	71	79	87	97	109	125	151	206
	0.05	0.025	38	54	60	67	76	86	101	124	174
	0.10	0.050	27	40	46	52	60	69	82	103	149
	0.20	0.100	16	27	32	37	43	52	63	81	123
					$\pi_1 = 0.85$						
0.90	0.01	0.005	581	767	841	924	1021	1140	1300	1556	2098
	0.02	0.010	474	643	711	787	877	988	1137	1377	1889
	0.05	0.025	337	481	540	607	686	785	918	1135	1603
	0.10	0.050	237	361	412	470	540	628	748	945	1376
	0.20	0.100	144	243	285	335	394	469	574	747	1135
π^2	2-sided	1-sided	0.50	0.65	0.70	0.75	0.80	0.85	0.90	0.95	0.99
	α						Power $1-\beta$				

The cells of the table give the number of patients required *in each treatment arm*.

Table 3.1 Sample sizes for comparison of proportions *(continued)*.

π^2	α 2-sided	1-sided	0.50	0.65	0.70	0.75	Power 1–β 0.80	0.85	0.90	0.95	0.99
					$\pi_1 = 0.85$						
0.95	0.01	0.005	120	158	173	190	209	233	266	318	427
	0.02	0.010	98	132	146	162	180	202	232	281	385
	0.05	0.025	70	99	111	125	141	161	188	231	326
	0.10	0.050	49	74	85	97	111	129	153	193	280
	0.20	0.100	30	50	59	69	81	96	117	152	231
					$\pi_1 = 0.90$						
0.95	0.01	0.005	369	487	533	586	647	723	824	986	1329
	0.02	0.010	301	408	451	499	556	626	721	872	1197
	0.05	0.025	214	305	342	385	435	497	582	719	1015
	0.10	0.050	151	229	261	298	343	398	474	598	871
	0.20	0.100	92	154	181	212	250	298	363	473	719
π^2	α 2-sided	1-sided	0.50	0.65	0.70	0.75	Power 1–β 0.80	0.85	0.90	0.95	0.99

The cells of the table give the number of patients required *in each treatment arm*.

This article was first published in the British Journal of Dermatology and is reproduced by permission of Blackwell Science Ltd

PSYCHOLOGICAL DISTURBANCE IN ATOPIC ECZEMA: THE EXTENT OF THE PROBLEM IN SCHOOL-AGED CHILDREN

CM Absolon, D Cottrell,* SM Eldridge† and MT Glover‡

Department of Child Psychiatry, The Royal London Hospital, London, UK
* Department of Child Psychiatry, University of Leeds, UK
† Department of Epidemiology and Medical Statistics, Queen Mary and Westfield College, London, UK
‡ Department of Dermatology, Newham General Hospital and the Royal London Hospital, London, UK

Accepted for publication 21 March 1997
Correspondence: Dr MT Glover, Academic Department of Dermatology, St Bartholomew's and The Royal London Hospital School of Medicine and Dentistry, Queen Mary and Westfield College, 2 Newark Street, London E1 2AT, UK

British Journal of Dermatology 1997, **137**:241-245

SUMMARY

Although psychological factors are widely considered to be important in atopic eczema, there have been few controlled studies to assess the extent of disturbance in affected children and the problems experienced by their parents. This study was designed to find out the degree of psychological difficulty experienced by children with atopic eczema, whether their mothers show higher levels of mental distress than a comparison group, and whether the families of children with atopic eczema have less social support than the comparison group. We investigated 30 school-aged children with atopic eczema for psychological problems using the Rutter parent scale and compared them with 30 children with relatively minor skin lesions such as viral warts. Mental distress in mothers was assessed using the General Health Questionnaire. The Family Support Scale was used to get a measure of the social support experienced by the families.

We found twice the rate of psychological disturbance in children in the eczema group compared with the control group. This difference was statistically significant for children with moderately severe eczema and severe eczema, but not for children with very mild eczema. Levels of mental distress were no greater in mothers of children with eczema than in parents of the control group and there was no difference in the degree of social support experienced by their families. These findings indicate that school-aged children with moderate and severe atopic eczema are at high risk of developing psychological difficulties, which may have implications for their academic and social development.

Psychological problems are widely perceived as important in atopic eczema.[1] Affected adults have been found to have higher neuroticism scores than controls,[2] and several reports indicate a strong tendency to suppress emotions, especially aggression.[3–5] Although much of this work has focused on adults, there is no doubt that eczema can generate considerable emotional problems for children.[6] Pre-school children with atopic eczema show greater fearfulness and dependency on their parents than controls.[7,8] For children over 5 years old, problems include time off school and impaired performance because of sleep deprivation, which may become habitual, and so persist even when the eczema is less severe.[5] Atopic eczema may be associated with a poor self-image and lack of self-confidence that can interfere with social development.[9] Some children may learn that they can punish or control parents by scratching,[10] and there is evidence that mothers of children with eczema feel less efficient in their disciplining of the affected child than controls.[7] Attempts to identify characteristic mother-child relationships that might be relevant in atopic eczema have produced varied and sometimes conflicting results.[11–13] It appears that attention to emotional and behavioural problems can lead to improvement in atopic eczema,[14–16] but there is very little information to indicate what proportion of patients have psychological disturbance that might benefit from such intervention.

This study was designed to establish the rate of psychological disorder in children between the ages of 5 and 15 years with atopic eczema. Psychological disorder, identified by the Rutter A Questionnaire, was judged to be present when there was an abnormality of behaviour, emotions or relationships which were sufficiently marked and sufficiently prolonged to cause handicap to the child and/or distress and disturbance in the family and community. In order to try and assess whether there is a relationship between the presence of psychological disorder and the severity of eczema, children with all degrees of eczema, even very mild eczema, were included. Because maternal mood disorders are known to cause psychological problems in children,[17] and so might be a potential confounding variable, we assessed current mental distress in mothers using the General Health Questionnaire.[18] Parents of children with atopic eczema have to deal with disturbed sleep, time-consuming treatments, and sometimes a rather irritable

14

child. How well the parents cope will depend to some extent on the amount of support they have from family, friends, teachers and health care professionals. The Family Support Scale was used to assess the degree of social support experienced by families in this study.

PATIENTS AND METHODS

Consecutive children with atopic eczema attending the dermatology out-patient departments at three inner London hospitals were asked to take part. Children with any degree of atopic eczema, even very mild eczema, aged from 5 to 15 years, with at least one English-speaking parent, were included in the study. The comparison group consisted of consecutive children aged from 5 to 15 years attending the same clinics with minor skin problems, e.g. viral warts, molluscum contagiosum and benign melanocytic naevi. Two patients with eczema and eight comparison patients chose not to enter the study. Parents were told that the object of the study was to see if common dermatological problems in childhood could affect well–being.

The children were assessed for psychological difficulties by a child psychiatrist (CMA) using the Rutter A2 scale.[17] This is a well developed questionnaire widely used in child psychiatry [19] and is designed to detect children with a clinically-significant degree of psychological disturbance. It has been used in more than 80 studies in many countries. It consists of 31 statements about behaviour, e.g. does the child have temper tantrums, stammer or stutter, steal things, worry unduly about things, tend to be fearful of new situations, destroy property or belongings, frequently disobey, or tell lies or bully other children, with a choice of responses (at least once a week, occasionally or never, or no, mild or severe). Children having an overall score of 13 or more are considered to have a psychological disorder, defined as an abnormality of behaviour, emotions or relationships which is sufficiently marked and sufficiently prolonged to cause handicap to the child and/or the family or community. It is possible to extract from the questionnaire separate scores to identify the presence of emotional disorder, conduct disorder or hyperactivity.

The mothers were assessed for mental distress using the General Health Questionnaire (28 item version),[18] using the binary scoring system with a cut-off point of 5. Examples of questions include: 'Have you felt that you are ill?'; 'Have you lost much sleep over worry?': 'Have you felt constantly under strain?': 'Have you been thinking of yourself as a worthless person?'; and 'Have you had the idea of taking your own life?'. The respondent is asked to say whether each of these applies a great deal, somewhat or not at all, or more than usual. The same as usual, or less than usual. The degree of social support experienced by the family was assessed using the Family Support Scale,[20] which gives a measure of both quality and quantity of support. The parent is asked to rate the amount of help they experience from 18 sources such as relatives, friends and general practitioner, on a scale of 0–5.

Table 1

Demographic variables in the eczema group and the control group

	Eczema group	Comparison group
Age in years:		
mean	8.7	9.9
range	5.3–13. 7	5.5–14.5
Male	13 (43%)	16 (53%)
Female	17 (57%)	14 (47%)
Family size (mean.)	2.6	2.5
One or both parents in employment	23 (77%)	24 (80%)
Parent unemployed or on sickness benefit	7 (23%)	6 (20%)
Housing: mean number of people per room	0.96	0.86
Ethnic group		
White (E, S, W or I)*	12 (40%)	16 (53%)
Black	5 (17%)	4 (13%)
Asian	7 (23%)	6 (20%)
Other	6 (20%)	4 (13%)

*E, English; S, Scottish; W, Welsh; I, Irish.

Details of family size, housing conditions, employment status of parents and the general health of the child were also recorded. The psychiatrist was not informed of the child's dermatological diagnosis, but full 'blinding' of the psychiatrist was not possible as some children had eczema visible on exposed skin, and occasionally parents referred to the eczema during the interview. However, the psychiatrist had no information on the severity of the eczema.

Scores for eczema severity using a well established system [21] were given by a dermatologist (MG) who was not aware of the results of the psychological assessment. Scoring sheets were used showing the front and back of the body divided into 20 zones of approximately equal area. A score from 0 to 3 was given for each zone in respect of severity of erythema and surface damage, and combined with an estimate of surface area affected within each zone. A score of 1 was given where the area affected was <33%, a score of 2 for an area of 34–66% and 3 where the area was >67%. The severity score was then multiplied by the respective area score to provide an adjusted score for that zone. The resulting scores were added to provide a total body score, up to a maximum of 180, for each of the two clinical features. Children with scores of less than 10 were classified as having mild eczema, scores from 10 to 34 as moderate, and 35 or more as severe. Results for the eczema group were compared with the non-eczema group using the x^2 test.

RESULTS

Thirty children with atopic eczema and 30 comparison children were enrolled in the study. The children with eczema and the comparison group were well matched in terms of age, gender, family size, employment status of parents and ethnic background (Table 1). The severity of eczema varied enormously between children (erythema score: range 1–113, median 15; surface damage score: range 0.6–108, median 15). The children with eczema were significantly more likely than the comparison group to have asthma (47% compared with 10%; $x^2 = 9.9$; $P = 0.002$). Hay fever was also more prevalent among children with eczema, although the difference was not statistically significant at the 5% level (40% compared with 20%, $x^2 = 2.9$; $P = 0.091$). Forty per cent of parents of children with eczema had eczema themselves, compared with only 3% of parents of the comparison group.

The rate of psychological disturbance, defined by a Rutter score of 13 or more, was 50% in the eczema group compared with 27% in the comparison group ($P = 0.063$; 95% CI for the difference is –6% to +48%.) One-third of the children were rated as having very mild eczema with severity scores of 10 or less. This subgroup had a rate of psychological disturbance of 30% which is very similar to the comparison group. In contrast, the rate of psychological disorder was 53% in children with moderate eczema ($n = 15$), and 80% in children with severe eczema ($n = 5$). The rate was 60% in children with moderate and severe eczema combined, more than twice the rate in the comparison group ($x^2 = 5.6$; $P = 0.018$).

Using the subdivisions in the Rutter Questionnaire to assess the children according to whether they exhibited disorders of conduct, emotion or hyperactivity, 80% of the children with eczema scoring above the Rutter cut-off point of 13 were identified as having an emotional disorder manifesting as excessive worries in 10 children, excessive fears in three children, frequent stomach aches in 11 children, frequent tears on arrival at school in two children, and difficulty getting to sleep and frequent waking at night in 12 children. Only 20% of the children with eczema scoring above the cut-off point were identified as having conduct disorders such as stealing (one child), destroying property (two children), frequent disobedience (eight children), telling lies (seven children) and bullying (four children). In the comparison group there were equal numbers of children identified as having emotional disorder and conduct disorder (excessive worries, four; excessive fears, five; frequent stomach aches, three; frequent tears on arrival at school, one; sleeping difficulty, four: stealing, two: destroying property, two; frequent disobedience, five: telling lies, four; and bullying, none). There was no difference in the hyperactivity rates between the two groups, with 11 children from each group scoring above the cut-off point for the summed hyperactivity score.

In the Rutter Questionnaire, the parent is asked whether their child has difficulty sleeping, if the difficulty is mild or severe, and whether the problem is in getting to sleep, waking during the night or waking early in the morning. On this basis, sleep disturbance was a problem in 67% of all children with atopic eczema in this study, compared with 13% of controls ($P = 0.001$). Because problems with sleep may be due to itch rather than to psychological factors in children with eczema, and because the scores for sleep disturbance were so high in children with eczema and might be having an undue effect on the total score, the Rutter scores were examined with the section on sleep excluded. This made no difference to the results, with all the same children still scoring above the cut-off point of 13 despite the removal of the sleep scores.

Degree of mental distress in mothers assessed with the General Health Questionnaire was very similar for the two groups (54%, for the eczema group and 43%, for the comparison group ($P = 0.35$). The degree of maternal distress was not related to the severity of eczema (Spearman Rank = 0.11; $P = 0.58$). There was no difference in the numbers of social supports for the two groups of families. Both groups had an average of eight sources of informal support each and they rated these supports as similarly helpful.

DISCUSSION

In this study of 30 school-aged children with atopic eczema attending hospital, we found the rate of psychological disturbance to be twice that of a comparison group, as measured by the Rutter A Questionnaire with the standard cut-off point of 13. We included children with all degrees of eczema in this study because the relationship between severity of eczema and rates of psychological disturbance has not been explored. We found that children with very mild eczema have rates of disturbance similar to those in the comparison group. For children with moderate and severe eczema, the rate of psychological disturbance was 60%, significantly higher than the comparison group. Exclusion of scores for sleep disturbance, which is a very common effect of eczema, had no effect on the results, with all the same children still scoring above the cut-off point.

Direct comparison of our results with other studies is difficult as some have included a parent interview or a teacher questionnaire as well. Using the Rutter Questionnaire a rate of psychological disturbance of 6% was found in children from the general population on the Isle of Wight,[22] and a rate of 12% in an inner London borough.[17] Garralda et al. found a rate of 23% in children attending their GP[23] which is similar to the rate in our comparison group and less than half the rate of 50% that we found in our eczema group as a whole. Using similar questionnaires disturbance was evident in 55% of children with hemiplegia,[24] 38% of children with leukaemia,[25] 28.6% of children with uncomplicated epilepsy and 58.3%, of children with brain-stem lesions causing fits.[26] Although links between atopic conditions and attention deficit disorder and hyperactivity have been reported,[27] we found no increase in symptoms of hyperactivity in this group of children with eczema compared with controls.

The rates of maternal mental distress were high in both groups (54%, and 43%). The Jarman indices for the three London boroughs included in this study show

14

them all to have high rates of deprivation which may account for these findings. The failure to find an association between the mother's distress and the severity of atopic eczema may in part be an effect of the General Health Questionnaire which, because it focuses on mood in the previous 4 weeks compared with usual, may fail to identify long-standing mental distress. There was no demonstrable difference in the degree of social support experienced by the families of children with eczema and those without. It seems, therefore, that the high rate of psychological disturbance evident in the eczema group cannot be attributed to maternal mood or lack of social support for the family.

This study does not enable us to determine how psychological problems are initiated. It is possible that the relationship is a cyclical one. Psychological disturbances might exacerbate eczema through difficulties with treatment, increased scratching and heightened emotions, which in turn may lead to deterioration in behaviour. Successful management in such cases will need to include attention to both physical and psychological aspects. Simple manoeuvres such as the use of star charts for applying topical treatments may be sufficient, but sometimes more input is necessary in the form of family therapy or individual therapy for children.

This study has revealed rates of psychological disturbance in children with atopic eczema which are similar to or greater than those that have been found in children with epilepsy and leukaemia, who frequently have psychological input as part of their management. Our findings suggest that psychological input should be considered more frequently as part of the management of children with atopic eczema.

ACKNOWLEDGEMENT

We would like to thank David Wright of the Department of Epidemiology and Medical Statistics, Queen Mary and Westfield College for help with statistical analysis.

References

1 Champion RH, Parish WE. Atopic dermatitis. In: *Textbook of Dermatology* (Champion RH, Burton JL, Ebling FJG, eds), 5th edn, Vol. 1. Oxford: Blackwell Scientific Publications, 1992; 589–610.

2 Geiler U, Ehlers A, Hohler T, Burkard G. The psychosocial status of patients with endogenous eczema. *Hautarzt* 1990; **41**: 416–23.

3 White A, Horne DJ, Varigos GA. Psychological profile of the atopic eczema patient. *Aust J Dermatol* 1990; **31**: 13–16.

4 Kuypers B. Atopic dermatitis: some observations from a psychological viewpoint. *Dermatologica* 1967; **136**: 387–94.

5 Fritz G. Psychological aspects of atopic dermatitis: a viewpoint. *Clin Pediatr* 1979; **18**: 360–4.

6 Lewis-Jones M, Finlay A. The Children's Dermatology Quality of Life Index: initial validation and practical use. *Br J Dermatol* 1995; **132**: 942–9.

7 Daud L, Garralda M, David TJ. Psychosocial adjustment in preschool children with atopic eczema. *Arch Dis Child* 1993; **69**: 670–6.

8 Golding J, Peters T. Eczema and hay fever. In: *From Birth to Five* (Golding J. ed.). Oxford: Pergamon Press, 1986.

9 Cotterill J. Psychiatry and the skin. *Br J Hosp Med* 1989; **42**: 401–4.

10 Miller H, Brauch D. A study of hostility in allergic children. *Am J Orthopsychiatry* 1950; **20**: 506–9.

11 Ring J, Palos E. Psychosomatic aspects of parent-child relations in atopic eczema. *Hautarzt* 1986; **37**: 609–17.

12 Gil M, Keefe F, Sampson H *et al.* The relation of stress and family environment to atopic dermatitis symptoms in children. *J Psychosom Res* 1987; **31**: 673–84.

13 Vaughan V. Emotional undertones in eczema in children. *J Asthma Res* 1966; **3**: 193–7.

14 Allen K, Harris F. Elimination of a child's excessive scratching by training the mother in reinforcement inhibition of scratching. *Behav Res Ther* 1966; **4**: 79–84.

15 Melin L. Frederiksen T, Noren E Swebilius B. Behaviour treatment of scratching in patients with atopic dermatitis. *Br J Dermatol* 1986; **115**: 467–74.

16 Koblenzer C, Koblenzer P. Chronic intractable atopic eczema. *Arch Dermatol* 1988; **124**: 1673–7.

17 Rutter M, Cox A, Tupling C *et al.* Attainment and adjustment in two geographical areas. I. The prevalence of psychiatric disorder. *Br J Psychiatry* 1975; **126**: 493–509.

18 Goldberg D. *Manual of The General Health Questionnaire*. Windsor: NEFR Publishing Company, 1978.

19 Elander J, Rutter M. An update on the status of the Rutter parent's and teacher's scales. *Psychol Psychiatry Rev Child* 1996; **1**: 31–5.

20 Dunst C, Jenkins V, Trivette C. The Family Support Scale: reliability and validity. *J Individual Family Commun Wellness* 1984; **1**: 45–52.

21 Sheehan M, Atherton D. A controlled trial of traditional Chinese medicinal plants in widespread non-exudative atopic eczema. *Br J Dermatol* 1992; **126**: 179–84.

22 Rutter M, Tizard J, Whitmore K. *Education, Health and Behaviour*. London: Longman, 1970.

23 Garralda M, Bailey D. Children with psychiatric disorders in primary care. *J Child Psychol Psychiatry* 1986; **27**: 611–24.

24 Goodman R, Graham P. Psychiatric problems in children with hemiplegia: cross sectional epidemiological survey. *Br Med J* 1996; **312**: 1065–9.

25 Maguire P. Psychological and social consequences of cancer. In: *Recent Advances in Clinical Oncology*. Edinburgh: Churchill Livingstone, 1982: 375–84.

26 Rutter M. A neuropsychiatric study in childhood. In *Clinics in Developmental Medicine*, Vol. 35/36. London: Heinemann/Spastics International Medical Publications, 1970.

27 Roth N. Coincidence of attention deficit disorder and atopic disorders in children: empirical findings and hypothetical background. *J Abnorm Child Psychol* 1991; **19**: 1–13.

14

This article was first published in the International Journal of Epidemiology and is reproduced with permission of Oxford University Press

AN EMPIRICAL STUDY OF CLUSTER RANDOMIZATION

Allan Donner

(Department of Epidemiology and Biostatistics, University of Western Ontario, London, Canada N6A 5137).

International Journal of Epidemiology 1982, **11**: 283–286.

Increasing attention has been given recently to the methodological issues associated with randomization of clusters rather than individuals in lifestyle intervention trials. These issues are explored through an empirical study of the 'effective sample size' imposed by randomization of three experimental units frequently considered in epidemiological research: the spouse pair, the general practice, and the large geographic area (county). The measurement of within-cluster dependence for a dichotomous outcome variable is also discussed, and a relationship shown between Fleiss's kappa and Cornfield's inflation factor.

There has been considerable attention given recently [1-4] to the problems of randomizing clusters rather than individuals in controlled trials of preventive measures and health care innovations. Although the use of randomization units larger than the individual may reduce the power to detect a real intervention effect, it may not always be feasible or economic to randomize individuals. For example, in a trial of dietary modification among adults, adherence to the experimental dietary regime would be more likely if all members of the household were enrolled. Thus the preferred unit of randomization for such a trial is often the family or spouse pair, while randomization units of larger size might be selected in other studies. For example, in a current trial [5,6] of the value of hypertension screening and compliance-enhancing management in general practice, it would be very difficult to randomize patients *within* practices to experimental and control groups. Having set up a programme in a practice for screening and treatment procedures, the efficient functioning of the programme would be severely compromised by the requirement that some patients and not others be entered into it. Thus in this study, it is the practice which is the unit of randomization.

In yet other studies the most appropriate unit of randomization is an entire community, as for example, in controlled trials of water fluoridation for the prevention of dental caries.[7] Except in isolated rural communities, water supplies are public, and it is therefore virtually impossible to deliver fluoridated water to randomly selected individuals and non-fluoridated water to other individuals in the same community.

In spite of growing awareness of the statistical issues raised by cluster randomization, there is very little empirical evidence to illustrate its impact on sample size requirements. As pointed out by Cornfield,[2] appropriate sets of data will need to be analysed to determine the actual increases in sample size requirements associated with randomization units of different size. In this paper we study these requirements empirically for three experimental units frequently considered in epidemiological research: the spouse pair, the general practice, and the large geographic area (county). To facilitate the comparison of results among the units of different size, data on the same subject population is used in each analysis.

STATISTICAL THEORY

The consequence of cluster randomization is a reduction in effective sample size. This occurs because the individuals within a cluster cannot be regarded as independent. For example, patients in a particular practice might tend toward slenderness because the physician is an avid believer in weight-control. Only rarely, however, will the dependence among members of the experimental unit be total. Thus the effective sample size, although not equal to the total number of individual subjects in the trial, will be somewhat greater than the number of experimental and control clusters.

The precise effect of cluster randomization on sample size requirements depends on both the size of the cluster and the degree of within-cluster dependence. In this paper we focus on the case of binary outcome data, since dichotomous variables are used more frequently than continuous variables in the planning of sample size requirements for intervention trials (for a discussion of the more straightforward case of a continuous outcome variable, see Donner et al [3]).

Consider a sample of k clusters, with the size of the ith cluster denoted by n_i, i= 1, 2, . . . ,k. Each of these clusters may be thought of as having its own proportion of subjects P_i, i= 1, 2, . . . ,k, with the characteristic in question, i.e. its own proportion of 'successes'. The degree of within-cluster dependence may be measured by a version of the kappa statistic originally derived by Cohen [8] and further developed by Fleiss and Colien.[9] This version, most recently described by Fleiss,[10] is given by

$$\hat{\kappa} = 1 - \frac{\sum_{i=1}^{k} n_i P_i(1-P_i)}{k(\bar{n}-1)\,\bar{P}\,(1-\bar{P})}, \quad (1)$$

where $\bar{n} = \sum_{i=1}^{k} n_i/k$ and $\bar{P} = \sum_{i=1}^{k} n_i P_i / \sum_{i=1}^{k} n_i$.

Suppose that $k/2$ of the clusters are randomly allocated to each of two groups. Then a simple extension of results derived by Cornfield[2] for the case of equal-sized clusters shows that the relative efficiency of randomization by cluster is given by

$$R = \frac{\bar{P}(1-\bar{P})}{\bar{n}\,\sigma^2},$$

where $\sigma^2 = \dfrac{n_i(P_i - \bar{P})^2}{k\bar{n}^2},$ \quad (2)

Expression (2) is the variance of the difference between the overall proportion of successes in the two groups achieved by individual randomization relative to the variance achieved by cluster randomization. It implies that the usual estimate of the required number of individuals in each group should be multiplied by an inflation factor IF=1/R to provide the same statistical power under cluster randomization as would be obtained under individual randomization.

METHOD

The data analysed were obtained from the study [5] referred to above on the value of hypertension screening and management in general practice. Patients aged 20–65 were grouped into spouse pairs, general practices (each associated with a single physician) and counties (roughly adjacent in the province of Ontario, Canada) according to information obtained from each patient's chart at the time of registration into the study. While the number of practices and counties in each analysis was 20 and 4, respectively, the number of spouse pairs varied

according to the information available for the characteristic in question. These characteristics, selected because of their potential interest as outcome variables in lifestyle intervention trials, were as follows: hypertension (diastolic blood pressure ≥ 90 mmHg), smoking (current smoker of cigarettes, pipe or cigar), drinking (average number of drinks consumed per day ≥ 1) and body fatness (ponderal index < 12.5). Information on the first of these variables was obtained from office charts, and on the remaining variables from a questionnaire administered in the physicians's office. Detailed definitions of the variables are given in the appendix.

RESULTS

The results of the analyses are shown in Table 1. As one might expect, the value of kappa, which measures the degree of within-cluster dependence, declines with the size of the corresponding unit. However, the value of the inflation factor does not follow this pattern, and, in fact, is always lowest for the spouse pair and highest for the county. This occurs because an observation recorded on a member of a spouse pair, although correlated with that taken on his mate, is statistically independent of all other observations in the study. If four large counties are randomized, on the other hand, the outcome on any one individual is correlated with a full quarter of the study population. Thus the sample size inflation factor is much higher in the latter case, even though the absolute degree of correlation between any two members is considerably lower.

As an example of how these results may be used, suppose a trial is being planned for which the proposed unit of randomization is the spouse pair, and the principal outcome variable is hypertension status. Then the number of subjects enrolled in the trial must be multiplied by a factor of 1.14 to obtain the same statistical power as would be obtained by the randomization of individuals. The corresponding inflation factors for practices is 6.28 and for counties is

Table 1

Variable*	Randomization unit	Number of units in analysis	Average unit size	Kappa	Inflation factor
Hypertension	Spouse pair	6376	2	0.14	1.14
	Practice	20	637.6	0.0076	6.28
	County	4	3188.0	0.0043	16.42
Smoking	Spouse pair	2893	2	0.25	1.25
	Practice	20	289.3	0.0026	1.47
	County	4	1446.5	0.0003	1.72
Drinking	Spouse pair	2865	2	0.22	1.22
	Practice	20	286.5	0.0062	4.62
	County	4	1432.5	0.0056	12.54
Body fatness	Spouse pair	2770	2	0.11	1.11
	Practice	20	277.0	0.013	6.04
	County	4	1385.0	0.0071	12.84

*See appendix for definitions.

16.42. These results show that a failure to account for randomization by cluster can drastically reduce the planned power of a trial, especially if the clusters are fairly large.

The value of the inflation factor given by the reciprocal of formula (2) depends on cluster size and thus for these data is comparable across characteristics only for the spouse pair. The value of kappa, on the other hand, is comparable across characteristics for each of the three experimental units. Thus the characteristic showing the greatest degree of within-family resemblance is smoking ($\hat{\kappa}$=.25). and that showing the greatest degree of within-practice resemblance is body fatness ($\hat{\kappa}$=.013). However the absolute degree of within-cluster resemblance for practices and for counties is very small for all characteristics studied. It is the *size* of these units which accounts for the magnitudes of their associated inflation factors.

It is also worth noting that the inflation factor for smoking shows the least variation of any characteristic among the three different units of randomization. This occurs because the value of kappa for smoking declines very steeply with unit size. In fact, the degree of within-cluster resemblance for practices and counties is smaller for smoking than for any other characteristic, while, as mentioned above, the degree of spouse-pair resemblance with respect to smoking, which depends on both unit size and the degree of within-cluster resemblance, is relatively stable across the three units.

Interpretation of Kappa

The version of kappa given by expression (1) essentially results from the application to dichotomous data of the standard formula [11] for the coefficient of intraclass correlation, widely used to measure the degree of within-cluster resemblance with respect to a continuous variable. If the underlying trait of interest has an approximate normal distribution, then this coefficient has the same clear-cut interpretation as the ordinary product-moment correlation between two randomly selected cluster members. If the underlying trait is dichotomous, however, the interpretation of the intraclass correlation (and hence kappa) is not as clear, except under special conditions. For the case of small, relatively homogeneous clusters of fixed size, such as spouse pairs or sibships, Donner *et al* [3] have shown that kappa may be interpreted directly in terms of the underlying cluster concordancy rate, where a concordant cluster is defined as one in which the responses of all members are identical (i.e., all 'successes' or all 'failures'). In this case, kappa estimates $(P_c-P_E)/(1-P_E)$ where P_c is the true concordance rate in the underlying population of clusters, and P_E is the concordance rate expected under the assumption of independence. For clusters of larger size, which tend to be more heterogeneous, this interpretation will no longer hold, although $\hat{\kappa}$ still provides a measure of within-cluster resemblance. Furthermore, for any cluster of fixed size n, it is easy to show that IF = 1 +(n–1)$\hat{\kappa}$, a

relationship which may be useful in the planning of studies for which prior information concerning, kappa is available. The values of kappa in Table 1 may also be used for this purpose, but should preferably be obtained from previous studies as similar as possible to those being planned. An additional complication is that the experimental units in many studies will be of variable size, in which case no simple relationship holds between $\hat{\kappa}$ and IF. However, if the variation is not too great, the formula above may be used as approximation with $\hat{n}$=n, where $\hat{n}$ is the average cluster size. For the data presented in Table 1, there is considerable variation in both practice size and county size, and thus the approximation is only roughly accurate for these two units.

ANALYSIS CONSIDERATIONS

As remarked by Cornfield,[2] 'randomization by cluster accompanied by an analysis appropriate to randomization by individual is an exercise in self-deception and should be discouraged'. For the case of small homogenous units such as sibship pairs or families, Donner *et al* [3] have discussed one approach to the comparison of two proportions arising from cluster randomization. For larger units, such as hospitals or counties, the approach suggested by Cornfield[2] should be used. The essential feature of both these approaches is the development of a variance expression for the difference between the two proportions which takes into account between-cluster variation. The application of standard inference techniques to data arising from cluster randomization may result in spurious statistical significance, since they ignore this source of variation.

FINAL REMARKS

The main purpose of this paper has been to illustrate the impact of cluster randomization on sample size requirements for lifestyle intervention trials. The sample size inflation factor associated with a particular unit of randomization will depend on both its size and nature. However two general conclusions are suggested by the results of the analyses above:

1. Although the degree of within-cluster resemblance tends to decline with cluster size, the magnitude of the corresponding inflation factor may not. This is because the relative efficiency of a given randomization unit declines rapidly with unit size, for any positive degree of within-cluster correlation. For very large units, such as counties, the relative efficiency may be less than 10%.

2. The selection of a randomization unit will often involve a choice between improved statistical power and a reduced risk of contamination. For example, if individuals within a neighbourhood or family practice were randomly allocated to an experimental programme of smoking, drinking or exercise modification, it is highly possible that some of the subjects allocated to the control group would become aware of the existence of the experimental groups, and attempt to receive its perceived benefits,

15

either directly or indirectly. The risk of this contamination can be reduced by randomizing neighbourhoods or practices rather than individuals. However the results in Table 1 suggest that this may involve a very substantial loss of statistical power for a given total number of subjects. Complicating the issue further is the fact that the loss in power may usually be estimated in advance, while the risk of bias may be very difficult to assess.

Ultimately it may be issues relating to feasibility and cost that play the decisive role in the choice of an experimental unit. However an appreciation of the statistical consequences of this choice is crucial if the study is to be properly planned.

ACKNOWLEDGEMENTS

Dr Donner's work was supported by National Health Research Scholar Award (Canada) and an Ontario Ministry of Health Demonstration Model Grant. The author is grateful to Drs Martin Bass, Carol Buck and Ms Shelley Bull for their helpful comments.

(Revised version received 4 March 1982)

APPENDIX
Definition of Outcome Variables
Hypertension

A patient is classified as hypertensive if (a) two diastolic blood pressure readings exceeding 90 mmHg are recorded on his/her office chart or (b) the patient is receiving antihypertensive drug therapy.

Body fatness

A patient is classified as having excess body fat if his/her ponderal index [height (in)/weight 1/3 (lbs)] is below 12.5.

Smoking

A patient is classified as a smoker if he/she replies yes to the following question:
'Do you smoke now (cigarettes, pipe or cigar)?'

Drinking

A patient is classified as a drinker if he/she replies: 'at least one drink a day' to the following question:
How many drinks of beer, wine and/or liquor do you consume in an average day?'
A 'drink' = 1 bottle of beer
or 4–5 oz. of wine or
$1/2$ oz, of spirits (whiskey, gin, rum, vodka, etc.)

References

1 Sherwin R. Controlled trials of the diet-heart hypothesis: some comments on the experimental unit. *Am J Epidemiol* 1978; **108**: 92–9.

2 Cornfield J. Randomization by group: a formal analysis. *Am J Epidemiol* 1978; **108**: 100–2.

3 Donner A, Birkett N, and Buck C. Randomization by cluster: sample size requirements and analysis. *Am J Epidemiol* 1981; **114**: 906–14.

4 Buck C and Donner A. The design of controlled experiments in the evaluation of non-therapeutic interventions. *J Chron Dis* (in press).

5 McWhinney IR, Donner A and Bass M. Hypertension screening and management in general practice. *Prev Med* 1978; 7: 112

6 Bass M, Donner A and McWhinney IR. The effectiveness of the family physician in hypertension screening and management. *Can Fam Phys* (in press).

7 Ast DB and Schlesinger ER. The conclusion of a ten-year study of water fluoridation. *Am J Pub Health* 1956; **46**: 265–71.

8 Cohen J. A coefficient of agreement for nominal scales. *Ed Psych Meas* 1960; **20**: 37–46.

9 Fleiss JL and Cohen J. The equivalence of weighted kappa and the intraclass correlation coefficient as a measure of reliability. *Ed Psych Meas* 1973; **33**: 613–19.

10 Fleiss JL. Statistical Methods for Rates and Proportions (2nd edn.) New York, Wiley, p. 227, 1981.

11 Snedecor GW and Cochran WG. Statistical Methods (7th edn.) Ames, Iowa State, p. 243, 1980.

This article was first published in Family Practice and is reproduced by permission of Oxford University Press

TRIALS WHICH RANDOMIZE PRACTICES I: HOW SHOULD THEY BE ANALYSED?

Sally M Kerry and J Martin Bland[a]

Received 5 August 1997; Accepted 3 October 1997. Division of General Practice and Primary Care and [a]Department of Public Health Sciences, St George's Hospital Medical School, Cramner Terrace, London SW17 0RE, UK.

Family Practice 1998; **15**: 80–83.

Background. In some general practice intervention trials, patients must be randomized in practices rather than individually, and this must be taken into account in the analysis.

Objectives. In this article we aim to show how failure to do this may lead to spurious statistical significance and CIs which are narrower than they should be, and to describe the use of summary measures for each practice as a simple method of analysis.

Method. The statistical issues are demonstrated by an example of a trial in general practice.

Discussion. The choice of unit of analysis will be most important where there are large numbers of patients recruited from each practice or a high degree of variability between practices.

Keywords. General practice, randomized controlled trials, statistical analysis.

INTRODUCTION

Randomized intervention studies have become accepted as the gold standard method for comparing new treatments with existing therapies. Randomization is used to remove any systematic bias due to other factors which might influence the outcome. The observed difference between the treatment groups can then be attributed to the intervention and not to confounding factors.

Experimental units

Randomized trials can be used to evaluate the effectiveness of a care package, new technology, the introduction of guidelines or a health education initiative. All patients in the same practice may need to be in the same intervention group and hence the need to randomize practices. In general, groups of individuals such as patients in a practice can be called clusters and the trials referred to as cluster randomized trials. Other examples of clusters may be areas of residence, hospitals and schools, but in this article we shall refer to practices.

In the Family Heart Study[1] of cardiovascular screening in general practice, practices were randomly allocated to screening or control. Cluster randomization was used here as patients attending the same practice might have interacted with one another and in this way the control group could have become contaminated.

However, there is a price to be paid for cluster randomization at the analysis stage. We can no longer think of our trial subjects as independent individuals. People within a practice will be more alike than a random sample of people from the study areas subject to the same intervention and hence we have two sources of variation, that between people attending a practice and that between practices. We must perform an analysis which takes account of variation at the level of the unit of randomization, namely the practice. This leads to a loss of power compared with a screening study involving the same number of subjects which randomizes the subjects individually to intervention or control. The larger the clusters, the more important this issue becomes. This feature of the design is often not appreciated by researchers. In a review of 16 non-therapeutic intervention trials employing cluster randomization, Donner *et al.* [2] that found only eight accounted for between-cluster variation in the analysis.

The question of the experimental unit also arises when the treatment is applied to the GP or nurse rather than to the patient directly. For example, in a study of GP care of the long-term mentally ill, practices were randomly assigned to two intervention groups. The GPs in the intervention group practices were taught a structured assessment schedule to use with their long-term mentally ill patients every 6 months for 2 years.[3] One of the outcome measures was the proportion of patients whose psychiatric medication had been changed during the study period of 2 years (Table 1). This was obtained by examination of the notes of all patients with long-term mental illness in the intervention and control practices. The patients were used to assess changes in the doctors' prescribing behaviour. The primary experimental unit was the GP, not the patient.

Patients can be regarded as repeat measurements of the GP, and are analogous to repeat measurements on a single patient in a trial. In general, a trial will produce more convincing evidence for the effectiveness of a treatment if 60 different people are recruited than if six people are measured on 10 occasions. In the latter example, the analysis must take into account that we have repeat measurements on the same people. One way of doing this is to form a summary statistic for each

16

Table 1

Number of patients whose psychiatric drugs were changed for each practice in the intervention and controls groups

Intervention group			Control group		
No. of patients			No. of patients		
Changed	Total	Percentage changed	Changed	Total	Percentage changed
11	23	47.8	4	14	28.
7	12	58.3	10	28	35.7
23	38	60.5	20	48	41.7
13	19	68.4	4	8	50.0
16	23	69.6	14	24	58.3
15	20	75.0	16	27	59.3
23	30	76.7	16	25	64.0
15	19	79.0	11	15	73.3
Total 123	184		95	189	
		Mean 66.9			Mean 51.4
		SD 10.6			SD 15.2

person, as recommended by Matthews *et al.*[4] Likewise, in a cluster-randomized trial we can construct a summary statistic for each cluster. In the long-term mental illness trial this was the proportion of patients who had their medication changed for each practice.

STATISTICAL ANALYSIS

In this paper we use the data of Table 1 to demonstrate the summary statistic method applied to the long-term mental illness study and compare this to analysis of the same data using the patient as the unit of analysis. We demonstrate that ignoring the between-cluster variability underestimates the standard error of the difference between the intervention groups and increases the apparent statistical significance of the observed differences.

Statistical analysis: individual randomization

If we had randomly assigned individual patients to intervention groups then we would test the observed difference in proportions between the two groups using a Normal approximation, equivalent to a chi-square test.[5] In the intervention group, 123 (66.9 %) of the 189 patients had changes made to their medication compared with 95 (50.3 %) out of 184 patients in the control group (Table 1). The difference in percentage of patients where changes were mide is 16.6. In order to carry out the test of significance we need the standard error of this difference. If we ignore the variation between practices, the standard error is 5.0 and the significance test for the difference in two proportions gives $P = 0.001$. The corresponding 95 % CI for the difference between proportions is 6.7–26.4 %.

Statistical analysis: cluster randomization

The above analysis is only correct if the observations are independent. Patients treated by the same doctor are

more likely to have similar changes made to their medication than a random sample of patients from the same intervention group. Thus we cannot assume that they are independent and must use a different method of analysis. The percentage of patients whose medication was changed was calculated for each practice. These are shown in Table 1.

The mean percentages were 66.9 (SD 10.6) for the eight practices in the intervention group and 51.4 (SD 15.2) for the eight practices in the control group. Hence the difference in the mean percentage conforming was 15.5. The pooled variance estimate is $(7 \times 10.6^2 + 7 \times 15.2^2)/14 = 171.7$ and the standard error of the difference is

$$\sqrt{171.7 \times (1/8 + 1/8)} = 6.6$$

Assuming that the data are normally distributed, and that the two groups have uniform variance, a *t*-test can be used to test the difference between the mean proportions. The *t*-test gives $P = 0.033$ and the 95% CI is 1.5–29.6 %. (In this example the test assumptions are only approximately true, but the *t*-test is robust to departures from normality for two equal-sized samples.[5] When the *t*-test assumptions are clearly violated the data might be transformed or a non-parametric test used.)

It is evident that the standard error is larger than before, due to the variability between the practices. The degree of discrepancy will be greater where there is high variability between practices compared with that between patients attending the same practice, and where there is a small number of practices. The CIs are wider and the statistical significance of the difference decreased.

In this example, two methods give slightly different estimates of the difference between the groups: 16.6 when the patient is the unit of analysis and 15.5 when the practice is the unit of analysis. This is because the number of patients per practice varied (Table 1). Studies where equal numbers of subjects are included from each practice will give the same estimate of the difference between the groups whether individual subjects or clusters are used as the unit of analysis, but the standard error and hence the levels of significance and the width of the CIs will differ.

The method of analysis using a summary statistic described above gave equal weight to all practices regardless of how many patients on their list had long-term mental illness. The summary statistics based on larger numbers of patients will be more precise estimates of that practice's performance than those based on smaller numbers. If the number of patients in each practice is used to weight the summary statistics, we will obtain the same estimates of the difference as in a by-patient analysis, but not the same standard errors. This gives an estimate of 16.6 for the difference between the groups and a CI of 12–29.9, $P = 0.018$. Using the numbers of patients as the weightings has the additional advantage that it gives more weight to those practices most involved in the care of the long-term mentally ill.

DISCUSSION

The consequences of cluster randomization as opposed to individual randomization are often poorly understood by researchers. This is perhaps understandable, as standard textbooks on medical statistics often confine discussion of clinical trials to those which randomize individuals. We have shown that analyses which ignore clusters will tend to underestimate the standard error of the treatment effect, and this in turn can lead to spurious statistical significance. This is due to two factors, the variability between clusters and the number of subjects within each cluster.

Practices are geographically based and therefore patients tend, to have similar socio-economic circumstances. Patients also choose which GP or practice to attend. It is known, for example, that patients from the ethnic minorities are more likely to attend a GP from the ethnic minorities. Patients are also subject to the same doctors beliefs and practices and likely to be given similar advice or prescriptions. A more general discussion of the reasons for similarity of individuals within a cluster is given by Donner.[2]

In studies which recruit few patients per practice and have little variation in outcome from practice to practice, the difference between using patient or practice as the unit of analysis may be negligible, and analysis by patient may be acceptable. For example, in a randomized trial of the effects of co-ordinating care for terminally ill patients,[6] 168 practices were randomly allocated so that patients in the intervention practices received the assistance of two nurse co-ordinators. The intervention was delivered directly to the 554 patients in the study and so the variability between practices was small compared with the variability between patients. As the number of patients per practice was also small it was reasonable to ignore the practice in the analysis. If the number of patients per practice had been large, as in a screening study, then even a small variability between practices may have been important and an analysis which took account of cluster variation would have been required.

In this paper we have demonstrated a simple approach to the analysis, which constructs a summary measure for each practice. There are other methods of analysis available, such as repeated measures analysis of variance, which are appropriate, but are not so easy to use or require more sophisticated software.

As there will be some loss of power due to the variability between practices, sample size calculations need to take this into account and consider not only the number of patients but the number of practices as well. In the following paper we show how to calculate sample sizes for practice randomized designs and discuss the implications of the loss of power, particularly for study designs where practice randomization is not strictly necessary.

References

1   Family Heart Study Group. Randomised controlled trial evaluating cardiovascular screening and intervention in general practice: principal result of British family heart study. *Br Med J* 1994; **304**: 313–320.

2   Donner A, Brown KS, Brasher P. A methodological review of non-therapeutic intervention trials employing cluster randomisation 1979–1989. *Int J Epidemiol* 1990; **19**: 795–800.

3   Kendrick T, Burns T, Freeling P. Randomised controlled trial of teaching general practitioners to carry out structured assessments of their long term mentally ill patients. *Br Med J* 1995; **311**: 93–98.

4   Matthews JNS, Altman DG, Campbell MJ, Royston R. Analysis of serial measurements in medical research. *Br Med J* 1990; **300**: 230–235.

5   Bland M. *An Introduction to Medical Statistics.* 2nd edn. Oxford: Oxford University Press, 1995.

6   Addington-Hall JM, MacDonald LD, Anderson HR *et al.* Randomised controlled trial of effects of coordinating care for terminally ill cancer patients. *Br Med J* 1992; **305**: 1317–1322.

16

This article was first published in Family Practice and is reproduced by permission of Oxford University Press

TRIALS WHICH RANDOMIZE PRACTICES II: SAMPLE SIZE

Sally M Kerry and J Martin Bland[a]

Division of General Practice and Primary Care and [a]Department of Public Health Sciences, St George's Hospital Medical School, Cramner Terrace, London SW17 0RE, UK.

Received 5 August 1997; Accepted 3 October 1997.

Family Practice 1998; **15**: 84–87

Background. When practices are randomized in a trial and observations are made on the patients to assess the relative effectiveness of the different interventions, sample size calculations need to estimate the number of practices required, not just the total number of patients.
Objective. Our aims were to introduce the methodology for appropriate sample size calculation and discuss the implications for power.
Method. A worked example from general practice is used.
Discussion. Designs which randomize practices are less powerful than designs which randomize patients to intervention groups, particularly where a large number of patients is recruited from each practice. Studies which randomize few practices should be avoided if possible, as the loss of power is considerable and simple randomization may not ensure comparability of intervention groups.
Keywords. General practice, randomized controlled trials, sample size, statistical analysis.

INTRODUCTION

Many randomized trials in general practice require all patients who attend the same practice to receive the same intervention. For example, in recent years evaluation of guidelines has given rise to several randomized trials where practices are randomized to receive guidelines or to act as controls. Patients from practices using the guidelines are compared with patients from the control group of practices.[1,2] These trials can be analysed using a summary statistic, usually a mean or a proportion, of observations from that practice.[3] This paper gives a worked example of the associated sample size calculations and discusses some of the implications for study design that arise from randomizing practices.

SAMPLE SIZE CALCULATIONS
Variability between practices

We will denote by s_w^2 the variance of observations taken from one practice, the within practice variance, and assume this is the same for all practices. If there are m subjects selected from each practice then the variance of a single sample mean is s_w^2/m.[4] The practice means or percentages (unknown) will vary from practice to

practice. We will denote their variance by s_c^2, the between practice variance. The observed variance of the outcome variable will be made up of the variability between practices and the variability due to taking a sample of patients from that practice, i.e. variance of outcome = $s_c^2 + s_w^2/m$. This can be used to replace the variance in the conventional sample size formula [5,6] for the difference between two means in order to obtain the number of practices, n, required in each intervention group. If the difference to be detected is d, using a significance level of 5% and a power of 90% the number of practices required in each group is given by

$$n = \frac{21(s_c^2 + s_w^2/m)}{d^2}$$

If the summary statistic is a percentage, p, we replace s_w^2 by, $p(100-p)$.

Example

In a proposed study of a behavioural intervention to lower smoking rates in general practice, practices were to be randomized into two groups, one to offer health promotion using a behaviourial approach by specially trained practice nurses and the other to usual general practice care. The outcome measure would be smoking rates in patients from each practice 1 year later. Smoking rates were obtained from a study of nine practices in the South-West Thames Region [7] and gave an overall prevalence of 22%, with a between practice variance, s_c^2, of 14. The minimum difference considered to he clinically relevant was 5 percentage points, that is if the smoking rate fell to 17% in the intervention group. The within practice variance could be estimated using the usual formula, $p(100-p)$ for the variance of a percentage. This is 1716 when the prevalence is 19.5%, the average of the two percentages expected in the control and intervention groups. If we aimed to recruit 100 patients per practice using the formula above we would need 25 practices in each group. Table 1 shows the number of practices required for different values of m, and the sample size required for individual randomization. In all situations the total number of subjects required is greater than if simple random allocation has been employed.

Table 1

Total number of practices in each group required to detect a difference of 5 percentage points in smoking levels where the control is 22% at the 5% significance level and 90% power

No. of patients per practice (m)	Total[a] standard deviation	Total[b] number of practices in each group	Total number of patients in each group	Design effect
10	13.08	144	1440	1.09
25	8.76	65	1625	1.22
50	6.73	39	1950	1.47
100	5.45	25	2500	1.89
500	4.14	15	7500	5.67
No. of subjects required using individual randomization[c]			1322	

[a] Total standard deviation $s = \sqrt{\dfrac{1570}{m} + 14}$.

[b] Total number of practices $= 21 \dfrac{s^2}{d^2}$ where d is the difference of interest.

[c] Calculated as $\dfrac{21 \times (1570 + 14)}{5^2}$

Design effect

The design effect, also known as the inflation factor, is the ratio of the total number of subjects required using cluster randomization to the number required using individual randomization. It can also be calculated as

$$Design\ Effect = 1 + (m - 1) \frac{s_c^2}{(s_c^2 + s_w^2)}$$

The term $s_c^2 / (s_c^2 + s_c^2 + s_w^2)$ is also known as the intracluster correlation coefficient (ICC). The design effect will always be greater than one, although it may take values close to one. As the number of patients per practice, m, increases, so does the design effect. For the behaviourial intervention trial the design effect is small when m is less than 10 (Table 1). However, this would involve recruiting a total of 288 practices and the nature of the intervention and difficulties in recruiting practices would make this impractical. If we chose to use 30 practices, then we would need 500 patients from each practice and the design effect would be 5.7. This design would require nearly six times as many patients as a patient-randomized design with the same power.

The above example has an intervention aimed directly at the patient and an outcome measurement for which the between-practices variance is low compared with the variability within practices, leading to a relatively small design effect. Studies where the intervention is aimed at changing the doctor's behaviour may have a greater design effect. For example, in a trial of feedback to improve the quality of cervical smears, the variability between doctors was likely to be higher because the outcome variable was more dependent on the doctor's behaviour than the patient.[8] Referral rates have also been reported to vary widely between general practices.[9]

The main difficulty in calculating sample size for cluster-randomized studies is obtaining an estimate of the between-cluster variation. Estimates of variation between individuals can often be obtained from the literature, but even studies that use cluster as the unit of analysis do not publish their results in such a way that the between-cluster variation can be estimated. Recognizing this problem, Donner[10] recommends that authors publish the cluster-specific event rates observed in their trial.

Our method calculates the number of practices required for a given number of patients per practice. In situations where the number of subjects recruited from each practice is not fixed we may wish to know how many subjects to choose from each practice as well as how many practices. A useful first step may be to calculate the sample size ignoring the clusters to give a minimum total sample size required. This will require only an estimate of the variance between individuals, which is usually the easier variance to obtain. If the intervention is applied to the individual subjects directly, then a small increase in sample size of 10% may suffice when only a few subjects are recruited per cluster. On the other hand, where the number of subjects per cluster is large, an estimate of the variability between clusters will be very important.

Small studies

If the unit of randomization is the practice or a district then the study may only be able to recruit a small number of clusters. Randomization of small numbers of clusters may not produce clusters that are similar with respect to factors which might be thought to influence outcome. Altman[11] gives a full discussion of the problems of a small number of randomization units in

17

trials which randomize individuals. Techniques such as stratification and minimization can also be applied to practices and may be useful in order to produce groups of practices which are similar with respect to several prognostic factors, while still retaining the benefits of randomization.

Alternatively, we might select pairs of clusters which are thought to be similar and randomly allocate one of each pair to the intervention and the other to the control group. In the Family Heart Study,[12] two practices were selected in each of 15 towns and one practice in each town was allocated to receive the intervention while the other practice acted as a control. Sample size calculations not only depend on the variability within clusters and the variability between clusters but the closeness in the matching of the pairs. If the pairs are well matched, then effect of the variability between clusters is reduced. Thus a paired design can in some way compensate for the loss of power introduced by cluster randomization compared with individual randomization.[13]

DISCUSSION

As the power of a trial is reduced by cluster randomization, such an approach needs to be justified.[10] In some situations individual randomization may be possible, but the groups may contaminate each other and thus reduce the observed intervention effect. This may arise when the same medical staff are treating both groups or when the subjects themselves may interact. The recruiting of staff specifically for the project to administer the intervention may reduce the contamination of the groups. The Family Heart Study[12] showed that for a lifestyle intervention using nurses specifically recruited and trained for the study there was no evidence of contamination of the groups when the intervention was compared with a control group from the same practice. If there is likely to be little contamination, then randomizing individual patients may be preferable in order to maximize the power of the study as in the OXCHECK[14] study.

In planning intervention trials the advantages of a design which randomizes clusters of individuals must be weighed against the disadvantages in terms of statistical power. Studies which randomize few clusters should be avoided, if possible, as the loss of power is considerable. More importantly, the two experimental groups may not be comparable with respect to factors which might influence outcome. Where randomization of clusters can be justified, when one is calculating the sample size, one needs to consider the number of clusters required, not just the total number of patients.

References

[1] Oakeshott P, Kerry SM, Williams JE. Randomized controlled trial of the effect of the Royal College of Radiologists' guidelines on general practitioners' referrals for radiographic examination. *Br J Gen Pract* 1994; **44**: 197–200.

[2] Feder G, Griffiths C, Highton C, Eldridge S, Spence M, Southgate L. Do clinical guidelines introduced with practice based education improve care of asthmatic and diabetic patients? A randomised controlled trial in general practices in east London. *Br Med J* 1995; **311**: 1473–1478.

[3] Kerry S, Bland M. Trials which randomize practices. 1. How should they be analysed? *Fam Pract* 1998; **15**: 80–83.

[4] Bland M. *An Introduction to Medical Statistics.* 2nd edn. Oxford: Oxford University Press, 1995.

[5] Florey C du V. Sample size for beginners. *Br Med J* 1993; **306**: 1181–1184.

[6] Lemeshow S, Hosmer DW, Klar J, Lwanga SK. *Adequacy of Sample Size in Health Studies.* Chichester: John Wiley and Sons, 1990.

[7] Ochera J, Hilton S, Bland JM, Jones DR, Dowell AC. Patients' experiences of health checks in general practice: a sample survey. *Fam Pract* 1994; **11**: 26–34.

[8] Buntix F, Knottnerus JA, Crebolder HFJM, Seegers T, Essed GGM, Schouten H. Does feedback improve the quality of cervical smears? A randomised controlled trial. *Br J Gen Pract* 1993; **43**: 194–198.

[9] Fertig A, Roland M, King H, Moore T. Understanding variation in rates of referral among general practitioners: are inappropriate referrals important and would guidelines help reduce rates? *Br Med J* 1993; **307**: 1467–1470.

[10] Donner A, Brown KS, Brasher P. A methodological review of non-therapeutic intervention trials employing cluster randomisation 1979–1989. *Int J Epidemiol* 1990; **19**: 795–800.

[11] Altman D. *Practical Statistics for Medical Research.* London: Chapman and Hall, 1991: Chapter 15.

[12] Family Heart Study Group. Randomised controlled trial evaluating cardiovascular screening and intervention in general practice: principal result of British family heart study. *Br Med J* 1994; **304**: 313–320.

[13] Shipley MJ, Smith PG, Dramaix M. Calculation of power for matched pair studies when randomisation is by group. *Int J Epidemiol* 1989; **18**: 457–461.

[14] Imperial Cancer Research Fund OXCHECK Study Group. Effectiveness of health checks conducted by nurses in primary care: results of the OXCHECK study after one year. *Br Med J* 1994; **308**: 308–312.

This article was first published by the Society of Teachers of Family Medicine and is reproduced by permission of Family Practice

LEARNING AS A FUNCTION OF LECTURE LENGTH

Charles L Bryner Jr, MD

Fam Med 1995;27:379–82

From the Naval Hospital, Jacksonville, Fla.

Background: The purpose of this study was to compare the learning of family practice residents after lectures of differing lengths (either 20 or 50 minutes' duration). Immediate and delayed recall were measured by written quizzes administered at the conclusion of each lecture and 2 weeks later:

Methods: A total of 390 quizzes, 220 immediate and 170 delayed, were completed by residents from all three year groups attending didactic lectures (is part of the regular training program curriculum at Naval Hospital Jacksonville. The completed quizzes were divided almost equally between 20- and 50-minute lectures.

Results: No significant difference was found when the Student's t test was used to compare the quiz scores following the contrasting lecture lengths at either the immediate post-lecture period (P=.294) or 2 weeks later (P=.5443).

Conclusion: This study shows that a 20-minute lecture was equal to the classic 50-minute lecture in terms of information retained by residents. If future studies confirm this study's findings, medical educators will need to reevaluate the length of lectures to improve efficiency of teaching.

It is said that lectures are periods of time when the notes of the lecturer are transferred to the note books of the students without going through the brains of either. Yet, academic lectures remain an important method of instruction [1-8] in family practice residency programs.

Faculty members in residency programs generally have little or no formal instruction in education or curriculum development.[9] Instead, faculty generally teach as they were taught, bringing all the habits learned as students into their teaching. Faculty expend efforts to stay abreast of clinical information, yet are often unaware of educational research. In short, faculty frequently prepare for what they teach but not how they teach.

A literature review using MEDLINE and ERIC databases and the Science Citation Index identified numerous publications about lecturing and its effectiveness in relation to time of day,[10] the material's knowledge density,[11] and speaker dynamism.[12-16] One topic was conspicuously underrepresented: how long should a lecturer talk?

Studies that correlated information retained after a lecture with the time during a lecture when the information was presented were reported by McLeish [17] and Thomas.[18] Both studies examined university lectures of approximately 50 minutes in length presented to adult students. In each study, the information retained was proportionately high in the early minutes of a lecture and dropped steadily thereafter to a trough at approximately 40 minutes into the lecture period. The last few minutes of the lecture show a sharp rise to a higher retention level (Figure 1). Bligh[19] and Stuart[20] independently confirmed that students' attentions wane quickly after the first 15–20 minutes of a lecture.[21,22]

Interactive learning methods that require active participation by the attendees might decrease this loss,[16,23-27] but in family medicine education, where so much must be learned in so little time, the lecture is still perceived as useful for presenting information efficiently.[1,17,25,27,28]

The lecturer's and students' performances follow a strikingly similar pattern.[17,21] Since the lowest points in performance of both the lecturer and the students occur simultaneously, perhaps a simple solution would be to eliminate the portion of the lecture where this occurs. A compressed lecture of 20 minutes' duration would theoretically tag the terminal upsurge in performance onto the initial high level of retention, avoiding the drop in performance for both lecturer and students. This should result in increased efficiency in presenting material and should be demonstrable by measuring retention of the information presented.

This study was designed to test the efficiency of lectures in two contrasting formats already in use at a residency training program. Specifically, this study addresses the question of whether residents learn as much from a 20-minute lecture as they do from a 50-minute lecture, assuming the lectures are given by the same individual.

METHODS

Lectures

A series of 20 lectures during a period of 90 days was given to residents enrolled in the Naval Hospital Jacksonville's family practice residency training program. The lectures were presented as part of the regularly

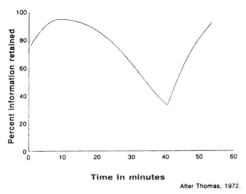

After Thomas, 1972.

Figure 1 *Retention Level During University Lectures*

Graph depicts learners' retention of lecture content according to when, during a 50-minute lecture, the information was presented. Note that maximal retention occurs early and late in the lecture.

scheduled lunchtime academic series. Specific dates of the lectures evaluated in this study were selected based solely on availability of dates at the time the research project was conceived. The dates were distributed among the five weekdays. The attendees had no previous knowledge of which lectures were to be part of the study.

Ten presenters were recruited to give lectures. The lecturers were from varied hospital departments and the local community and approximated the mix of lecturers normally participating in the conference curriculum. Each lecturer agreed to deliver two lectures covering different topics in his or her field of expertise. The topics chosen by the lecturer were deemed about equal in factual content and difficulty of comprehension. Each lecture was to be initially prepared to fill a lecture time slot of 50 minutes. The lecturer then selected one of each pair of presentations to be compressed by removing some supporting discussion but leaving factual content intact. The compressed lecture was to be presented in a 20-minute time limit. By pairing a compressed lecture with a regular lecture given by the same presenter, those components of learning that were

functions of lecturer identity were assumed to cancel out. Ten regular lectures and 10 compressed lectures were presented on different days but at the same approximate time of day and in the same location. Presenters were free to choose their own presentation style and audiovisual support, as long as both lectures were presented in a similar fashion.

Attendees at these lectures included residents representing each of the three year levels of training. During this study, availability of any specific resident varied with the clinical rotation assigned. Because rotation schedules change frequently, the overall mix of residents remained fairly constant. Staff physicians and medical students were not part of the study population. All residents were told in advance that a research project about lecture methods and learning effectiveness was being conducted, but the research question was not revealed.

Assessment of Learning

Each presenter selected facts and concepts from each lecture on which quiz questions were to be fashioned but did not know which items would ultimately be tested. All quizzes were written by the author prior to lecture length being assigned to the topic to ensure equal difficulty for quizzes given for both the compressed and regular length lectures. For each lecture, approximately half the testing points were incorporated into a quiz given immediately following the lecture. A second or "delayed" quiz was given 2 weeks after the lecture to each resident who completed the first quiz. The delayed quiz included all questions from the first quiz and the second half of the selected testing points not used in the first quiz. The quizzes consisted of short-answer completion. true/false, matching, multiple choice, and multiple-multiple choice (Type K) questions. The residents were briefed before the start of this lecture series to complete each quiz without reference to notes, handouts, texts, or other sources of information. The quiz scores were kept entirely confidential and not used for residents' evaluations.

Table 1

Comparison of Scores on Quizzes That Followed Compressed and Regular Lectures

	Immediate* Quiz		Delayed** Quiz			
			Repeat Questions		New Questions	
	Number of Responses	Average Score on Quiz	Number of Responses	Average Score on Quiz	Number of Responses	Average Score on Quiz
Compressed (20-minute format)	104	75.8%	81	65.7%	81	52.7%
Regular (50-minute format)	116	75.8%	89	63.6%	89	56.6%
Totals	220		170		170	
P values comparing compressed and regular		.294		.5443		.6756

* Immediate refers to the quiz given immediately following the lecture
** Delayed refers to the quiz given 2 weeks after a lecture

Lectures were monitored by a faculty member to ensure that all quiz questions had been addressed in the lecture. Only those residents present for the entire duration of the lecture were tested. Delayed quizzes were offered only to those who had completed and returned the immediate quiz for a specific lecture. A time limit of 48 hours was allotted for completion and return of the delayed quiz. Quizzes that did not meet this deadline were not included in the study.

Data Analysis

The scores from the immediate quizzes of the regular and compressed lectures were compared to measure short-term learning. The scores from the delayed quizzes of the regular and compressed lectures were compared as a measure of long-term retention of the information presented. The scores from the delayed quizzes were also broken down to compare scores on those questions previously given in the immediate quizzes vs those questions that were "new" on the delayed quizzes.

Mean scores were compared using Student's t test. The sample size was shown by power analysis to be sufficient to demonstrate a statistical significance if there was a 15-point average difference between quiz scores from compressed and regular lectures.

RESULTS

A total of 390 completed quizzes were returned. Of this total, 220 had been administered at the conclusion of a lecture (immediate quizzes, of which 100% were returned), and 170 were completed and returned 2 weeks after the lecture (delayed quizzes. of which 77% were returned). Completed quizzes in both immediate and delayed categories were approximately equally divided between compressed and regular lectures (Table 1). The quizzes were completed by 29 different individuals. The number of respondents varied from five to 15 for any single lecture.

The mean quiz scores following regular and compressed lectures were compared in each of three categories (Table 1): immediate quizzes, the portion of the delayed quizzes comprised of questions repeated from the immediate quiz (delayed repeat), and the portion of the delayed quizzes comprised of questions not appearing in the immediate quiz (delayed new). There was no significant difference in the average scores between quizzes from compressed and regular lectures (Student's t test).

DISCUSSION

This study was undertaken to measure the effect of lecture length on residents' learning. The results showed that the compressed, 20-minute lecture taught as much as the classic-length, 50-minute lecture when objective quiz scores were used to measure learning. Comparing quiz scores from two lectures on different topics could have biased the results. However, pairing lectures from the same discipline should theoretically have provided equally difficult lectures on which to base the testing. The paired lectures from the same presenter should theoretically have cancelled out any lecturer effects. An alternative design would have been a comparison between the same lecture topics presented twice, once in each format, by the same lecturer to separate audiences. Given the limited number of residents in most programs, and the fact that the audiences would then be different, this design is logistically not feasible.

Quizzes were fashioned without foreknowledge of which lecture format was to be used for the given topic. Thus, equally difficult quizzes were created for both formats. While no measures were made of the quizzes' validity as a measure of learning or knowledge acquisition, this method of measure was chosen because of its simplicity and because it is similar to the way some programs measure resident learning.

To avoid biasing the score of the delayed quizzes by reinforcement from quizzes given immediately after a lecture, the delayed quizzes were split into two portions, questions identical to those of the immediate quiz (delayed repeat) and questions not included in the immediate quiz (delayed new). As expected, delayed repeat questions were answered correctly at a higher rate than delayed new questions but at a lower rate than immediate quiz questions (Table 1).

The implications of this study are straightforward. The classic-length lecture failed to show any advantage over a compressed lecture in terms of immediate recall or long-term retention of the information presented. If lectures were shortened to 20-minute presentations, more time could be available for other educational activities.

Further research is required to replicate this study's findings; the future study design needs to eliminate some of the confounders mentioned above. While this limited project represents only a first step at questioning current methods in residency education, if future studies confirm its findings, medical educators will need to re-evaluate the length of lectures to improve efficiency of teaching.

Acknowledgments: This research was conducted in conjunction with a faculty development fellowship at the University of North Carolina School of Medicine's Department of Family Practice. Special thanks to Steven Ornstein, MD, and Frank Stritter, PhD, who served as research mentors and Alfred Reid who guided data analysis.

Corresponding Author: Address correspondence to Dr Bryner, 606 Chivas Court, Orange Park, FL 32073–4227.

18

References

1 Cashin WE. *Improving lectures.* Manhattan, Kan: Kansas State University: Center for Faculty Evaluation and Development, 1985.

2 Beard RM. *Motivating students.* London: New York: Routledge & Kegan Paul, 1980.

3 Beard RM. *Teaching and learning in higher education,* 4th ed. London: Harper & Row, 1984.

4 Irby DM. Evaluating instruction in medical education. *J Med Educ* 1983;**58**:844–9.

5 Zolty TC. Improving undergraduate lectures: the sender, the message, and the receiver. *Political Science Teacher* 1990;**3**(4):6–8.

6 DaRosa DA. Evaluating the effectiveness of the lecture versus independent study. *Eval Program Plann* 1991; **14**(3): 141–6.

7 Sade RM, Stroud MR. Medical student attendance at lectures: effect on medical school performance. *J Med Educ* 1982;**57**(3):191–2.

8 Riggs JW, Blanco JD. Is there a relation between student lecture attendance and clinical science subject examination score? *Obstet Gynecol* 1994;**84**(2):311–3.

9 DeRemee RA. The great pyramid of medicine: a case for the rotating internship. *Bull N Y Acad Med* 1982;**58**:628–35.

10 Holloway PJ. The effect of lecture time on learning. *Br J Educ Psychol* 1966;**36**(3):255–8.

11 Russell IJ. Hendricson WD, Herbert RJ. Effects of lecture information density on medical student achievement. *J Med Educ* 1984;**59**:881–9.

12 Coats WD. Smidchens U. Audience recall as a function of speaker dynamism. *J Educ Psychol* 1966;**57**:189–91.

13 Ware JE, Jr Williams RG. The Dr Fox effect: a study of lecturer effectiveness and ratings of instruction. *J Med Educ* 1975;**50**:149–56.

14 Kaplan RNI. Reflections on the Dr Fox paradigm. *J Med Educ* 1974;**49**:310–2.

15 Kirby DM. Clinical teacher effectiveness in medicine. *J Med Educ* 1978;**53**:808–15.

16 Abrami PC. Leventhal L, Perry RP. Educational seduction. *Review of Educational Research* 1982;**52**(3):446–64.

17 McLeish J. The lecture method. In: Gage NL, Rehage KJ, eds. *The psychology of teaching methods.* Chicago: National Society for the Study of Education: University of Chicago Press, 1976:252–30 1.

18 Thomas EJ. The variation of memory with time for information appearing during a lecture. *Studies in Adult Education* 1972;**4**:57–62..

19 Bligh DA. *What's the use of lectures?* Harmondsworth, England: Penguin. 1972.

20 Stuart J. Rutherford RJ. Medical student concentration during lectures. *Lancet* 1978;**2**(8088):514–6.

21 Maddox H. Hoole E. Performance decrement in the lecture. *Educational Review* 1975;**28**:17–30.

22 Johnstone AH, Percival F. Attention breaks in lectures. *Education in Chemistry.* 1976; **13**(2):49–50.

23 Gray, JA. Continuing education: what techniques are effective? *Lancet* 1986:2(8504):447–8.

24 Beard RM. Research into teaching methods in higher education, mainly in British universities, 4th ed. Guildford, England: Society for Research into Higher Education, 1978.

25 Davies IK. *Instructional technique.* New York: McGraw Hill, 1981.

26 Schwartz PL. Active, small-group learning with a large group in a lecture theater: a practical example. *Med Teach* 1989;**11**(1):81–6.

27 Barker SP. Comparison of effectiveness of interactive videodisc versus lecture-demonstration instruction. *Phys Ther* 1988;**68**(5):699–703.

28 Dunnington G, Witzke D, Rubeck R, Beck A, Mohr J, Putnam C. A comparison of the teaching effectiveness of the didactic lecture and the problem-oriented small group session: a prospective study. *Surgery* 1987;**102**(2):291–6.

This article was first published in the BMJ and is reproduced by permission of the BMJ

RANDOMISED CONTROLLED TRIAL COMPARING HOSPITAL AT HOME CARE WITH INPATIENT HOSPITAL CARE. II: COST MINIMISATION ANALYSIS

BMJ 1998;**316**:1791-1796 (13 June)

Sasha Shepperd, *research officer, Division of Public Health and Primary Health Care,*
University of Oxford, Institute of Health Sciences, Headington, Oxford OX3 7LF.

Diana Harwood, *research assistant, Health Services Research Unit, Division of Public Health and Primary Health Care,*
University of Oxford, Institute of Health Sciences.

Alastair Gray, *director, Health Economics Research Centre, Division of Public Health and Primary Health Care,*
University of Oxford, Institute of Health Sciences.

Martin Vessey, *professor of public health and head of department, Division of Public Health and Primary Health Care,*
University of Oxford, Institute of Health Sciences, Headington, Oxford OX3 7LF.

Patrick Morgan, *consultant in public health medicine,*
Northamptonshire Health Authority, Northampton NN1 5DN.

Correspondence to: Sashashepperd@dphpc.ox.ac.uk

ABSTRACT

Objectives: To examine the cost of providing hospital at home in place of some forms of inpatient hospital care.
Design: Cost minimisation study within a randomised controlled trial.
Setting: District general hospital and catchment area of neighbouring community trust.
Subjects: Patients recovering from hip replacement (n=86), knee replacement (n=86), and hysterectomy (n=238); elderly medical patients (n=96); and patients with chronic obstructive airways disease (n=32).
Interventions: Hospital at home or inpatient hospital care.
Main outcome measures: Cost of hospital at home scheme to health service, to general practitioners, and to patients and their families compared with hospital care.
Results: No difference was detected in total healthcare costs between hospital at home and hospital care for patients recovering from a hip or knee replacement, or elderly medical patients. Hospital at home significantly increased healthcare costs for patients recovering from a hysterectomy (ratio of geometrical means 1.15, 95% confidence interval 1.04 to 1.29, P=0.009) and for those with chronic obstructive airways disease (Mann-Whitney U test, P=0.01). Hospital at home significantly increased general practitioners' costs for elderly medical patients (Mann-Whitney U test, P<0.01) and for those with chronic obstructive airways disease (P=0.02). Patient and carer expenditure made up a small proportion of total costs.
Conclusion: Hospital at home care did not reduce total healthcare costs for the conditions studied in this trial, and costs were significantly increased for patients recovering from a hysterectomy and those with chronic obstructive airways disease. There was some evidence that costs were shifted to primary care for elderly medical patients and those with chronic obstructive airways disease.

INTRODUCTION

There is little evidence to justify the widespread adoption of hospital at home on the basis of cost. A review of the subject identified only one randomised controlled trial that compared the cost of hospital at home with inpatient hospital care.[1] This trial, based in the United States, recruited patients with a terminal illness and found no difference in overall healthcare costs.[2] There is conflicting evidence from non-randomised studies.[3,4]

We report the results of a prospective economic evaluation, in the context of a randomised controlled trial, of the cost of providing hospital at home as a substitute for some forms of inpatient hospital care. The three questions addressed by the economic evaluation were

- Does substituting hospital at home care for hospital care result in a lower cost to the health service?
- Does hospital at home care, compared to hospital care, increase the cost to general practitioners?
- Does hospital at home care increase the cost borne by the patients and their families compared with hospital care?

METHODS

We describe patient recruitment and randomisation in our accompanying paper.[5] This economic evaluation took the form of a cost minimisation analysis, as the health outcomes of the two arms of the trial did not differ. Our primary interest was the cost to the health service, but we also examined the costs incurred by patients and families, as they could influence the acceptability of a hospital at home scheme.

We recruited five groups of patients: patients recovering from a hip replacement, a knee replacement,

19

Key messages

- Hospital at home schemes are a popular alternative to standard hospital care, but there is uncertainty about their cost effectiveness

- In our randomised controlled trial we compared the cost of hospital at home care with that of inpatient hospital care for patients recovering from hip replacement, knee replacement, and hysterectomy; elderly medical patients; and those with chronic obstructive airways disease

- There were no major differences in health service costs between the two arms of the trial for patients recovering from hip or knee replacement and elderly medical patients

- Hospital at home care increased healthcare costs for patients recovering from hysterectomy and for those with chronic obstructive airways disease

- Hospital at home care resulted in some costs shifting to general practitioners for elderly medical patients and those with chronic obstructive airways disease

or a hysterectomy; patients with chronic obstructive airways disease; and elderly patients with a mix of medical conditions. All patients were aged 60 years or over, except those recovering from a hysterectomy, who were aged 20-70 years.

Data collection

The box lists the uses of health service resources on which data were collected. We obtained cost data for hospital care and hospital at home care from the respective trusts' finance departments for the financial year 1994-5, apportioned on the basis of activity for 1993-4. Details of the unit costs are available from the authors.

Hospital costs

The cost of hospital care included staffing costs, all non-staff running costs, and capital costs. Patient dependency scores were developed by hospital nursing and medical staff to reflect the marginal costs incurred during a patient's episode of hospital care (and hence the marginal savings of early discharge). [3 6] These scores were used to weight the costs for each day that a patient was in hospital. The costs of physiotherapy and occupational therapy were calculated according to the amount of time spent with a typical patient for each clinical group, and included a cost for non-contact time. Equipment costs (based on ward records), the cost of items not directly related to levels of patient care, and capital charges for land and buildings (based on valuation and including interest and depreciation) were divided by the number of ward bed days for the year 1994-5 to arrive at a charge per bed day. The cost of prescribed drugs was obtained from the hospital pharmacy department.

The time profile for costing hospital care differed for each clinical group. The costs for surgical patients excluded the costs of the operation, as these costs do not alter with different rehabilitative care. For patients having a hip or knee replacement, costs were calculated from the fourth postoperative day. For patients having a hysterectomy, costs were calculated from the first postoperative day. Cost data for medical patients were collected for the duration of their hospital stay.

Hospital at home costs

The cost of hospital at home care included all staffing and non-staff running costs. The costs of nurses, physiotherapists, and occupational therapists were based on the amount of time spent with patients, and included a cost for non-contact time. The following non-staff costs were included: central administration, travel, training, telephones and pagers, equipment, and office space. Medical supplies and equipment costs were depreciated over a 10 year period with a discount rate of 6%.[7] These costs were apportioned on an equal basis to each patient receiving hospital at home care, assuming costs were payable in advance at the start of the year. Administration and travel costs were apportioned according to the volume of patients. The cost of prescribed drugs was obtained from the hospital's pharmacy department.

General practitioner costs

Research nurses visited each practice to record the number of general practitioners' home visits and number of patients' visits to the surgery. The community trust providing the hospital at home care reimbursed general practitioners visiting hospital at home patients at a rate of £100 per patient and £25 for each visit. General practitioner costs for the hospital care group were calculated with unit costs developed by the Personal Social Services Research Unit, Kent.[8]

Uses of health service resources that were recorded for cost minimisation analysis

Hospital care
- Number of inpatient days
- Number of inpatient days due to a hospital readmission related to the trial diagnosis
- Medication

Hospital at home care
- Number of hospital at home days
- Number of hospital at home visits (including duration of visit and grading of staff)
- Medication

Hospital transport
- Number of journeys made by ambulance or a health service car

General practitioner visits
- Number of visits to doctor's surgery
- Number of home visits

Carer costs

Carers were asked to record all expenditures related to the trial diagnosis (including equipment and adaptations, consumables, and travel) in a diary for one month, and any loss of earnings and days off work due to caring for their patient. Carers were also asked to record the number of hours a day they spent caring for the patient.

Statistical analysis

We describe the sample size calculations in our accompanying paper.[5] Analysis was done on an intention to treat basis. When appropriate, data with non-normal distribution was log transformed before further parametric analysis was done. The Mann-Whitney U test was used for continuous variables that did not approximate a normal distribution after log transformation.

Sensitivity analyses were conducted for areas that could possibly restrict the generalisability of the trial results. These were the trial rate of reimbursing general practitioners, patients' duration of hospital at home care observed in the trial, and the use of average costs per inpatient day instead of dependency adjusted hospital costs.

RESULTS

Results are presented by clinical condition for both arms of the trial. Inpatient hospital care and hospital at home care accounted for most of the healthcare costs. Tables 1, 2, and 3 show health service resources and costs for each patient group.

Early discharge of patients after elective surgery

Patients allocated to hospital at home care after a hip or knee replacement or a hysterectomy spent significantly fewer days in hospital (tables 1 and 2). However, they received significantly more days of health care with the addition of hospital at home. For patients recovering from a hip or knee replacement, the total costs to the health service were not significantly different between the two groups. For patients recovering from a hysterectomy, total health service costs were significantly higher for those allocated to hospital at home care. Of the total numbers of patients undergoing these procedures during the study period, we recruited about 20% of all those having hip replacements, 25% of those having knee replacements, and 35% of those undergoing hysterectomy.

Table 1

Health service resources and costs consumed at 3 months after hospital admission by patients allocated to hospital at home care or inpatient hospital care: orthopaedic patients recovering from hip or knee replacement

	Hospital at home	Hospital	Difference (95% CI)
Hip replacement:	(n=36*)	(n=49)	
Mean (SD) days in hospital care	8.11 (5.52)	11.87 (4.52)	-3.75 (-5.92 to-1.58)
Mean (SD) days in hospital at home care	6.58 (4.26)	–	–
Mean (SD) total days of care	14.69 (5.13)	11.87 (4.57)	2.84 (0.75 to 4.93)
Median (interquartile range) days of readmission	0 (0.00-0.00)	0 (0.00-0.00)	P=0.39†
Mean (SD) hospital costs including readmission (£)	515.42 (473.20)	776.30 (364.53)	-260.87 (-441.56 to -80.19)P<0.01
Mean (SD) hospital at home costs (£)	351.24 (240.58)	–	–
Median (interquartile range) GP costs: home and surgery visits (£)	42.84 (0.00-64.61)	15.49 (0.00-45.19)	P=0.06†
Mean (SD) total health service costs (£)	911.39 (563.76)	815.70 (347.99)	Ratio of geometric mean 1.05 (0.87 to 1.27) P=0.59
Knee replacement:	(n=46‡)	(n=39)	
Mean (SD) days in hospital care	10.28 (4.60)	13.31 (4.57)	-3.02 (-5.01 to -1.04)
Mean (SD) days in hospital at home care	5.72 (4.98)	–	–
Mean (SD) total days of care	16.00 (5.44)	13.31 (4.57)	2.69 (0.50 to 4.88)
Median (interquartile range) days of readmission	0 (0.00-0.00)	0 (0.00-0.00)	P=0.23†
Mean (SD) hospital costs including readmission (£)	1092.24 (615.27)	1348.35 (625.94)	-256.11 (-524.61 to -12.38) P=0.06
Mean (SD) hospital at home costs (£)	348.16 (275.25)	–	–
Median (interquartile range) GP costs: home and surgery visits (£)	15.49 (0.00-57.15)	15.49 (0.00-30.98)	P=0.22†
Mean (SD) total health service costs (£)	1461.62 (666.61)	1375.36 (637.76)	Ratio of geometric mean 1.05 (0.88 to 1.26) P=0.55

GP= general practitioner. *No data available for 1 patient. †Mann-Whitney U test. ‡No data available for 1 patient.

19

Table 2

Health service resources and costs consumed at 3 months after hospital admission by patients allocated to hospital at home care or inpatient hospital care: patients recovering from hysterectomy

	Hospital at home (n=111*)	Hospital (n=123†)	Difference (95% CI)
Mean (SD) days in hospital care	4.34 (1.86)	5.79 (2.98)	-1.44 (-2.09 to -0.79)
Mean (SD) days in hospital at home care	3.11 (2.64)	–	–
Mean (SD) total days of care	7.45 (2.59)	5.79 (2.98)	1.66 (0.94 to 2.39)
Median (interquartile range) days of readmission	0 (0.00-0.00)	0 (0.00-0.00)	P=0.21‡
Mean (SD) hospital costs including readmission (£)	487.43 (350.20)	647.77 (496.27)	Ratio of geometric mean 0.76 (0.67 to 0.87) P<0.01
Mean (SD) hospital at home costs (£)	250.18 (273.54)	–	–
Median (interquartile range) GP costs: home and surgery visits (£)	30.98 (15.49-61.96)	30.98 (15.49-61.96)	P=0.70‡
Mean (SD) total health service costs (£)	771.78 (408.72)	679.39 (439.83)	Ratio of geometric mean 1.15 (1.04 to 1.29) P<0.01

GP=general practitioner. *No data available for 3 patients. †No data available for 1 patient. ‡Mann-Whitney U test.

Table 3

Health service resources and costs consumed at 3 months after hospital admission by patients allocated to hospital at home care or inpatient hospital care: elderly medical patients and patients with chronic obstructive airways disease

	Hospital at home	Hospital	Difference (95% CI)
Elderly medical:	**(n=50)**	**(n=44*)**	
Mean (SD) days in hospital care	12.84 (14.69)	13.20 (14.19)	-0.36 (-6.30 to 5.57)
Mean (SD) days in hospital at home care	9.04 (7.79)		
Mean (SD) total days of care	21.88 (18.30)	13.20 (14.19)	8.67 (1 90 to 15.45)
Median (interquartile range) days of readmission	0 (0.00-1.00)	0 (0.00-0.00)	P=0.08†
Median (interquartile range) hospital costs including readmission (£)	913.76 (243.31-2045.68)	1366.16 (629.08-2033.50)	P=0.21†
Mean (SD) hospital at home costs (£)	793.45 (811.36)		
Median (interquartile range) GP costs: home and surgery visits (£)	67.84 (45.19-172.83)	45.19 (15.49-82.95)	P<0.01†
Median (interquartile range) total health service costs (£)	1705.32 (913.83-3121.55)	1388.76 (645.06-2094.88)	P=0.09†
Chronic obstructive airways disease:	**(n=15)**	**(n=17)**	
Mean (SD) days in hospital care	6.93 (3.39)	12.12 (7.49)	-5.18 (-9.48 to -0.89)
Mean (SD) days in hospital at home care	5.33 (3.94)	–	–
Mean (SD) total days of care	12.27 (3.69)	12.12 (7.49)	0.15 (-4.21 to 4.51)
Median (interquartile range) days of readmission	5.00 (0.00-10.0)	0.00 (0.00-3.00)	P=0.08†
Median (interquartile range) hospital costs including readmission (£)	1389.53 (821.65-1993.97)	1198.53 (712.00-1508.24)	P=0.56†
Mean (SD) hospital at home costs (£)	710.61 (526.50)	–	–
Median (interquartile range) GP costs: home and surgery visits (£)	115.38 (25.00-214.30)	15.49 (0.00-91.02)	P=0.02†
Median (interquartile range) total health service costs (£)	2379.67 (1458.09-2759.05)	1247.64 (772.50-1619.19)	P=0.01†

GP=general practitioner. *No data available for 2 patients. †Mann-Whitney U test.

19

Elderly medical patients and patients with chronic obstructive airways disease

No significant difference was detected between the two groups of elderly medical patients in the number of days spent in hospital, but, with the addition of hospital at home care, the total days of health care for the hospital at home group was significantly higher (table 3). Patients with chronic obstructive airways disease in the hospital at home group spent significantly fewer days in hospital, but this reduction was offset by the time spent in hospital at home care so there was no significant difference between the two groups for the total days of health care (table 3). For elderly medical patients, total costs to the health service were not significantly different between the two groups. Patients with chronic obstructive airways disease allocated to hospital at home care incurred significantly greater healthcare costs than did those receiving only hospital care. About 1% of all patients admitted for medical conditions during the study period were recruited to either the elderly medical or chronic obstructive airways disease groups. Nineteen of these patients were recruited by general practitioners, of whom nine were allocated to hospital care. However, only two of these patients received acute hospital care.

General practitioner costs

For patients discharged early after elective surgery, no significant differences in general practitioner costs were detected between the two groups. However, for elderly medical patients and those with chronic obstructive airways disease, the costs of general practitioner services were significantly higher for the patients allocated to hospital at home care compared with those in the hospital groups.

Costs to patients and carers

Patients' and carers' expenses made up a small proportion of total costs. There were no significant differences between the two groups for any of the categories of patients, and inclusion of these costs did not alter the results. The median cost for all patient groups was £0. The greatest expense was incurred by patients with chronic obstructive airways disease: median cost for the hospital at home group was £0 (interquartile range £0-£19.8) and for the hospital group was £0 (£0-£0). There were no significant differences between the two groups of carers in the time spent caring for the patient, although this was a substantial element in both groups. Few carers reported loss of earnings from caring for the patient, as most of the carers were retired. Further details of these costs will be published elsewhere.

Sensitivity analysis

Table 4 shows the results of the sensitivity analyses. Reducing length of stay in hospital at home care changed the difference in total healthcare costs for patients recovering from a hysterectomy and for those with chronic obstructive airways disease. A one day

reduction eliminated the difference in cost for patients recovering from a hysterectomy, while a two day reduction altered the results so that hospital at home care became significantly less costly than hospital care for these patients. Costs remained significantly more expensive for patients with chronic obstructive airways disease when duration of hospital at home care was reduced by one day, but a reduction of two days resulted in a non-significant difference between the two groups.

Using average hospital costs instead of dependency adjusted costs reduced the difference in cost between hospital at home care and hospital care for all groups of patients except for the elderly medical patients. Using standard general practitioner costs[8] for both arms of the trial altered the results only for patients recovering from a hip replacement, and general practitioner costs for these patients became significantly more expensive (Mann-Whitney U test P=0.03).

DISCUSSION

Many believe that hospital at home schemes will contain healthcare costs by reducing the demand for acute hospital beds. Our findings indicate that this is not the case. Instead, hospital at home care increased health service costs for some groups of patients, while for others there were no net differences in costs. This is perhaps not surprising, as patients who were discharged early to hospital at home care went home when their hospital care was least expensive. Once in hospital at home care some patients, particularly elderly patients with a medical condition, required 24 hour care. Furthermore, hospital at home increased the overall duration of an episode of health care. This pattern has been observed elsewhere.[4] It may be possible to decrease the amount of time patients spend in hospital at home, and thus reduce cost. However, this could have an adverse effect on patient outcomes. For elderly medical patients and those with chronic obstructive airways disease, hospital at home care increased general practitioner costs, providing evidence that some costs were shifted within the health service.

Perhaps surprisingly for a service that is intended to reduce the pressure on acute hospital beds, the proportion of patients eligible for hospital at home care was low. Other evaluations have also described a relatively low volume of eligible patients.[2 4 9-12] This contrasts with the numbers described by some service providers (Harrison V, Intermediate Care Conference, Anglia and Oxford NHS Executive, Milton Keynes, October, 1997). An increased volume of patients would not, however, alter the costs substantially as only a small proportion of hospital at home costs are fixed. It is possible that patients who would otherwise agree to use hospital at home are deterred by an evaluation. An alternative explanation may be that hospital at home provides extra care in the community but not necessarily care that would otherwise be carried out in a hospital setting.

19

Table 4

Sensitivity analysis: comparing costs of hospital care, dependency adjusted costs and average costs, with costs of hospital at home care after reducing lengths of stay by one or two days

	Hip replacement HaH (n=36) v hospital (n=49)	Knee replacement HaH (n=46) v hospital (n=39)	Hysterectomy HaH (n=111) v hospital (n=123)	Elderly medical HaH (n=50) v hospital (n=44)	Chronic obstructive airways disease HaH (n=15) v hospital (n=17)
Trial results: difference in total healthcare costs using dependency adjusted hospital costs					
Difference in cost (£)	Mean 95.68	Mean 86.26	Mean 92.40	Median 316.56	Median 1132.03
Ratio of geometric mean (95% CI)	1.05 (0.87 to 1.27)	1.05 (0.88 to 1.26)	1.15 (1.04 to 1.29)	—	—
P value	0.59	0.55	0.009	0.09	0.01
Sensitivity analysis: difference in total healthcare costs using average hospital costs					
Difference in cost (£)	Mean -36.80	Mean 35.23	Mean 60.85	Median 518.35	Median 741.36
Ratio of geometric mean (95% CI)	0.89 (0.73 to 1.09)	1.004 (0.82 to 1.22)	1.06 (0.98 to 1.23)	—	—
P value	0.27	0.96	0.10	0.05	0.02
Sensitivity analysis: length of stay in hospital at home care reduced by 1 day					
Difference in cost (£)	Mean 58.32	Mean -8.01	Mean -21.75	Median 227.25	Median 840.26
Ratio of geometric mean (95% CI)	1.02 (0.84 to 1.23)	1.002 (0.84 to 1.19)	0.99 (0.90 to 1.11)	—	—
P value	0.87	0.99	0.99	0.17	0.04
Sensitivity analysis: length of stay in hospital at home care reduced by 2 days					
Difference in cost (£)	Mean 10.61	Mean -49.10	Mean -80.48	Median 103.37	Median 757.23
Ratio of geometric mean (95% CI)	0.95 (0.78 to 1.15)	0.96 (0.81 to 1.15)	0.88 (0.78 to 0.99)	—	—
P value	0.59	0.68	0.03	0.38	0.06

HaH=hospital at home.

Just as inappropriate admissions are a problem for acute hospitals, there is no reason to believe they do not pose a problem for services such as hospital at home. We found that some patients allocated to hospital care were never admitted to hospital and stayed at home with no extra services. This has been found elsewhere (A Wilson, personal communication) and suggests that hospital at home schemes could potentially provide care to patients who would otherwise not be receiving healthcare services. Alternatively, hospital at home may be viewed as supplementing existing services, which may be an acceptable policy option for some groups of patients, particularly elderly medical patients who prefer this form of care.

The extent to which hospital at home care can substitute for hospital care in the United Kingdom is limited. This can partly be explained by the speed at which hospital at home schemes have been set up. Purchasers and providers have responded quickly to initiatives, usually supported by "ring fenced" monies, designed to ease the pressure on hospital beds. Schemes have usually been grafted onto primary care services, with minor alterations to the mix of skills already available. They may become out of date with changes in hospital practice. This is a particular problem for schemes admitting patients who are discharged early from hospital. As hospital lengths of stay decrease, the number of days that can be transferred into the community is correspondingly reduced.

Conclusions

The results of this trial suggest that simply shifting services from one location to another is unlikely to reduce health service costs. Patients discharged early after elective surgery go home at a time when they use least resources. When an inpatient stay involves relatively high nursing costs, as with elderly medical patients, early discharge to hospital at home is unlikely to be significantly cheaper than hospital based care as most of these nursing costs still have to be incurred. Hospital at home care may be cost effective for patients who are relatively independent but who require technical support, such as those receiving intravenous antimicrobial therapy. However, there is little evidence to support or refute this.[13] Service developments, as much as clinical interventions, need to be evidence based. Arguments for diverting resources away from hospital beds should be viewed in the light of the available evidence.

Acknowledgments

We thank the Rockingham Forest NHS Trust, Kettering General Hospital NHS Trust, Northamptonshire Health Authority, and local general practitioners for supporting this research. We also thank Jean Pugh and Angela Howe for their diligent work as research nurses, Helen Doll for statistical advice, and Dr Henry McQuay and Dr JA Muir Gray for their support during the planning of this trial.

Contributors: SS defined the research question, collaborated in designing the trial, coordinated the trial, analysed the data, and was the principal writer of the paper. DH contributed to the running of the trial, maintained the databases, and helped with writing the paper. AG discussed core ideas and participated in analysing and interpreting the data and writing the paper. MV collaborated in designing the trial, solving problems that occurred during the trial, and writing the paper. PM assisted with the study design, implementing the trial, and writing the results. SS is guarantor for the paper.

Funding: R&D Programme NHS Executive Anglia and Oxford and the National R&D Programme, Primary Secondary Care Interface, NHS Executive North Thames.

Conflict of interest: None.

References

1   Shepperd S, Iliffe S. Hospital at home compared with in-patient hospital care [review]. In: Bero L, Grilli R, Grimshaw J, Oxman A, eds. *The Cochrane library. Cochrane Collaboration; Issue 1*. Oxford: Update Software, 1998(Updated quarterly.)

2   Hughes SL, Cummings J, Weaver F, Manheim L, Braun B, Conrad K. A randomised trial of the cost effectiveness of VA hospital–based home care for the terminally ill. *Health Serv Res* 1992; **26**: 801-817.

3   Hollingsworth W, Todd C, Parker M, Roberts JA, Williams R. Cost analysis of early discharge after hip fracture. *BMJ* 1993; **307**: 903-906.

4   Hensher M, Fulop N, Hood S, Ujah S. Does hospital at home make economic sense? Early discharge versus standard care for orthopaedic patients. *J R Soc Med* 1996; **89**: 548-551.

5   Shepperd S, Harwood D, Jenkinson C, Gray A, Vessey M, Morgan P. Randomised controlled trial comparing hospital at home care with inpatient hospital care. I: three month follow up of health outcomes. *BMJ* 1998; **316**: 1786-1791.

6   Jonsson B, Lindgren B. Five common fallacies in estimating the economic gains of early discharge. *Soc Sci Med* 1980; **14**: 27-33.

7   Drummond MF, O'Brien B, Stoddart GL, Torrance GW. *Methods for the economic evaluation of health care programmes*, 2nd ed. Oxford: Oxford University Press , 1997.

8   Netten A, Dennett J. *Unit costs of health and social care 1996*. Canterbury: Personal Social Services Research Unit , 1996.

9   Adler MW, Waller JJ, Creese A, Thorne SC. Randomised controlled trial of early discharge for inguinal hernia and varicose veins. *J Epidemiol Community Health* 1978; **32**: 136-142.

10 Ruckley CV, Cuthbertson C, Fenwick N, Prescott RJ, Garraway WM. Day care after operations for hernia or varicose veins: a controlled trial. *Br J Surg* 1978; **65**: 456-459.

11 Martin F, Oyewole A, Moloney A. A randomised controlled trial of a high support hospital discharge team for elderly people. *Age Ageing* 1994; **23**: 228-234.

12 Donald IP, Baldwin RN, Bannerjee M. Gloucester hospital at home: a randomised controlled trial. *Age Ageing* 1995; **24**: 434-439.

13 Gilbert DN, Dworkin RJ, Raber SR, Leggett JE. Outpatient parenteral antimicrobial drug therapy. *N Engl J Med* 1997; **337**: 829-838.

(Accepted 15 April 1998)

19

This article was first published by the BMJ and is reproduced by permission of the BMJ

ENVIRONMENT OF INFANTS DURING SLEEP AND RISK OF THE SUDDEN INFANT DEATH SYNDROME; RESULTS OF 1993-5 CASE-CONTROL STUDY FOR CONFIDENTIAL INQUIRY INTO STILLBIRTHS AND DEATHS IN INFANCY

BMJ 1996;**313**:191-195 (27 July)

Peter J Fleming, Peter S Blair, Chris Bacon, David Bensley, Ian Smith, Elizabeth Taylor, Jem Berry, Jean Goulding, John Tripp, Confidential Enquiry into Stillbirths and Deaths Regional Coordinators and Researchers

Peter J Fleming, *professor of infant health and developmental physiology*, Foundation for the Study of Infant Deaths Research Unit, Institute of Child Health, Royal Hospital for Sick Children, Bristol BS2 8BJ.

Peter S Blair, *medical statistician*, Foundation for the Study of Infant Deaths Research Unit, Institute of Child Health, Royal Hospital for Sick Children, Bristol BS2 8BJ.

Chris Bacon, *consultant paediatrician*, Friarage Hospital, Northallerton, North Yorkshire DL6 1JG.

David Bensley, *statistician*, Operational Research Division, NHS Executive, Quarry House, Leeds LS2 9UA.

Iain Smith, *senior lecturer*, Nuffield Institute for Health, Leeds LS2 9PL.

Elizabeth Taylor, *consultant senior lecturer in paediatrics*, Sheffield Children's Hospital, Sheffield S10 2TH.

Jem Berry, *professor of paediatric pathology*, University of Bristol, St Michael's Hospital, Bristol BS2 8EG.

Jean Golding, *professor of paediatric and perinatal epidemiology*, Institute of Child Health, Royal Hospital for Sick Children, Bristol BS2 8BJ.

John Tripp, *consultant paediatrician*, Department of Child Health, Postgraduate Medical School, Royal Devon and Exeter Hospital, Exeter EX2 5DW.

Confidential Enquiry into Stillbirths and Deaths Regional Coordinators and Researchers

The regional coordinators and researchers of the confidential inquiry into stillbirths and deaths in infancy are given at the end of this article.

Correspondence to: Professor Fleming.

ABSTRACT

Objective: To investigate the role of sleeping arrangements as risk factors for the sudden infant death syndrome after a national risk reduction campaign.

Design: Two year population based case-control study. Parental interviews were conducted for each infant who died and for four controls matched for age and date of interview.

Setting: Three regions in England with a total population of 17 million people.

Subjects: 195 babies who died and 780 matched controls.

Results: Prone and side sleeping positions both carried increased risks of death compared with supine when adjusted for maternal age, parity, gestation, birth weight, exposure to smoke, and other relevant factors in the sleeping environment (multivariate odds ratio = 9.00 (95% confidence interval 2.84 to 28.47) and 1.84 (1.02 to 3.31), respectively). The higher incidence of side rather than prone sleeping led to a higher population attributable risk (side 18.4%, prone 14.2%). More of the infants who died were found with bed covers over their heads (21.58; 6.21 to 74.99). The use of a dummy had an apparent protective effect (0.38; 0.21 to 0.70). Bed sharing for the whole night was a significant risk factor for infants whose mothers smoked (9.25; 2.31 to 34.02). No protective effect of breast feeding could be identified on multivariate analysis.

Conclusions: This study confirms the importance of certain risk factors for the sudden infant death syndrome and identifies others—for example, covers over the head, side sleeping position–which may be amenable to change by educating and informing parents and health care professionals.

INTRODUCTION

Despite the fall in the incidence of sudden unexpected deaths in infancy in the United Kingdom, particularly that which followed the "Back to Sleep" campaign in 1991, such deaths remain one of the largest single group of deaths in infancy.[1]

Previous studies have drawn attention to the importance of several features of the environment in which infants sleep–for example, sleeping position, bedding, use of dummies–as factors affecting the risk of the sudden infant death syndrome.[2 3] Other factors, such as breast or bottle feeding and bed sharing, have not consistently been found to be associated with risk of death.[4][5][6] No large scale studies have yet been published of the impact on such factors of the major national campaign aimed at reducing risk.

The study of sudden unexpected deaths in infancy was established as a part of the national confidential inquiry into stillbirths and deaths in infancy (CESDI), with funding from the Department of Health. The aim was to conduct a detailed case-control study of all sudden unexpected deaths in infancy in the participating regions of the United Kingdom combined with a confidential inquiry into such deaths over a two year period starting one year after the national risk reduction campaign. A summary of the preliminary results of this study and data relating to mattress covers have been published.[7][8]

In this paper we present the results of a detailed analysis of several aspects of the infant's sleeping environment and the risk of the sudden infant death syndrome.

METHODS

Study design, case notification, and selection of controls

The study aimed to include all deaths from the syndrome in infants aged 7 to 364 days inclusive in two NHS regions in the United Kingdom (Southwest and Yorkshire) from February 1993 and a third region (Trent) from September 1993 until January 1995 inclusive, the total population of the study area being about 17 million. Cases were ascertained through a communication network of professionals and lay organisations who reported all sudden unexpected deaths within 24 hours.

Data were collected on a standard questionnaire by research interviewers, consistency of approach being maintained by regular training meetings. The interviewers visited each bereaved family twice. On the first occasion, usually within five days of the death, after obtaining informed consent they took a standardised semistructured history, including a narrative account of events leading up to and surrounding the infant's final sleep. On the second visit, a few days later and usually within two weeks of the death, they completed the full questionnaire.

The questionnaire contained over 600 items, including demographic and social data; the medical history of the infant and other family members; use of cigarettes, alcohol and drugs; the precise sleeping arrangements for the infant; and full details of the events preceding and the circumstances surrounding the death. Information was collected both with regard to the family's usual practices by day and by night and to the period when the baby died. Most of these data were obtained by parental interview, the remainder were derived from medical and nursing records.

Four controls for each case were selected by the method previously used in Avon.[2] The health visitor for the index case was asked to identify the two babies on her list next older and the two babies next younger, within two weeks of the age of the index baby. In the few instances where the family thus identified was not available or declined to be interviewed or when the health visitor thought inclusion inappropriate–for example, because of recent bereavement–then the family with the next closest baby in age was substituted. If a health visitor did not have four suitable babies on her own list she drew from the list of her nearest colleague.

This method of control selection gave a high compliance rate and allowed rapid collection of control data. The geographical matching inherent in this system, however, may lead to an underestimate of the significance of factors relating to socioeconomic status.[9]

The interviewer visited each control family within a week of the death to collect the same data as for the index case. A period of sleep (the "reference sleep") was identified in the control infant's life in the 24 hours before the interview corresponding to that in which the index baby had died, particular importance being given to the index parents' view of whether it had been a night or a daytime sleep. Data were collected for this period equivalent to those collected for the index baby.

Regional confidential review committee

All available information on each case was reviewed in detail by a multidisciplinary confidential review committee. Only those deaths that were unexpected by history and for which no sufficient cause was determined by thorough investigation, including a full paediatric postmortem examination and review of the circumstances of the death, were attributable to the sudden infant death syndrome.[10][11][12] The methodology has previously been used and validated in studies in Avon.[2][5][9][11]

Statistical analysis

For both the univariate and the multivariate analysis the matching was taken into account by using conditional logistic regression. This was carried out with version 6 of the SAS package,[13] and results have been verified against similar procedures available in SYSTAT, GLIM, and EGRET. Odds ratios are quoted for categorical variables adjusted for the matching, P values are used for

Table 1

Sleeping position in babies who died from the sudden infant death syndrome and matched controls

Detail	No (%) of babies who died	No (%) of controls	Odds ratio (95% confidence interval)
Position put down:			
Back	82 (43.6)	509 (65.8)	1.00
Side	76 (40.4)	241 (31.1)	2.01 (1.38 to 2.93)
Front	30 (16.0)	24 (3.1)	9.58 (4.86 to 18.87)
No with data available	188	774	
Position found:			
Back	67 (35.8)	618 (81.9)	1.00
Side	43 (23.0)	92 (12.2)	4.51 (2.65 to 7.66)
Front	77 (41.2)	45 (6.0)	21.36 (11.67 to 39.08)
No with data available	187	755	

continuous variables, and the unadjusted Fisher's exact test was utilised for small cell frequencies. Centiles at birth were computed by using z scores from the FOX-PRO package.[14] Population attributable risk was calculated by using the multivariate odds ratio and percentage of exposed among the index group.[15]

The multivariate model included all effect modifiers that were significant in the univariate analysis (P<0.05) and remained significant in the multivariate analysis when we controlled for the other effect modifiers and variables being tested. These were maternal age, parity (defined as the number of liveborn children at the time of interview), gestation in weeks, birth weight adjusted for gestation and sex, and a measure for socioeconomic status. A number of markers of socioeconomic status were collected, including social class, parental education, weekly income, whether the family received any income support, and several questions regarding housing conditions. Detailed analysis has shown all of these factors to be significant,[7] the most significant being family income supplement, a means tested benefit which takes account of the family needs as well as income. This has therefore been used throughout this report as an indicator of socioeconomic deprivation.

Smoking was found to be an important risk factor and was also entered into the model, a detailed analysis of the data on smoking is included in the accompanying paper.[16]

RESULTS

Quality of data and collection

Ascertainment of cases and controls

During the study period 266 sudden unexpected deaths in infancy were identified. Subsequent checking with statutory notifications revealed five such deaths in the study regions which had not been identified during the study period. Of the potential control families, 57 could not be used (21 were not available, 23 were thought unsuitable, and 13 refused). Replacements were immediately found so that ascertainment of controls was 100%. Most of the deaths (216 (81.2%)) were attributable to the sudden infant death syndrome; seven index families could not be interviewed, either because they were subject to a police investigation or could not be traced, and 12 families refused interview, which gives a consent rate of 94.3%. In two further cases no controls were taken because the index family lived outside the study area. This analysis therefore deals with 195 cases and their 780 matched controls.

Time to first interview

The median time from the discovery of the death until the first interview of the index parents was 4.5 days; 82% of families were interviewed within 14 days and 95% within 28 days of the death.

Matching for age

Over two thirds of the controls were matched within two weeks and over 90% within one month of the age of the index baby.

Univariate results adjusted for matching

Sleeping position

Table 1 shows the positions in which the babies who died and the controls were put down to sleep and found after sleep for the last or reference sleeps. The prone position was the least common sleeping position in which infants were put down, but it carried the greatest risk. An important new observation in these data is that the side sleeping position carried a significantly increased risk when compared with supine (odds ratio = 2.01; 95% confidence interval 1.38 to 2.93), regardless of whether the lower arm was extended forward or not. A change in position during the reference sleep from side to prone was rare among the controls (9/238 (3.8%)) compared with the babies who died (29/74 (39.2%)), while conversely the change from side to supine was rare among the babies who died but

Table 2

Tog values of bedding used for babies who died from the sudden infant death syndrome and matched controls

	No (%) of babies who died	No (%) of controls	Odds ratio (95% confidence interval)	
Tog value			Not adjusted	Adjusted*
Usually by night:				
<6 togs	81 (42.0)	391 (50.2)	1.00	1.00
6-9 togs	80 (41.5)	318 (40.8)	1.27 (0.86 to 1.87)	1.27 (0.83 to 1.95)
≥=10 togs	32 (16.6)	70 (9.0)	2.27 (1.32 to 3.90)	1.65 (0.90 to 3.04)
No with data available	193	779		
Usually by day:				
<6 togs	135 (70.0)	643 (82.6)	1.00	1.00
6-9 togs	43 (22.3)	117 (15.0)	2.00 (1.26 to 3.15)	2.07 (1.24 to 3.46)
≥=10 togs	15 (7.8)	18 (2.3)	4.32 (1.97 to 9.46)	3.94 (1.64 to 9.49)
No with data available	193	778		
When put down:				
<6 togs	90 (47.1)	456 (58.5)	1.00	1.00
6-9 togs	68 (35.6)	263 (33.8)	1.50 (0.99 to 2.26)	1.52 (0.96 to 2.42)
≥=10 togs	33 (17.3)	60 (7.7)	3.38 (1.94 to 5.87)	2.78 (1.49 to 4.16)
No with data available	191	779		
When found:				
<6 togs	112 (58.9)	556 (71.4)	1.00	1.00
6-9 togs	51 (26.8)	183 (23.5)	1.61 (1.05 to 2.47)	1.57 (0.97 to 2.54)
≥=10 togs	27 (14.2)	40 (5.2)	4.41 (2.20 to 7.62)	3.52 (1.74 to 7.11)
No with data available	190	779		

*Controlled for socioeconomic status (with family income supplement).

common among the controls. The major risk factor was for infants put down on their sides and found prone (21.69; 8.84 to 53.20) rather than for infants who remained on their sides or rolled to supine (1.21; 0.79 to 1.87).

Thermal environment

Significantly more of the mothers of control infants than of babies who died worried about their babies becoming too hot (0.47; 0.28 to 0.76). Twice as many babies who died (21.8%) as controls (11.9%) slept in rooms in which the heating was on for the whole duration of the last or reference sleep (2.14; 1.33 to 3.15). Table 2 shows the thermal resistance (tog value) of bedding and clothing for sleep, usually and during the last or reference sleep for babies who died and controls. The babies who died were more heavily wrapped than the controls, both usually and during the last or reference sleep, the risk increasing as the tog value increased. A small but significant proportion of babies who died wore a hat to sleep, both usually at night (3.1% v 0.1% controls; P<0.0003) and for the last or reference sleep (5.2% v 1.8% controls; P<0.015) (Fisher's exact test). Data from the Meteorological Office showed no difference between the outdoor temperatures in the 24 hour periods preceding the deaths and those preceding the interviews of the controls.

Arrangement of bedding

Table 3 shows the type of bedding, how the bedding was arranged, where the infant was put in the bed, and whether the infant was usually found or found after the last or reference sleep with covers over the head. Very few babies who died or control infants were put down for the last or reference sleep at the bottom of the bed; this reflected usual practice. Significantly more babies who died (9.0% v 3.2%) were found at the bottom of the bed after the last or reference sleep (3.02; 1.42 to 6.25). More babies who died than controls were found with covers over their heads, and of these, more were sleeping under duvets (64% v 33% controls).

Bed sharing and room sharing

Routine bed sharing with parent(s) (two or more nights a week) was commoner among babies who died (26%) than controls (14.2%) (2.04; 1.36 to 3.07). During the last or reference sleep this difference was significant only for those who had been in bed with the parent(s) for more than one hour (25.7% v 15.3% controls; 1.86; 1.23 to 2.81) or for the whole night (14.9% v 4.0%; 4.12; 2.30 to 7.40). For most this was their usual practice; very few did so because the baby seemed unwell. More of these index mothers had consumed three or more units of alcohol in the preceding 24 hours (44.8%) compared with the control mothers (19.3%),

20

Table 3

Arrangement of bedding in babies who died from the sudden infant death syndrome and matched controls

Detail of bedding	No (%) of babies who died	No (%) of controls	Odds ratio (95% confidence interval)
Duvet used for last or reference sleep:			
No	112 (57.7)	602 (77.3)	1
Yes	82 (42.3)	177 (22.7)	2.82 (1.95 to 4.08)
No with data available	194	779	
Bedding for last or reference sleep:			
Tucked in or no bedding	82 (44.3)	467 (60.3)	1
Lying loosely over	103 (55.7)	307 (39.7)	1.92 (1.35 to 2.73)
No with data available	185	774	
Where in bed:			
Top or middle	169 (98.3)	689 (98.1)	
Bottom	3 (1.7)	13 (1.9)	P = 1.0*
No with data available	172	702	
Usually found with covers over head:			
Sometimes or never	181 (94.3)	763 (97.9)	
Often or always	11 (5.7)	16 (2.1)	2.72 (1.11 to 6.77)
No with data available	192	779	
Found with covers over head after last or reference sleep:			
No	148 (81.3)	747 (97.6)	
Yes	34 (18.7)	18 (2.4)	18.93 (8.05 to 44.48)
No with data available	182	765	

*Fisher's exact test.

although bed sharing was still significant among those who did not consume alcohol (2.92; 1.44 to 5.87). Most of the index mothers who shared their bed also smoked (86.2% v 35.5% controls). In a subgroup analysis the risk associated with bed sharing was not significant for non-smoking mothers (2.55; 0.80 to 8.19) but highly significant for mothers who smoked (17.57; 7.58 to 40.72). There was no difference in the proportions of babies who died and control infants sharing a room with an adult or another child usually or during the last or reference sleep.

Use of dummies

There was no difference in the proportion of the babies who died and controls who routinely used a dummy, but for the last or reference sleep there was a significant excess of control infants (52.8%) who used a dummy compared with babies who died (39.8%) (0.59; 0.42 to 0.84).

Breast feeding or bottle feeding

More of the control infants (60.3%) than the babies who died (45.1%) had ever been breast fed (0.50; 0.35 to 0.71), but the protective effect did not increase with increasing duration of breast feeding. Breast feeding was significant independently of dummy use, the cumulative protective effect of both being additive (0.26; 0.15 to 0.44). Bottle feeding was strongly associated with lower socioeconomic status and with smoking. When breast feeding was adjusted for socioeconomic status its apparent protective effect became non-significant (0.69; 0.47 to 1.02).

Multivariate model

From the univariate analysis various factors seem to be associated with an increased or decreased risk of the sudden infant death syndrome. To examine their significance, however, we need to look at their relation to each other and to control for other significant risk factors. Table 4 shows how the significance of the variables associated with the sleeping environment changes when they are put in the multivariate model with each other and how it changes further when we control for other significant risk factors.

The risk associated with prone sleeping, side sleeping, and covering of the head by bedding and the protective effect of using a dummy remained significant when we controlled for other factors. Bed sharing also remained significant, but a subgroup analysis showed that the associated risk was significant only among smokers (multivariate odds ratio 9.25; 2.51 to 34.02) rather than non-smokers (2.27; 0.41 to 12.54). The risks associated with heating and using a duvet were significant among the factors associated with the sleeping environment but just failed to reach significance when we controlled for other risk factors. No protective effect of breast feeding was identifiable when we controlled for all other factors.

DISCUSSION

The results of this, the first large scale case-control study of the sudden infant death syndrome after the national risk reduction campaign, demonstrate the effects of the changes introduced and shed new light on the aetiology and epidemiology of the syndrome.

Sleeping position and bed sharing

The significance of the prone sleeping position as a risk factor for the syndrome has been confirmed. A new finding is that the side sleeping position, previously recommended as a safer alternative to prone sleeping, is itself associated with a significantly increased risk of death when compared with supine. This added risk seems to result mainly from the tendency of babies placed on their sides to roll prone and was not influenced by the position of the infant's arm. The higher prevalence of side sleeping than prone sleeping in the present population means that the population attributable risk from side sleeping (18.4%) is higher than that of prone sleeping (14.2%) despite a much lower odds ratio.[15]

Interpretation of the effects of bed sharing on the risk of death is complicated by the interactions with several other factors. Mothers who habitually take their babies into bed with them are not homogeneous but come from disparate ethnic, social, and cultural groups with very different approaches to child care, breast feeding, smoking, and alcohol misuse. The data confirm the conclusion of the New Zealand study[17] that there is a significant risk from bed sharing if the parents smoke and support a previous suggestion (not borne out in the New Zealand study) that bed sharing is a risk if the mother has recently consumed alcohol.[18] There is no suggestion that taking the baby into bed for a short time for feeding or for comfort poses any risk–except that the mother may then fall asleep and keep the baby in her bed all night long.

Thermal environment

Thermal stress emerges in the present study as a smaller independent risk factor for the syndrome than previously reported.[2] This might be expected from the known interaction between heavy wrapping and prone sleeping, the prevalence of which has sharply declined. It is postulated that the interaction may arise from a reduction in heat loss from the face of a baby lying prone.[19]

In the present study most babies slept supine or on their sides so that adverse effects of heavy wrapping would be less likely, unless the head became totally covered and heat loss from both face and scalp was prevented. Total covering by the bedding emerged from the multivariate analysis as the most potent of all risk factors. The fact that babies who died had been previously found totally covered more often than the controls suggests that the way the bedding is usually arranged might be partly responsible. This lends support to the recent "Feet to Foot" initiative from the Foundation for the Study of Infant Deaths, which advocates that a baby's bedding should be made up so that the baby's feet are at the foot of the cot and risk of slipping beneath the covers is reduced. Our finding that

Table 4

Multivariate analysis of significant factors in sleeping environment for risk of the sudden infant death syndrome. Figures are odds ratios (95% confidence intervals)

Variable*	Univariate	Multivariate Sleeping†	All factors††
Prone sleeping	9.58 (4.86 to 18.87)	10.03 (4.33 to 23.24)	9 (2.84 to 28.47)
Side sleeping	2.01 (1.38 to 2.93)	2.16 (1.36 to 3.43)	1.84 (1.02 to 3.31)
Infant found with covers over head	18.93 (8.05 to 44.48)	31.38 (10.4 to 95.0)	21.58 (6.21 to 74.99)
Tog value (6-9 togs)	1.5 (0.99 to 2.26)	0.95 (0.55 to 1.63)	0.89 (0.45 to 1.76)
Tog value ($\geq = 10$ togs)	3.38 (1.94 to 5.87)	1.04 (0.44 to 2.46)	0.94 (0.31 to 2.83)
Wearing hat	P = 0.015§	6.21 (0.74 to 51.93)	4.13 (0.22 to 77.89)
Heating on all night	2.14 (1.30 to 3.50)	3.14 (1.60 to 6.17)	2.37 (0.96 to 5.84)
Whether mother ever breast fed	0.5 (0.35 to 0.71)	0.42 (0.26 to 0.67)	1.06 (0.57 to 1.98)
Bed sharing with parents all night	4.12 (2.30 to 7.40)	4.06 (1.78 to 9.23)	4.36 (1.59 to 11.95)
Using dummy	0.59 (0.42 to 0.84)	0.44 (0.27 to 0.70)	0.38 (0.21 to 0.70)
Using duvet	2.82 (1.95 to 4.08)	1.88 (1.14 to 3.12)	1.72 (0.90 to 3.30)
Loose bed covering	1.92 (1.35 to 2.73)	1.25 (0.79 to 1.99)	1.07 (0.61 to 1.89)

*All variables are for last or reference sleep except for breast feeding.

† Controlled for all sleeping environment factors listed in table.

†† Controlled for maternal age, parity, gestation, birth weight, whether family received family income supplement, exposure to tobacco smoke, and factors in sleeping environment that remain significant.

§ Fisher's exact test, hence odds ratio not given.

20

very few mothers, index or control, practised this technique during the study, which preceded the initiative, suggests that there is a large potential for change. Duvets or quilts were associated with added risk both in themselves and through their propensity to total covering; this reinforces the advice that the use of duvets or quilts should be strongly discouraged for infants under 1 year.

Breast feeding and dummy use

As in the Avon study,[5] no independent protective effect was identified from breast feeding when we controlled for other significant factors. In the univariate analysis the lack of any "dose-response" effect from breast feeding suggests that it is acting as a marker of the lifestyle of mothers who breast feed rather than showing a biological effect in itself. The loss of significance when account is taken either of smoking or of socioeconomic status supports this interpretation, as does the very small protective effect among the infants of nonsmoking mothers. There are of course other good reasons to continue recommending breast feeding.

The apparent protective effect of a dummy is in agreement with the observation in New Zealand,[3] but in that study a high proportion of infants were sleeping prone. Dummy use is more common in the more socioeconomically deprived groups in the United Kingdom and is the only factor over-represented in these groups that is associated with a significantly reduced risk of the syndrome. It is not clear whether use of a dummy is a marker of a particular pattern of infant care in this group. These findings should not be used to claim that dummies prevent cot death, but it may not be appropriate for health care professionals routinely to discourage the use of dummies in young infants. Further research is needed to identify any adverse effects of dummy use, in particular the reported adverse effects on breast feeding.[20]

The regional coordinators of the confidential inquiry into stillbirths and deaths in infancy were Ms Lesley Anson (Yorkshire); Mrs Rosanne Sodzi (South Western, 1993-5); Mrs Rosie Thompson (South Western, from 1995); Ms Sue Wood (Trent). The research health visitors of the inquiry were Mrs Christine Ahronson, Mrs Lindsay Cansfield, Mrs Carmel Davis, Mrs Margaret Griffin, Mrs Pat Johnson, Mrs Lynette Lovelock, Mrs Lynne Middleton, Mrs Pam Mueller, Mrs Shirley Stephenson, Mrs Dawn Taylor, Mrs Lorraine Wright, and the research midwives were Mrs Chris Laws and Mrs Rosie McCabe.

Funding: National Advisory Body for the confidential inquiry into stillbirths and deaths in infancy.

Conflict of interest: None.

References

1 Wigfield R, Fleming PJ. The prevalence of risk factors for SIDS: impact of an intervention campaign. In: Rognum TO, ed. *Sudden infant death syndrome: new trends in the nineties.* Oslo: Scandinavian University Press, 1995:124-8.

2 Fleming PJ, Gilbert RE, Azaz Y, Berry PJ, Rudd PT, Stewart A, *et al.* The interaction between bedding and sleeping position in sudden infant death syndrome: a population based case-control study. *BMJ* 1990;**301**:85-9.

3 Mitchell EA, Taylor BJ, Ford RPK, Stewart AW, Becroft DMO, Thompson JMD, *et al.* Dummies and the sudden infant death syndrome. *Arch Dis Child* 1993;**68**:501-4.

4 Klonoff-Cohen H, Edelstein SL. Bed sharing and the sudden infant death syndrome. *BMJ* 1995;**311**:1269-72.

5 Gilbert RE, Wigfield RE, Fleming PJ, Berry PJ, Rudd PT. Bottle feeding and the sudden infant death syndrome. *BMJ* 1995;**310**:88-90.

6 Ford RPK, Taylor BJ, Mitchell EA, Enright SA, Stewart AW, Becroft DMO, *et al.* Breastfeeding and the risk of sudden infant death syndrome. *Int J Epidemiol* 1993;**22**:885-90.

7 National Advisory Body for CESDI. *Annual report for 1994.* London: Department of Health, 1996.

8 Blair P, Fleming P, Bensley D, Smith I, Bacon C, Taylor E. Plastic mattresses and sudden infant death syndrome. *Lancet* 1995;**345**:720.

9 Wigfield RE, Fleming PJ, Berry PJ, Rudd PT, Golding J. Can the fall in Avon's sudden infant death rate be explained by the observed sleeping position changes? *BMJ* 1992;**304**:282-3.

10 Taylor EM, Emery JL. Categories of preventable infant deaths. *Arch Dis Child* 1990;**63**:535-9.

11 Gilbert RE, Rudd PT, Berry PJ, Fleming PJ, Hall E, White DG, *et al.* Combined effect of infection and heavy wrapping on the risk of sudden infant death. *Arch Dis Child* 1992;**67**:272-7.

12 Cordner SM, Willinger M. The definition of the sudden infant death syndrome. In: Rognum TO, ed. *Sudden infant death syndrome, new trends in the nineties.* Oslo: Scandinavian University Press, 1995.

13 SAS Institute. *SAS user's guide.* Version 6. 4th ed. Cary, NC: SAS Institute, 1989.

14 Microsoft Corporation. *Fox-Pro.* Redmond, Washington: Microsoft Corporation, 1995.

15 Bruzzi P, Green SB, Byar DP, Brunton LA, Schaiver C. Estimating the population attributable risk for multiple risk factors using case control data. *Am J Epidemiol* 1985;**122**:904-14.

16 Blair PS, Fleming PJ, Bensley D, Smith I, Bacon C, Taylor E, *et al.* Smoking and the sudden infant death syndrome: results from 1993-5 case-control study for confidential inquiry into stillbirths and deaths in infancy. *BMJ* 1996;**313**:195-8.

17 Scragg R, Mitchell EA, Tayloret B, Stewart AW, Ford RPK, Thompson JMD, *et al.* Bed sharing, smoking and alcohol in the sudden infant death syndrome. *BMJ* 1993;**307**:1313-8.

18 Norvenious SG. Sudden infant death syndrome in Sweden in 1973-1977 and 1979. *Acta Paediatr Scand Suppl* 1987;**333**:1-138.

19 Fleming PJ, Levine MR, Azaz Y, Wigfield R. The development of thermoregulation and interactions with the control of respiration in infants: possible relationship to sudden infant death. *Acta Paediatr Scand* 1993;**389**(suppl):57-9.

20 Barros FC, Victora CG, Semer TC, Filho ST, Tamosi E, Weiderpass E. Use of pacifiers is associated with decreased breastfeeding duration. *Pediatrics* 1995;**95**:497-9.

This article was first published in the International Journal of Epidemiology and is reproduced by permission of Oxford University Press

ALCOHOL, FISH, FIBRE AND ANTIOXIDANT VITAMINS INTAKE DO NOT EXPLAIN POPULATION DIFFERENCES IN CORONARY HEART DISEASE MORTALITY

Daan Kromhout,* Bennie PM Bloemberg,* Edith JM Feskens,* Michael GL Hertog,* Alessandro Menotti[†] and Henry Blackburn[†]

International Journal of Epidemiology 1996, **25**: 753–759.

* Division of Public Health Research, National Institute of Public Health and Environment, PO Box 1, 3720 BA Bilthoven, The Netherlands.

[†] Division of Epidemiology, School of Public Health, University of Minnesota, Minneapolis, Minnesota 55455, USA.

Background. Within the Seven Countries Study data we investigated whether population differences in 25-year mortality rates from coronary heart disease could be explained by population differences in alcohol, fish, fibre and antioxidant intake.

Methods. Baseline surveys were carried out between 1958 and 1964, on 12 763 middle-aged men constituting 16 cohorts in seven countries. In 1987 and 1988 equivalent food composites representing the average food intake of each cohort at baseline were collected locally and analysed for their fibre and antioxidant content in one central laboratory. The vital status of all participants was verified at regular intervals over 25 years.

Results. Alcohol and fish intake were inversely related to 25-year mortality from coronary heart disease in univariate analyses. These associations became non-significant when the confounding effects of saturated fatty acids, flavonoids and smoking were taken into account. Fibre and antioxidant vitamins intake were not related to coronary heart disease mortality in either uni- or multivariate analysis.

Conclusion. These cross-cultural analyses show that alcohol, fish, fibre and antioxidant vitamins do not explain population differences in coronary heart disease mortality, independently of saturated fatty acids and flavonoids intake and cigarette smoking.

Keywords: alcohol, fish, fibre, antioxidants, vitamins, coronary heart disease

Recent reports of the Seven Countries Studies showed that population differences in long-term coronary heart disease mortality (CHD) can largely be explained by differences in saturated fatty acids and flavonoids intake and cigarette smoking.[1,2] Other cross-cultural studies suggest that the average population intake of alcohol, fish, fibre and antioxidant vitamins is also associated with CHD mortality rates.[3–6] To get a fuller perspective on diet, alcohol and smoking in population differences in CHD the associations are investigated between population intakes of alcohol, fish, fibre and antioxidant vitamins in relation to 25-year mortality rates from CHD. Results are discussed in the light of knowledge on the role of diet, alcohol and smoking in the development of athero-thrombotic complications.

METHODS

Between 1958 and 1964, 12 763 men aged 40–59 were enrolled in the Seven Countries Study. In these countries 16 cohorts were established, 11 in rural areas in Finland, Italy, Greece, the former Yugoslavia and Japan, two cohorts of railroad employees in the USA and Italy, one of workers in a large cooperative in Serbia, one of university professors in Belgrade and one of inhabitants of a small commercial market town in the Netherlands. The characteristics of these cohorts have been described in detail.[7–9]

Information on smoking was collected by questionnaire and the percentage of cigarette smokers per cohort was calculated. Between 1959 and 1964 dietary information was collected in small random samples of 14 of the 16 cohorts.[10] In the other two cohorts dietary information was gathered around 1970. The weighed record method was used in all dietary surveys. In 1985 and 1986 the original dietary, data of all these cohorts were coded by one dietitian in a standardized way. The average intake of different foods consumed in the 16 cohorts was calculated and summarized in 16 food groups including fish and alcoholic beverages.

In 1987, equivalent food composites representing the average food intake of each cohort at baseline were collected from local markets by two dietitians. These foods were transported in cooling boxes to the laboratory of the Department of Human Nutrition, Agricultural University, Wageningen, The Netherlands (Head: M B Katan). The foods were cleaned and

21

equivalent food composites prepared according to the average consumption patterns of the cohorts. Oxalic acid was added to the equivalent food composites in order to preserve the vitamin C content. The foods were homogenized and frozen at −20°C until chemical analyses of the different nutrients took place.

In 1987 and 1988, total lipids were isolated according to Osborne and Voogt [11] and fatty acids were determined by gas chromatography. [12] Dietary cholesterol was determined by the method of Jonker *et al.* [13] The total flavonoid content was quantified by high-performance liquid chromatography as the sum of quercetin, kaempferol, myricetin, luteolin and apigenin. [14] Alcohol was determined by the method of Boehringer-Mannheim. [15] Total dietary fibre was determined with an enzymatic-gravimetric method. [16] b-carotene was determined by high-performance liquid chromatography and spectrophotometry, [17] vitamin C by a fluorimetric method, [18] and vitamin E by high-performance liquid chromatography with spectrofluorescence detection. [19]

The vital status of all men was checked roughly every 5 years. Over 25 years 5973 men (47%) died. Only 56 men (0.4%) were lost to follow-up. The underlying cause of death of the men who died was established centrally by Blackburn and Menotti during the first 10 years of follow-up and after 10 years of follow-up by Menotti. The causes of death were coded using the 8th revision of the International Classification of Diseases (ICD). Mortality from CHD was defined as ICD 410–414. Age-adjusted mortality rates were calculated using the age distribution of all participants in the Seven Countries Study as a standard.

The dietary intake variables represent the average for each cohort. The intake of alcohol and fish was skewed to the right and therefore the logarithm was used. Adjustment for energy intake was not made, because, at the population level, energy intake is not associated with CHD mortality. Analyses concern only inter-cohort comparisons. Because of the limited degrees of freedom, the multiple regression models never included more than four independent variables. Only two-sided *P*-values are reported.

RESULTS

The population average absolute alcohol intake varied between 2 g/day in Finland and 91 g/day, in Dalmatia (Croatia) (Table 1). Also a large variation was observed in fish consumption. No fish was consumed in Velika Krsna (Serbia) but the men in the fishermen's village of Ushibuka (Japan) consumed 207 g/day. A threefold difference in fibre intake was noted. Men in Ushibuka (Japan) consumed 21 g/day compared with 57 g/day among their counterparts in Corfu (Greece). The intake of b-carotene and vitamin C was very low in Velika Krsna (Serbia). The highest b-carotene and vitamin C intake was found in Dalmatia (Croatia) and the USA rail workers respectively. Intake of vitamin E was highest in the cohorts with a high intake of olive oil (e.g. Crete and Corfu, Greece) and was low in the Japanese cohorts (Ushibuka and Tanushimaru).

Population average alcohol intake was significantly and inversely related to 25-year mortality rates from CHD (Figure 1). After multivariate analyses, including saturated fatty acids and flavonoid intake and the prevalence of smoking, alcohol was no longer statistically significantly associated with long-term CHD mortality (Table 2). This was due to a significant inverse relation between saturated fatty acids and alcohol intake (Table 3). Fish consumption was significantly inversely

Table 1

Average population intake of alcohol (100%), fish, fibre and antioxidant vitamins in the Seven Countries Study.

Cohort	Alcohol (g/d)	Fish (g/d)	Fibre (g/d)	β-carotene (mg/d)	Vit C (mg/d)	Vit E (mg/d)
US Railroad	4.7	3	22.5	2.6	142	11.8
East Finland	1.8	58	50.0	1.4	80	11.2
West Finland	1.9	7	43.0	2.1	65	10.7
Zutphen, Netherlands	2.6	12	25.2	2.9	110	11.6
Crevalcore, Italy	46.5	22	25.3	1.2	50	16.5
Montegiorgio, Italy,	37.4	35	27.6	2.9	44	14.5
Rome, Italy,	37.8	30	26.5	2.6	53	14.9
Dalmatia, Croatia	91.1	96	30.1	4.2	60	17.8
Slavonia, Croatia	12.3	35	36.7	3.4	41	13.1
Velika Krsna, Serbia	8.7	0	38.8	0.6	17	9.5
Zrenjanin, Serbia	9.5	7	34.8	2.2	112	13.9
Belgrade, Serbia	3.9	19	25.6	1.7	71	20.9
Crete, Greece	10.8	18	43.1	1.8	136	23.3
Corfu, Greece	16.2	60	57.2	2.2	125	32.8
Tanushimaru, Japan	11.9	93	24.3	1.9	39	7.2
Ushibuka, Japan	14.0	207	21.0	1.4	45	8.6

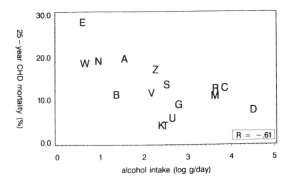

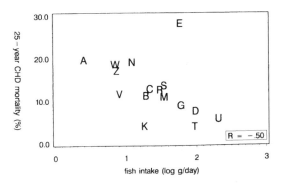

Figure 1 *Relation between alcohol (100%) intake at baseline and 25-year mortality from coronary heart disease*

Figure 2 *Relation between fish intake at baseline and 25-year mortality from coronary heart disease*

related with 25-year CHD mortality (Figure 2), but this association also became non-significant after adjustment for saturated fatty acids and flavonoid intake and the prevalence of cigarette smoking (Table 2). The population average intake of fibre, b-carotene, vitamin C and vitamin E was unrelated to 25-year mortality rates from CHD (Table 2).

DISCUSSION

In the present study, dietary data collected around 1960 were related to mortality from CHD during the subsequent 25 years. The chemical analyses of alcohol, fibre and antioxidant vitamins were carried out 25 years later in equivalent food composites representing the average food consumption pattern of each cohort. This delay could have biased the estimate of average population intake of the different dietary variables. However, strong correlations were observed between fatty acid determinations carried out 25 years apart.[1] We suspect that alcohol, fibre and vitamin content of foods and beverages probably did not change much over the 25 years. Therefore we believe that the results of the chemical analyses carried out in 1987 and 1988 are probably a good indicator of the average population intake of these variables at the beginning of the Seven Countries Study.

In studying the relations between dietary variables and long-term CHD mortality it is important to know what changes occurred in the intake of these variables over the 25-year period. Chemical analyses of food composites were not carried out repeatedly during 25 years of follow-up. However, results of analyses using food balance sheet data from 1961–1965 and 1975–1977 of the seven countries showed strong, correlations for the relevant foods (e.g. alcoholic beverages, fish, cereals, vegetables, fruits, and fats and oils).[10] These results suggest that the relative position of the cohorts in the distribution of different foods was maintained. Therefore, the average intake of chemically-determined dietary variables in the equivalent food composites represent the average food consumption pattern at baseline and can be used for studying associations with long-term CHD mortality rates.

The strength of the present study is the standardized methodology for data collection and the prospective design. The weakness is that only 16 cohorts were included in the study with limited possibilities for multivariate analyses. The small number of cohorts may also influence the stability of the associations. In such situations the selection of cohorts is of utmost importance. In the Seven Countries Study, qualitative differences in dietary patterns between the cohorts in the late 1950s formed the primary reasons for their selection. The large differences in food and nutrient intake between the cohorts made the Seven Countries

Table 2

Regression coefficients for population averages of different dietary variables and 25-year mortality from CHD in the Seven Countries Study

Dietary variable	Coronary heart disease			
	UV	95% CI	MV	95% CI
Alcohol (log) (g)	-3.44	-5.76, -1.11*	-0.06	-1.44, 1.33
Fish (log) (g)	-6.65	-12.93, -0.37*	-1.03	-4.66, 2.61
Fibre (g)	0.13	-0.18, 0.44	-0.07	-0.20, 0.05
β-carotene (mg)	-0.18	-4.00, 3.64	0.51	-0.94, 1.97
Vitamin C (mg)	0.04	-0.05, 0.12	-0.00	-0.04, 0.03
Vitamin E (mg)	-0.28	-0.79, 0.22	-0.11	-0.33, 0.11

UV = univariate model, MV = multivariate model adjusted for intake of saturated fatty acids and flavonoids, and for smoking prevalence, CI = confidence interval.
* P < 0.05.

21

Table 3

Correlations among population averages of different dietary variables and prevalence of smoking in the Seven Countries Study

Dietary variable	Saturated fat (g)	Flavonoids (mg)	Smoking (%)
Alcohol (log) (g)	−0.58*	0.39	0.01
Fish (log) (g)	−0.49	0.66**	0.40
Fibre (g)	0.25	−0.48	−0.16
β–carotene (mg)	−0.00	0.30	0.06
Vitamin C (mg)	0.07	−0.42	0.06
Vitamin E (mg)	−0.22	−0.32	−0.31

*$P < 0.05$.
**$P < 0.01$.

Study appropriate for determining diet-disease associations at the population level.

In the present study, an inverse association was observed in univariate analysis between population average alcohol intake and 25-year mortality rates from CHD. In analyses using food balance sheet data from 18 and 21 developed countries, a similar inverse association was observed and mainly attributed to the consumption of wine.[3,20] In an analysis using 40 countries at different stages of economic development it was shown that this association was only present in countries with a high saturated fat and dietary cholesterol intake (e.g in economically developed countries).[6] These results suggest that alcohol intake is inversely related to CHD mortality in univariate analysis in economically developed countries.

In the present study, the association between alcohol intake and CHD mortality disappeared after multivariate analysis because of an inverse relation between saturated fatty acids and alcohol intake. In the 18-country-study of St Leger *et al.* alcohol, in contrast to fatty acids, remained inversely related to CHD mortality.[3] Multivariate analyses carried out by Criqui and Ringel and by Renaud and De Logeril showed that wine was inversely related to CHD mortality whereas animal and dairy fat were positively associated.[20,21] The heterogeneity of the results after multivariate analysis may result from a number of factors. The number and selection of countries differed between the different studies. The present study is the only one that is truly prospective. Dietary data were collected in random samples of cohorts of men followed for 25 years. Population average intake of different nutrients was chemically determined in one laboratory. In the other studies, food balance sheet data were used. These data represent the availability of foods per country and not the foods actually consumed and cannot be broken down by age, gender or socioeconomic status. Fatty acid intake was calculated from food tables, [3,6] or dairy, fat was used as a proxy for saturated fat. Probably for these reasons a stronger association was found between

saturated fatty acids and CHD mortality in the present study than in the other cross-cultural studies. Finally, full multivariate models that included saturated fatty acids, cigarette smoking and dietary antioxidants were not used in the other studies.

Comparisons between Eskimos and Danes suggest that differences in population CHD mortality rates may be explained by differences in seafood consumption. [22] In a cross-cultural study including 21 developed countries, a weak inverse relation was observed between fish consumption and CHD mortality.[4] This association disappeared when adjustment was made for milk products and meat, which are indicators of saturated fat intake. Similar results were obtained in the present study. The inverse relation between fish consumption and CHD mortality disappeared when saturated fatty acids, flavonoids and smoking were included in the multivariate model. Fish consumption was inversely associated with saturated fatty acids and positively with flavonoid intake and smoking. These results suggest that fish consumption is not important in explaining differences in CHD mortality rates between countries.

In univariate analyses using food balance sheets and mortality data for 40 countries at different stages of economic development, a strong inverse relation was observed between vegetable food consumption and CHD mortality ($r = -0.80$).[6] In this study, and also in a cross-cultural study using food balance sheet data for 20 economically developed countries, inverse associations were found between dietary fibre intake and CHD mortality.[5,6] In the present study dietary fibre intake was not associated with CHD mortality in either uni- or multivariate analysis. This may be for reasons similar to those mentioned in the discussion on the association between alcohol intake and CHD mortality.

In univariate analysis an inverse relation was found between vitamin E intake and mortality from CHD in the 40 countries study.[6] Also a strong inverse relation was observed between the per capita vitamin E consumption and CHD mortality, in 17 European countries.[23] Plasma vitamin E levels were inversely associated with mortality from CHD in 16 European countries participating in the WHO MONICA project.[24] In the present study the intake of antioxidant vitamins including vitamin E was not associated with long-term CHD mortality either in uni- or multivariate analysis. Several facts may explain these different results. Firstly, the use of food balance sheet data to estimate vitamin E intake is less reliable than chemical analysis of equivalent food composites. Secondly, plasma vitamin E is only weakly related to vitamin E intake.[25] Thirdly, potential confounders (e.g. saturated fatty acids, flavonoids intake and cigarette smoking) were not sufficiently taken into account. The results of the present study, suggest that flavonoids are more important than vitamin E in explaining differences in CHD mortality between countries. However, based on the results of other cross-cultural studies the role of vitamin E in explaining differences in CHD mortality rates cannot be ruled out.

The results of the Seven Countries Study have shown that cross-cultural differences in CHD mortality can largely be explained by differences in the intake of saturated fatty acids, flavonoids and smoking. [2] This is in agreement with current thinking about the aetiology of CHD, the 'final complication' of the athero-thrombotic process. Saturated fatty acids with 12–16 carbon atoms elevate low density lipoproteins (LDL) [26] and may down-regulate the LDL receptor. [27,28] In turn, these lipoproteins can be oxidized by cigarette smoking. [29] There is evidence from *in vitro* studies that vitamin E and flavonoids may inhibit LDL oxidation. [30,31] Saturated fatty, acids with 14 or more carbon atoms may promote arterial thrombosis. [32] There is some evidence that flavonoids influence the cyclo-oxygenase enzyme cascade and therefore arterial thrombosis. [33] This suggests that a lifestyle characterized by a high intake of saturated fatty acids, a low intake of antioxidants, and a high prevalence of smoking, will promote the development of athero-thrombotic complications.

This does not mean that alcohol. fish and fibre are unimportant in the aetiology of CHD. These dietary variables have been shown to be important determinants of CHD in individuals,[34–36] though they do not explain population differences in CHD. The effects of alcohol and fish were correlated with those of saturated fatty acids and flavonoids. Fibre was not associated with CHD mortality, either in uni- or multivariate analyses. These results support the point made by Rose that determinants of diseases at the individual level are not necessarily the same as those at the population level.[37]

The results of the Seven Countries Study show that low mortality rates from CHD occur with different diets. The most prominent examples are the Mediterranean and Japanese diets. Both of these eating patterns are low in saturated fatty, acids and high in antioxidants. In the classical Mediterranean diet, wine and fish are used in moderation.[38] In the Japanese diet fish plays an important role, but fish is not a panacea as illustrated by Eastern Finland. The average fish intake of Finnish men was 60 g/day, but they had the highest mortality rate from CHD presumably due to a high saturated fatty acid intake, a low intake of antioxidants and a high prevalence of smoking. Non-smoking and a healthy diet are prerequisites for low rates of CHD.

ACKNOWLEDGEMENTS

We are grateful to Annemarie Jansen, Esther Goddijn, Ronald Schlemper and Monique Verschuren for their contributions to the collection and preparation of the equivalent food composites, and to Martijn B Katan and his team at the Department of Human Nutrition, Agricultural University, Wageningen for preparation and macronutrient analyses of the equivalent food composites. We would also like to thank Peter C H Hollman and his team at the State Institute for Quality Control of Agricultural Products, Wageningen for the flavonoids and vitamins analyses of the equivalent food composites. The authors are also grateful to the principal investigators who initiated the Seven Countries Study and especially to Ancel Keys for his initiative and efforts in carrying out the study for more than 25 years. The mortality follow-up in Dalmatia and Slavonia was supported by a grant from the Netherlands Nutrition Foundation.

References

1. Kromhout D, Menotti A, Bloemberg B *et al*. Dietary saturated and trans fatty acids, cholesterol and 25-year mortality from coronary heart disease. The Seven Countries Study. *Prev Med* 1995; **24**: 308–15.

2. Hertog MGL, Kromhout D, Aravanis C *et al*. Flavonoid intake and long-term risk of coronary heart disease and cancer in the Seven Countries Study. *Arch Intern Med* 1995; **155**: 381–86.

3. St Leger A S, Cochrance A L, Moore F. Factors associated with cardiac mortality in developed countries with particular reference to the consumption of wine. *Lancet* 1979; **i**: 1017–10.

4. Crombie I K, McLoone P, Smith W C S, Thomson M. Tunstall Pedoe H. International differences in coronary heart disease mortality and consumption of fish and other foodstuffs. *Eur Heart J* 1987; **8**: 560–63.

5. Liu K, Stamler J, Trevisan M, Moss D. Dietary lipids, sugar, fibre and mortality from coronary heart disease–bivariate analysis of international data. *Atherosclerosis* 1982; **2**: 221–27.

6. Artaud-Wild S M, Connor S L, Sexton G, Connor W E. Differences in coronary mortality can be explained by differences in cholesterol and saturated fat intakes in 40 countries but not in France and Finland. A paradox. *Circulation* 1993; **88**: 2771–79.

7. Keys A, Aravanis C, Blackburn H W *et al*. Epidemiological studies related to coronary heart disease: characteristics of men aged 40–59 in seven countries. *Acta Med Scand* 1967; **460 (Suppl.)**: 1–392.

8. Keys A (ed). Coronary heart disease in seven countries. Circulation 1970; **41 (Suppl. 1)**: 1-211.

9. Keys A. *Seven Countries: a Multivariate Analysis of Death and Coronary Heart Disease*. Cambridge, MA: Harvard University Press, 1980.

10. Kromhout D, Keys A, Aravanis C *et al*. Food consumption patterns in the 1960s in seven countries. *Am J Clin Nutr* 1989; **49**: 889–94.

11. Osborne DR, Voogt P, Soxhlet method. In: *Analysis of Nutrients and Foods*. First edn. London, New York: Academic Press, 1978, pp. 155–56.

12. Metcalfe LD, Schmitz A, Pekka J R. Rapid preparation of fatty acid esters from lipids of gaschromatographic analyses. *Anal Chem* 1966; **18**: 514–15.

13. Jonker D, Hoek G D van der, Glatz J F C, Posthumus M A, Katan M B. Combined determination of free, esterified and glycosilated plant sterols in food. *Nutr Rep Int* 1985; **32**: 943–51.

14. Hertog M G L, Hollman P C H, Venema D P. Optimization of a quantitative HPLC determination of potentially anticarcinogenic flavonoids in vegetables and fruits. *J Agric Food Chem* 1992; **40**: 1591–98.

15. *Methoden der Bochemischen Analytik und Lebensmittelanalytik*. Mannheim: Boehringer-Mannheim, 1987, pp. 10–12.

16. Total dietary fiber in foods; enzymatic gravimetric method. Changes in methods. Williams S (ed.) *J Ass Off Anal Chem* 1985; **68**: 399.

17. Speck AJ, Temalilwa CR, Schrijver J. Determination of beta-carotene content and vitamin A activity of vegetables by High-Performance Liquid Chromatography and Spectrophotometry. *Food Chem* 1986; **19**: 65–74.

18 Roy RB, Conetta A, Salpeter J. Automated fuorimetric method for the determination of total vitamin C in food products. *J Ass Off Chem* 1976; **59**: 1244–50.

19 McMurray CH, Blanchflower WJ. Determination of alpha-tocopherol in animal foodstuffs using high-performance liquid chromatography with spectrofluorescence. *J Chromatogr* 1979; **176**: 488–92.

20 Criqui MH, Ringel BL. Does diet or alcohol explain the French paradox. *Lancet* 1994; **334**: 719–23.

21 Renaud S, De Logeril M. Wine, alcohol, platelets, and the French paradox for coronary heart disease. *Lancet* 1992; **339**: 1523–26.

22 Kromann N, Green A. Epidemiological studies in the Upernaerk district, Greenland. *Acta Med Scand* 1980; **208**: 401–06.

23 Bellizzi MC, Franklin MF, Duthie GG, James WPT. Vitamin E and coronary heart disease: the European paradox. *Eur J Clin Nutr* 1994; **48**: 822–31.

24 Grey KF, Puska P, Jordan P, Moser UK. Inverse correlation between plasma vitamin E and mortality from ischemic heart disease in cross-cultural epidemiology. *Am J Clin Nutr* 1991; **53**: 3265–3345.

25 Willett WC, Stampfer MJ, Underwood BA, Speitzer FE, Rosner BR, Hennekens CH. Validation of a dietary questionnaire with plasma carotenoid and alpha-tocopherol levels. *Am J Clin Nutr* 1983; **38**: 631–39.

26 Mensink R P, Katan M B. Effect of dietary fatty, acids on scrum lipids and lipoproteins: a meta-analysis of 27 trials. *Arterioscl Thromb* 1992; **12**: 911–19.

27 Brown MS, Goldstein JL. A receptor mediated pathway for cholesterol homeostasis. *Science* 1986. **232**: 34–47.

28 Spady DK, Dietschy JM. Interaction of dietary cholesterol and triglycerides in the regulation of hepatic low density, lipoprotein transport in the hamster. *J Clin Invest* 1988; **81**: 300–09.

29 Steinberg D, Parathasarathy S, Carew TE. Khoo JC, Witzum J L. Beyond cholesterol: modifications of low density lipoprotein that increase its atherogenicity. *N Engl J Med* 1989; **320**: 915–24.

30 Estebauer H, Dieber-Rotheneder M, Striegl G, Waeg G. Role of vitamin E in preventing the oxidation of low-density lipoprotein. *Am J Clin Nutr* 1991; **53**: 314S–21S.

31 De Whalley C V, Rankin S M, Hoult J R S, Jessup W, Leake D S. Flavonoids inhibit the oxidative modification of low density lipoproteins. *Biochem Pharmacol* 1990; **39**: 1743–49.

32 Renaud S, Dumont E, Godsey F, McGregor L, Morazin R. Effects of diet on blood clotting and platelet aggregation. In: Nutrition in the 1980's: Constraints on our knowledge. New York: AR Liss Inc., 1981 pp. 361–81.

33 Gryglewski RJ, Korbut R, Robak J, Swies J. On the mechanism of antithrombotic action of flavonoids. *Biochem Pharmacol* 1987; **36**: 317–21.

34 Beaglehole R, Jackson R. Alcohol, cardiovascular diseases and all causes of death: a review of the epidemiological evidence. *Drug Alcohol Rev* 1992; **11**: 275–90.

35 Shekelle RB, Stamler J. Fish and coronary heart disease: the epidemiologic evidence. *Nutr Metab Cardiovasc Dis* 1993; **3**: 46–51.

36 Anderson JW, Deakins DA, Floore TL, Smith BM, Whitis SE. Dietary fibre and coronary heart disease. *Rev Food Science Nutr* 1990; **29**: 95–147.

37 Rose G. Sick individuals and sick populations. *Int J Epidemiol* 1985; **14**: 32–38.

38 Fidanza F. The Mediterranean Italian diet: Keys to contemporary thinking. *Proc Nutr Soc* 1991; **50**: 519–26.

(Revised version received January 1996)

This letter was first published in the BMJ and is reproduced with permission of the BMJ

TH Lam, Professor, Department of Community Medicine and Unit for Behavioural Sciences, University of Hong Kong, Hong Kong

BMJ 1997;315:880 (4 October)

LETTERS

Relative risks are inflated in published literature

EDITOR

Relative risks are often reported incorrectly in medical journals. In a paper in the BMJ, Jian-Min Yuan and colleagues describe a relative risk of 3.72 for the relation between cancer of the upper aerodigestive tract and heavy drinking as a "3.7-fold increased risk"; this description is incorrect.[1] They also describe a relative risk of 1.30 for total mortality and heavy drinking as "a 30% excess risk"; this description is correct. They also write that "heavy drinking was associated with a significant 1.7-fold ... excess in risk of death from stroke"; the excess is 70%.

In an earlier paper by the same authors in JAMA there were similar problems.[2] A relative risk of 1.6 was correctly described as a "60% greater risk," while a relative risk of 2.3 was incorrectly described as a "2.3-fold excess risk." The paper also stated that "rates in Shanghai Chinese were 2-fold to 8-fold higher than in Los Angeles whites," but the rates in Shanghai were actually two to eight times those in Los Angeles whites. Such problems were not confined to the interpretation of relative risks. The sentence "In China, the yearly per capita consumption of cigarettes has increased 3-fold between the 1950s and 1987, from about 500 to 1748" is incorrect; the increase is actually twofold or 200%. Peto et al, in an accompanying editorial, stated "that heart attack mortality is five times lower, and that stroke mortality is five times higher."[3] This was a problem because the authors were referring to the ratio of 5.3 (366/69) and 1:4.2 (48/201) respectively.

I have found similar problems in reports by American, British, and Chinese authors (in alphabetical order). This problem is important when relative risks or differences of two measures are described. We have to be cautious about the confusing meaning of the suffix "-fold"; n-fold is equal to n times, and is equal to nx100%. Therefore, a relative risk of 3.5 is 2.5-fold, or 2.5 times, or a 250% increase or excess in risk, not 3.5-fold or a 350% increase or excess. I wonder how long we will continue to see such inadvertent inflation of relative risks in the literature.

References

[1] Yuan J-M, Ross RK, Gao Y-T, Henderson BE, Yu MC. Follow up study of moderate alcohol intake and mortality among middle aged men in Shanghai, China. *BMJ* 1997;**314**:18-23. (4 January.)

[2] Yuan J-M, Ross RK, Wang X-L, Gao Y-T, Henderson BE, Yu MC. Morbidity and mortality in relation to cigarette smoking in Shanghai, China: a prospective male cohort study. *JAMA* 1996;**275**:1646-50.

[3] Peto R, Chen Z, Boreham J. Tobacco—the growing epidemic in China. *JAMA* 1996;**275**: 1683-4

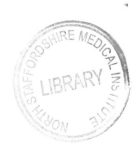

22